LIPPINCOTT'S HANDBOOK FOR PSYCHIATRIC NURSING AND CARE PLANNING

D1611688

LIPPINCOTT'S HANDBOOK FOR PSYCHIATRIC NURSING AND CARE PLANNING

Maryann Foley, RN, BSN
Clinical Consultant
Foley Consulting, LLC
Flourtown, Pennsylvania

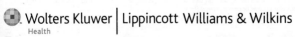
. Wolters Kluwer | Lippincott Williams & Wilkins
Health
Philadelphia · Baltimore · New York · London
Buenos Aires · Hong Kong · Sydney · Tokyo

Acquisitions Editor: Jean Rodenberger
Developmental Editor: Renee Gagliardi
Director of Nursing Production: Helen Ewan
Senior Managing Editor / Production: Erika Kors
Production Editor: Mary Kinsella
Art Director, Design: Joan Wendt
Art Director, Illustration: Brett McNaughton
Manufacturing Coordinator: Karin Duffield
Production Services / Compositor: Cadmus

First Edition

9 8 7 6 5 4 3 2

Printed in China

Library of Congress Cataloging-in-Publication Data

Foley, Maryann.
  Lippincott's handbook for psychiatric nursing and care planning/subject matter expert, Maryann Foley; reviewers, Jean S. Anthony ... [et al.].
    p. ; cm.
  Includes index.
  ISBN-13: 978-1-58255-730-4
  ISBN-10: 1-58255-730-6
  1. Psychiatric nursing—Handbooks, manuals, etc. 2. Nursing assessment—Handbooks, manuals, etc. I. Title. II. Title: Clinical and care planning guide for psychiatric nursing.
  [DNLM: 1. Mental Disorders—nursing—Handbooks. 2. Forensic Nursing—Handbooks.
3. Nursing Assessment—Handbooks. 4. Psychiatric Nursing—Handbooks. WY 49 F663L 2010]
  RC440.F535 2010
  616.89'0231—dc22

                                                                          2008045674

LWW.COM

SUBJECT MATTER EXPERT

Maryann Foley, RN, BSN
Clinical Consultant
Foley Consulting, LLC
Flourtown, Pennsylvania

REVIEWERS

Jean S. Anthony, PhD, MSN, RN
Assistant Professor
University of Cincinnati, College of Nursing
Cincinnati, Ohio

Joan C. Masters, EdD, RN
Assistant Professor of Nursing
Bellarmine University
Louisville, Kentucky

Gail Marlene Day, PhD, MSN, CNS Psy/MH, BC
Instructor and Advanced Practice Registered Nurse
San Antonio College
San Antonio, Texas

Marilyn S. Fetter, PhD, APRN
Assistant Professor
Villanova University
Villanova, Pennsylvania

Pamela J Nelson, PhD(c), MS, BSN, CNS, RN
Clinical Nurse Specialist
Mayo Medical Center
Rochester, Minnesota

PREFACE

Changes in healthcare and healthcare delivery demand that nurses have a sound knowledge base and be skillfully competent when providing care to clients, regardless of the underlying condition. This fact assumes even greater importance for the area of psychiatric–mental health nursing. Nurses need to be able to assess, plan, and intervene quickly and appropriately as part of an interdisciplinary team using evidenced-based knowledge.

Lippincott's Handbook for Psychiatric Nursing and Care Planning is an easy-to-use, portable, clinical reference designed to provide practicing nurses and nursing students with a quick reference approach to essential, need-to-know, critical information for clinical practice. Nursing students and new graduates will find this book to be a valuable resource for the mental health arena. The comprehensive coverage of key concepts and topics allows students to use this book regardless of the textbook used in class. In addition, the text provides a hands-on resource for students and nurses working in any setting, for example, the emergency department or medical-surgical area, when working with a client who may have a mental health issue or psychiatric disorder or a client who is prescribed some type of psychopharmacologic agent. Nurses returning to the clinical area will also find this handbook helpful as a review and refresher resource.

The book is divided into seven sections to provide the user with an organized framework. *Section One* includes two chapters that cover the foundational concepts of psychiatric-mental health nursing, including core concepts such as mental disorders and mental illness, neurotransmitters, theories and frameworks, defense mechanisms, and stress and anxiety as well as legal and cultural considerations specific to psychiatric-mental health practice.

Section Two addresses key aspects of assessment, interviewing, and communication. The nursing process is highlighted in conjunction with the nurse–client relationship, interviewing, and therapeutic and nontherapeutic communication techniques. Assessment is further emphasized with the inclusion of 35 of the most common, accepted, and reliable assessment tools that could be used to gather data about a client. These tools, organized by disorder or condition, are presented alphabetically to promote ease of use.

Section Three addresses therapeutic modalities that may be used with clients experiencing psychiatric-mental health disorders. This section includes two chapters that cover the various types of individual, group, and family therapies as well as integrative and somatic therapies. Throughout this section, extensive cross-referencing leads the reader to the page number where the disorder(s) typically associated with the use of the modality is (are) discussed.

Section Four covers psychopharmacology, with individual chapters highlighting major drug classes used. Each chapter follows a consistent format, providing general information about the drug class along with a summary of the various subclasses or groups and examples. Individual drug monographs follow, highlighting drug class, indications and dosages, half-life, common adverse reactions, key drug interactions, and nursing considerations. In all, seven major drug classes are presented, with a total of 83 individual drug monographs. Where appropriate, cross-referencing appears to lead the reader to the page where the indicated disorder is discussed.

Section Five presents a discussion of mental health and psychiatric disorders. It contains twelve chapters, each dealing with a specific group of disorders. Each chapter addresses the group of disorders and then goes on to describe the most common disorders for that group. The disorders are alphabetically arranged and employ the nursing process framework and an interdisciplinary approach. Assessment includes information about *DSM-IV-TR* diagnostic criteria, common history, physical assessment and psychosocial assessment findings, assessment tools (with a cross-reference to the page where it is presented in Chapter 4) if applicable, as well as laboratory and diagnostic test findings, if appropriate. Treatment modalities are highlighted in a box with cross references, where appropriate, to the pages where the modality or drug therapy is discussed. Nursing care planning is emphasized applying evidenced-based knowledge through the use of the most up-to-date North American Nursing Diagnosis Association (NANDA) taxonomy and incorporation of Nursing Outcomes Classification (NOC) and Nursing Interventions Classification (NIC). This information can be adapted to individualize client care.

Section Six addresses emergency situations such as anger and aggression, abuse and violence, suicide, and crisis and disaster. Incorporating the use of boxes and tables, this section provides essential information about each situation with an emphasis on the nurse's role.

Section Seven describes special situations including forensic clients, children and adolescents, older adults, and homeless clients. The chapter on forensic clients includes information about the characteristics of the forensic population, effects of incarceration, strategies to maintain boundaries, and the nurse's role. For children and adolescents, discussion focuses on developmental perspectives and the most common psychiatric and mental health disorders found in this population, emphasizing assessment and the nurse's role for each disorder. The chapters on older adults and homeless clients highlight key adaptations needed for assessment and the nurse's role in meeting the priority needs for these populations.

Lippincott's Handbook for Psychiatric Nursing and Care Planning is more than just a nursing diagnosis handbook or a reference for planning care. It provides an overall holistic approach with an emphasis on important clinical information. The extensive use of cross-referencing, alphabetical organization, and use of tables, boxes, and bulleted lists promotes ease of use, thereby providing nurses facing multiple demands on their time and energy with a valuable resource for information.

CONTENTS

Foundational Concepts of Psychiatric-Mental Health Nursing

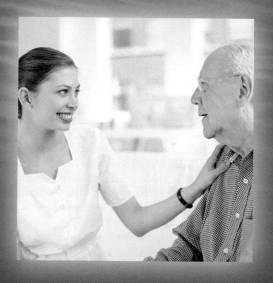

Core Concepts of Psychiatric-Mental Health Nursing

Mental Health

Mental health means the successful performance of mental function, resulting in productive activities, fulfilling relationships, and the ability to adapt to change and cope with adversity. Mental health provides people with a capacity for rational thought, communication, learning, emotional growth, resilience, and self-esteem. Individuals with emotional well-being (mental "healthiness") function comfortably in society and are satisfied with their achievements.

Mental health implies mastery and relative contentment in love, work, play, spirituality, and relationships. Mentally healthy people perform meaningful tasks, enjoy life, have a sense of humor, and are satisfied in their interpersonal dealings. They show optimism, benefit from rest and sleep, and work well alone and with others. They accept responsibility for actions, reach sound judgments, and express feelings in an inoffensive and contextually appropriate manner.

Elements of mental health that contribute to the preceding characteristics are as follows:

- *Self-governance*: Acting independently, dependently, or interdependently as the need arises without permanently losing autonomy
- *Progress toward growth or self-realization*: Being willing to move forward to maximize capabilities

- *Tolerance of the unknown*: Facing the uncertainty of life and the certainty of death with faith and hope
- *Self-esteem*: Being aware and accepting of personal abilities and limitations through lifelong self-reflection and feedback from others
- *Reality orientation*: Distinguishing fact from fantasy and behaving accordingly
- *Mastery of environment*: Interacting competently, effectively, and creatively with and influencing environmental contexts
- *Stress management*: Experiencing congruent emotions in daily life and tolerating stress-provoking situations in an adaptive, creative, and flexible way, knowing that any negative feelings are time limited

Mental Disorders and Mental Illness

Mental disorders are health conditions that cause distress, impair ability to function, or both and are marked by alterations in thinking, mood, or behavior. **Mental illness** is considered a clinically significant behavioral or psychological syndrome marked by distress, disability, or the risk of suffering, disability, or loss of freedom (American Psychiatric Association [APA], 2007). Problems result from brain function or dysfunction, and they cause the person distress, impairment, or both. Related symptoms must exceed expected reactions to everyday events, such as a death in the family. Additionally, the syndrome is not merely a cultural expectation.

Incidence and Etiology

Mental illness affects people of all ages and knows no racial, ethnic, gender, or socioeconomic barriers. Mental illness, including suicide, is the second leading cause of U.S. disability (heart disease is first), and it is the leading cause of disability for people 15 to 44 years old. The specific causes of mental illnesses are largely unidentified but generally involve enormously complex interactions among genetic predispositions and environmental factors.

Classification

The American Psychiatric Association developed a classification system for mental disorders more than 50 years ago. The current classification system, *Diagnostic and Statistical Manual of Mental Disorders,* 4th edition, text revision (*DSM-IV-TR*), now in its sixth revision, is most commonly accepted in the U.S. and Canadian clinical community. This multi-axial classification system groups disorders by symptom clusters and differentiates between normality and psychopathology on the basis of the duration and severity of symptoms (Box 1.1).

The *DSM* categorical classification lists diagnostic criteria for each mental disorder. Its five-axis system provides a comprehensive picture of the client's mental functioning. Each disorder's criteria describe its behaviors, symptoms, or signs; its duration; and sometimes other qualifiers (eg, severe, recurrent). The criteria, however, do not determine the diagnosis. Clinicians who use the criteria as guidelines decide on the diagnosis. Many clients have more than one diagnosis on the first three axes.

Neurotransmission

Neurotransmitters are a diverse group of chemical-transmitting substances. As a nerve impulse, or action potential, reaches the end of a presynaptic axon, neurotransmitter molecules are released into the synaptic space.

Originally, approximately six neurotransmitters were known; current research has revealed several dozen, and several hundred or thousands may remain undiscovered (Table 1.1).

box

1.1 *DSM-IV-TR* Classification System

- Axis I—Clinical disorders
- Axis II—Personality disorders and mental retardation
- Axis III—General medical conditions (eg, diabetes, asthma; if findings from the history and physical examination are normal, no diagnosis is given)
- Axis IV—Psychosocial and environmental problems
- Axis V—Global assessment of functioning (GAF; a hypothetical continuum of mental health–illness ranges from 100 [superior functioning)] to 1 [persistent danger of hurting self or others]), written as numbers (0 to 100) meaning "current functioning"/"highest level of functioning in past year" (*see p. 51 for the actual GAF*).

table

1.1. Some Neurotransmitters and Their Functions

Neurotransmitter	Presumed Function	Possible Implications for Mental Illness
Biogenic Amines: Catecholamines		
Dopamine	Involved in pleasurable feelings and complex motor activities	Schizophrenia
Norepinephrine	Regulates awareness of environment, attention, learning, memory, and arousal	Mood disorders
Epinephrine	Has limited presence in the brain; contributes to the "fight-or-flight" response	
Biogenic Amines: Indolamines		
Serotonin	Contributes to temperature regulation	*Low levels:* depression, aggression, suicidality, and impulsivity *High levels:* anxiety disorders (fearfulness, avoidance)
Histamine	Involved in allergic responses; role in CNS remains elusive	Weight gain associated with psychotropic medications

continued on page 6

table
1.1. **Some Neurotransmitters and Their Functions** *(continued)*

Neurotransmitter	Presumed Function	Possible Implications for Mental Illness
Biogenic Amines: Cholinergics		
Acetylcholine	Mediates cognitive functioning directly or by modulating another neurotransmitter indirectly; is the most widely used neurotransmitter in the body; contributes to sleep–wake cycles	Sleep disorders
Neuropeptides: endorphins and enkephalins, neurotensin, vasoactive intestinal peptide, cholecystokinin, and substance P	Appear to play a secondary messenger role and contribute to modulating the pain response	Alzheimer's disease, movement disorders
Amino Acids		
Excitatory: aspartic acid, glutamic acid, cysteic acid, and homocysteic acid	Sparse information available; high levels can be toxic	
Inhibitory: gamma-aminobutyric acid (GABA)	Slows down body activity	Dementia, schizophrenia, and anxiety disorders

Most neurotransmitters are synthesized and stored in the terminal region of the neuron, where they are released after electrical stimulation (an action potential) causes the neuron to fire (ie, become depolarized). Depolarization causes changes in the fluxes of particular ions across a cell membrane. The neurotransmitters then diffuse across the synaptic cleft to act on and attach to receptors in the membrane of the postsynaptic cell. This postsynaptic cell may be another neuron, a muscle cell, or a specialized gland cell.

Neurotransmitters can either inhibit or excite the receptor cell, making an axon discharge more or less likely. The nerve cell "decides" whether to send output as a result of the number of inhibitory or excitatory inputs it receives. Excitatory neurotransmitters are more likely to cause cells to become depolarized, whereas inhibitory neurotransmitters are less likely to cause cells to become depolarized (Table 1.2).

Although the specific contributions of neurotransmitters to mental illness are not known, recent evidence suggests that no single neurotransmitter is responsible for any one disorder. Current findings indicate that psychiatric illnesses are associated with alterations in several neurotransmitters. Moreover, the alterations may result not from a simple abundance or overabundance of neurotransmitters but from ratios of various neurotransmitters or any number of complex permutations (Table 1.3).

Psychopharmacotherapy involves blocking or enhancing certain neurotransmitters (see Section 4, *Psychopharmacology*). Although neurotransmitters are numerous, the three major neurotransmitter pathways essential to understanding certain psychiatric conditions and the actions of medications used to treat them are dopamine, norepinephrine, and serotonin.

Theories and Frameworks

Conceptual frameworks and theories are nothing more than *worldviews*—ideas about how the world works. Various theories in psychiatry represent worldviews and are a way of thinking about people and the world. They all offer different explanations for human behavior and promote interventions consistent with their tenets to help people with psychiatric disorders. No one theory adequately

table
1.2. **Neurotransmission**

Synthesis and Release.
Neurotransmitters are synthesized
in the presynaptic neuron, where
they are stored in the terminal
region. When a nerve impulse
stimulates the presynaptic neuron,
the neurotransmitters are released
into the synaptic cleft.

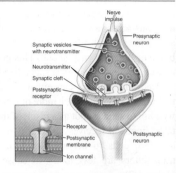

Binding. The neurotransmitters
then move across the synaptic
cleft to bind to receptors on the
postsynaptic neuron. The type of
receptor (inhibitory or excitatory)
determines the specific action of
the neurotransmitter.

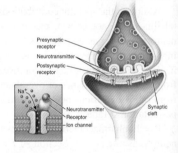

accounts for all human behavior or mental illness, although some
perspectives have more supporting research than others, and some
are completely unsupported from an evidence-based standpoint
(Table 1.4).

Defense Mechanisms

Defense mechanisms are unconscious measures that people use to
protect their personal stability against anxiety and threat resulting
from conflicts among the id, ego, and superego. Defense mechanisms

table
1.3.

Major Neurotransmitter Pathways in Mental Health

Dopamine. (1) *Nigrostriatal.* Extending from the substantia nigra to the basal ganglia, this pathway is part of the extrapyramidal nervous system and controls movement. Dopamine deficiencies here result in movement disorders (eg, Parkinson's disease) and contribute to certain side effects of antipsychotic medications. **(2)** *Mesolimbic.* This pathway is thought to be involved in pleasurable sensations and euphoria resulting from substance abuse. Overactivity of dopamine here is thought to contribute to hallucinations and delusions. **(3)** *Mesocortical.* This pathway begins in the midbrain and projects to the limbic cortex. It is thought to mediate both the negative and cognitive symptoms of psychosis. **(4)** *Tuberoinfundibular.* This pathway extends from the hypothalamus to the anterior pituitary and regulates prolactin secretion, which is inhibited by dopamine.

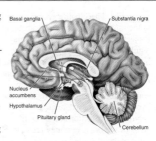

Norepinephrine. These pathways regulate cognitive mood, emotions, and movement. They originate in the locus ceruleus, which focuses attention on internal or external stimuli. Projections to the limbic cortex may mediate emotions, energy level, and psychomotor retardation, whereas projections to the cerebellum may mediate motor movements. Norepinephrine pathways also regulate autonomic functions. Projections to the brainstem control blood pressure, projections to the heart control heart rate, and projections to the urinary tract control bladder emptying. Deficiencies of norepinephrine may lead to impaired attention, concentration, and memory; delayed information processing; depression; psychomotor retardation; and fatigue.

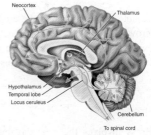

continued on page 10

table

1.3. **Major Neurotransmitter Pathways in Mental Health** *continued*

Serotonin. These pathways originate in the raphe nucleus of the brainstem. Projections to the frontal cortex may regulate mood, whereas those to the basal ganglia may regulate movement as well as obsessions and compulsions. Projections to the limbic areas may control anxiety and panic; those to the hypothalamus may regulate eating behaviors. Projections to different areas of the brainstem may regulate sleep and nausea and vomiting. Serotonin neurons that project down the spinal cord may control sexual responses such as orgasm and ejacula-tion. Last, receptors in the gut may regulate both appetite and gastroin-testinal functioning. Deficiencies in serotonin may lead to depressed mood, anxiety, panic, phobia, obsessions, compulsions, food cravings, and bulimia.

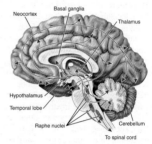

are not "real" and cannot be empirically observed, nor can they be "proven." Typically, defense mechanisms operate at the unconscious level, such that most people are unaware that they are using them. Examples of defense mechanisms are highlighted in Table 1.5.

Stress

Stress involves the everyday events, situations, and problems to which a person is exposed.

Stress is not a disorder—it is a normal part of everyday life and does not have good or bad connotations. The perception of stress depends on the individual; an event that one person views as threat-ening may be tolerated easily or enjoyed by others. Therefore, the feeling of stress as a negative emotional state is based substantially

table
1.4.

Theories and Frameworks

Theory or Model	Area of Focus	Key Concepts
Psychoanalytic Models		
Sigmund Freud	View of the human mind as conscious and unconscious processes Psychoanalysis: accessing unconscious via dreams and free association	• Human personality structure: id, ego, superego • Personality development as series of successive stages: oral, anal, phallic, latent, and genital • Object relations (psychological attachment to another person or object) • Anxiety (*see page 19*) and use of defense mechanisms • Transference and countertransference
Alfred Adler	Sense of inferiority as motivation for living	• Feelings of inferiority, if avoided, leading to unrealistic goals and strong desire for power and dominance • Inferiority intolerable, resulting in self-centered neurotic attitudes, overcompensation, retreat from real world
Carl Jung	Analytical psychology Two types of personalities: extroverted and introverted	• Extroverted: interest in others and external objects • Introverted: self-interest • Both present, but libido directs to one or the other • Persona (how person appears to others, not what person really is)
Behavioral Theories and Models • STIMULUS-RESPONSE THEORIES		
Edwin Guthrie	Conditioning as important in learning	• Specific stimulus with recurrent responses

continued on page 12

1.4. Theories and Frameworks *continued*

Theory or Model	Area of Focus	Key Concepts
Ivan Pavlov	Unconditioned stimulus leading to unconditioned response	• Connection between thought processes and physiologic responses • Classic conditioning
John Watson	Stimulus response Behaviorism Learning as classical conditioning Relationship between mind and body	• Reflexes (learning via classic conditioning) • Principle of frequency • Principle of recency
• REINFORCEMENT THEORIES		
B.F. Skinner	Reinforcement for behavior	• Respondent behavior due to specific stimuli • Operant behavior: learning as the consequence of a behavioral response via conditioning (behavior followed by reinforcement will recur)
Edward Thorndike	Problem solving and stimulus response	• Importance of effects after response or behavior reinforcement
Cognitive Theories and Models		
Albert Bandura	Social cognitive theory Acquisition of behaviors via learning from others	• Modeling (pervasive imitation) • Disinhibition (individual learned not to make a response then makes response when another makes inhibited response) • Elicitation (wanting to do the same as another without desire) • Self-efficacy (person's sense of own ability to deal effective with environment)

Aaron Beck	Relationship between cognition and mental health	• Cognitions (verbal or pictorial events in consciousness) • Beliefs (information-processing systems) • Faulty beliefs leading to errors in judgments becoming habitual errors in thinking
Kurt Lewin	Field theory Understanding of learning, motivation, personality, and social behavior	• Life space • Positive valences • Negative valences

Developmental Theories and Models

Erik Erikson	Psychosocial development model Developmental conflicts based on age	• Eight stages of development based on conflict • Specific tasks to be resolved • Success with resolution leading to strength and virtues
Jean Piaget	Intellectual development Intelligence as adaptation to environment	• Cognitive growth continually evolving with increasing differentiation over time • Four periods of intellectual growth to explain the development of and changes in knowledge
Carol Gilligan	Gender differentiation Female development and relationships	• Females learning to value relationships and becoming interdependent at earlier age than males • Female development based on experiences within relationships

Existential Theories and Models

Albert Ellis	Rational emotive therapy	• Eleven irrational beliefs used by individuals to make self unhappy • "Automatic" thoughts causing unhappiness in certain situations

continued on page 14

table
1.4.

Theories and Frameworks *continued*

Theory or Model	Area of Focus	Key Concepts
Fredrick Perls	Gestalt therapy	• Emphasis on feelings and thoughts in the "here and now" • Self-awareness leading to self-acceptance and responsibility for own thoughts and feelings
Interpersonal Theories and Models		
Harry Stack Sullivan	Interpersonal relationships significant to personality development	• Five life stages that focus on interpersonal relationships • Three developmental cognitive modes of experience: protaxic mode, parataxic mode, and syntaxic mode • Therapeutic community or milieu (establishment of satisfying interpersonal relationships); Milieu therapy *(see page 130)*
Hildegard Peplau	Therapeutic nurse–patient relationship	• Four phases in the nurse–patient relationship; patient to accomplish certain tasks and change relationships to foster healing • Nurse acting in roles of stranger, resource person, teacher, leader, surrogate, and counselor • Anxiety as initial response to psychic threat • Four levels of anxiety
Humanistic Theories and Models		
Abraham Maslow	Hierarchy of needs	• Basic drives or needs for motivation • Lower-level needs dominating until met; then next-level needs dominate • Self-actualization

| Carl Rogers | Client-centered therapy
Therapeutic relationships | • Client as the key to healing
• Each person experiencing world differently; each person with the best knowledge of own experience
• Client as the expert
• Promotion of self-esteem via unconditional positive regard, genuineness, empathetic understanding |

Nursing Theories and Models

Madeleine Leininger	Transcultural nursing	• Cultural care diversity and universality • Learning principles related to culture care, cultural assessments, the universality of cultural diversity, and the importance of fit between the client's healthcare values and services provided • Caring as culturally based
Ida Jean Orlando	Dynamic nurse–patient relationship	• Three areas of concern: nurse–patient relationship, nurse's professional role, identity, and development of nursing knowledge • Focus on entire client
Joyce Travelbee	Hope Expansion of concern to address long-term illnesses	• Suffering as a feeling of displeasure that ranges from simple, temporary upset to the extreme opposite • Despair as beyond the extreme suffering • Search for meaning in life and experiences
Jean Watson	Transpersonal caring Caring as the foundation of nursing	• Transpersonal caring-healing relationships • Clinical Caritas processes (10 processes) • Caritas Field • Sensitivity to self and others

continued on page 16

table

1.4. **Theories and Frameworks** *(continued)*

Theory or Model	Area of Focus	Key Concepts
Imogene King	Theory of goal attainment Systems model	• Three interacting systems: personal, interpersonal, and social • Individual's interaction with environment leading to perceptions that affect reactions and interactions • Goal-oriented, purposeful individual reacting to stressors and interacting as an open system with the environment and being affected by variables
Betty Neuman	Neuman systems model Expansion beyond illness model to include problem finding and prevention	• Nature of the relationship between the nurse and client • Client's response to stressors • Client as collaborator for goal setting and intervention identification • Nurse as intervener to help lessen client's encounter with stress to strengthen client's ability to deal with stressors
Dorothea Orem	Self-care Individuals being helped by nursing Promotion of individual independence and self-care	• Theory of self-care (independent activities by an individual to promote and maintain well-being) • Theory of self-care deficit (nursing to help individuals) • Five approaches to help meet self-care requisites: acting or doing for, guiding, teaching, supporting, and providing an environment to promote client's ability to meet current or future demands • Theory of nursing systems (actions used to meet individual's self-care requisites)

table
1.5.

Defense Mechanisms

Defense Mechanism	Description	Example from Popular Culture
Acting out	Expressing thoughts and feelings in actions rather than words	*Say Anything* (1989): Lloyd Dobler blasts a love song from a boom box outside his girlfriend's window to communicate his feelings for her.
Compensation	Emphasizing positive traits to make up for real or perceived weaknesses	*The Office* (2005): Michael Scott repeatedly calls attention to his humor and friendliness to distract people from his questionable management skills.
Denial	Refusing to recognize a reality that might be troublesome or traumatic	*The Sopranos* (1998): The family goes along with the idea that Tony, the husband and father, is in "waste management," instead of organized crime.
Devaluation	Maintaining an entirely negative view of another person by ignoring his or her virtues (the opposite is idealization)	*Eternal Sunshine of the Spotless Mind* (2004): Following a nasty breakup, Clementine refuses to acknowledge that her boyfriend had good traits or that they once were happy together.
Identification	Acting and behaving like someone else; taking on another's personality characteristics	*Seinfeld* (1990): George Costanza starts to imitate a new friend he wants to go into business with, constantly referring to himself in the third person.

continued on page 18

table
1.5.

Defense Mechanisms *continued*

Defense Mechanism	Description	Example from Popular Culture
Intellectualization	Using the powers of the intellect, thinking, and reasoning to blunt reality	*House* (2004): Dr. Gregory House argues, wisecracks, and logically tears apart his colleagues when they confront him about behavior or try to analyze his emotions.
Projection	Refusing to recognize behavior in oneself and instead "projecting" it or seeing it in someone else	*Friends* (1994): Ross insists that his ex-girlfriend Rachel (whom he still loves) is flirting with him and trying to reconcile.
Reaction formation	Doing the opposite of one's unconscious wishes	*It's a Wonderful Life* (1946): George Bailey becomes increasingly mired in the everyday affairs of his small town, despite desperately wanting to leave home to travel the world.
Regression	Going back to an earlier and happier time of development	*American Beauty* (1998): During a midlife crisis, Lester Burnham quits his job at an agency, starts working at a fast-food restaurant, and begins behaving like a teenager.
Repression	Involuntarily placing material of life experience out of the conscious	*The Bourne Identity* (2002): Jason Bourne cannot remember troubling episodes from his career as a spy.
Sublimation	Taking repressed feelings and transforming them into positive and constructive pursuits	*The Pursuit of Happyness* (2006): Chris Gardner represses his anger about separating from his wife and frustration over money troubles into overachieving at his internship.
Suppression	Wishing to put something unpleasant out of awareness and voluntarily doing so	*Lost* (2004): Hugo, a survivor of a plane crash, organizes a makeshift golf game to provide distraction from the harsh challenges of surviving on a deserted island.

on an individual's appraisal of the stressor and assessment of his or her ability to respond to it.

To cope effectively with stress, the brain initiates physiologic mechanisms that protect against injury and allow the individual to either fight or flee. The widespread effects of the "fight-or-flight response," mediated by the sympathetic nervous system, include the following:

- Heart rate and blood pressure increase.
- Blood flows to the muscles.
- Breathing rate increases.
- Perspiration increases.
- Blood clotting ability increases.
- Saliva production decreases.
- Digestion decreases.
- Immune response decreases.
- Energy-producing stored glycogen is released.

Anxiety

Feeling anxious is part of the human condition. All people experience some anxiety at some time in their lives. Most people are familiar with the feelings associated with anxiety and can verbalize that they are having them. Anxiety, largely rooted in fear, is best described as a sense of psychological distress. People may feel transient anxiety before a job interview, when a loved one does not arrive home as expected, or when they are alone on a dark street at night. Feeling anxious, frightened, uneasy, or worried is a normal response to various life experiences that people could perceive as disruptive, threatening, or dangerous.

Anxiety versus Stress

Anxiety is different from stress. Stressors are frequently cited as causes of anxiety, and when the mind interprets events as threatening, it responds accordingly, with symptoms of anxiety.

Response to Anxiety

In addition to the fight-or-flight stress response that occurs in stressful situations, the body also responds psychologically and cognitively. These responses may include:

- Feelings of nervousness
- Vague discomfort
- Uncertainty
- Self-doubt
- Apprehension, dread, or restlessness
- Difficulty concentrating
- Heightened sensation
- Upset appearance

The fight-or-flight reaction is life saving in the short term and is particularly effective against physical threats. Many people, however, feel anxious about long-term situations that they cannot influence, have feelings of anxiety with no known trigger, or worry helplessly about events taking an unlikely catastrophic turn. Others may experience panic attacks or feel extreme fear about items or creatures that most people take in stride. In these situations, anxiety can become debilitating and chronic, with the physiologic, psychological, and cognitive effects becoming chronic as well.

Levels of Anxiety

Anxiety can be mild, moderate, severe, or reach panic levels, affecting cognitive, psychological, and physical function accordingly. Each level affects the following areas differently:

- Sensation: the ways people perceive and process sensory input
- Cognition: the ability to concentrate, learn, and solve problems
- Verbal ability: speech content, form, rate, and volume

Mild anxiety results in improved functioning; however, as anxiety increases, an individual's ability to function decreases. Cognitive functioning becomes distorted, and bodies must endure extended periods of high physical alert. Table 1.6 summarizes the typical findings associated with each level of anxiety.

table
1.6. Levels of Anxiety

Anxiety Level	Psychological Responses	Physiologic Responses
Mild	Wide perceptual field Sharpened senses Increased motivation Effective problem solving Increased learning ability Irritability	Restlessness Fidgeting Gl "butterflies" Difficulty sleeping Hypersensitivity to noise
Moderate	Perceptual field narrowed to immediate task Selectively attentive Cannot connect thoughts or events independently Increased use of automatisms	Muscle tension Diaphoresis Pounding pulse Headache Dry mouth High voice pitch Faster rate of speech Gl upset Frequent urination
Severe	Perceptual field reduced to one detail or scattered details Cannot complete tasks Cannot solve problems or learn effectively Behavior geared toward anxiety relief and is usually ineffective Doesn't respond to redirection Feels awe, dread, or horror Cries Ritualistic behavior	Severe headache Nausea, vomiting, and diarrhea Trembling Rigid stance Vertigo Pale Tachycardia Chest pain
Panic	Perceptual field reduced to focus on self Cannot process any environmental stimuli Distorted perceptions Loss of rational thought Doesn't recognize potential danger Can't communicate verbally Possible defusions and hallucination May be suicidal	May bolt and run OR Totally immobile and mute Dilated pupils Increased blood pressure and pulse Flight, fight, or freeze

Normal versus Abnormal Anxiety

Anxiety becomes abnormal or pathological when people are anxious despite no real threat, when a threat has passed long ago but continues to impair functioning, or when people substitute adaptive coping mechanisms with maladaptive ones. Other indicators of a need for intervention or treatment include anxiety with the following characteristics:

• Is of greater-than-expected intensity based on the context
• Prevents fulfillment of professional, personal, or social roles
• Is accompanied by flashbacks, obsessions, or compulsions
• Curtails daily or social activities
• Lasts longer than expected given the precipitating stress

Unrelieved anxiety causes physical and emotional problems, and people may use various adaptive or maladaptive coping mechanisms to try to manage it (Box 1.2).

Short-term use of these coping mechanisms might be a natural response to a stressor and does not necessarily indicate a need for treatment. Persistent or recurrent anxiety, however, requires evaluation to determine whether a client has an anxiety disorder.

box
1.2 **Adaptive and Maladaptive Coping Mechanisms for Anxiety**

• Withdrawal: Retreat from anxiety-provoking experiences
• Acting out: Discharge of anxiety through aggressive behavior
• Psychosomatization: Visceral or physiologic expression of anxiety
• Avoidance: Management of anxiety-laden experiences through evasive behaviors
• Problem solving: Systematic method for addressing difficult situations

Legal and Cultural Considerations

Client Rights

Clients receiving psychiatric-mental health care have basic rights (Box 2.1). This issue calls for special attention, because the treatment of clients with mental illness tends to be more coercive, less voluntary, and less open to public awareness and scrutiny than are the admission and treatment of clients with other needs or disorders.

Informed Consent

Informed consent is the consent that a recipient of healthcare gives to treating providers after the recipient receives sufficient information that enables him or her to understand a proposed treatment or procedure. Sufficient information includes the following components:

- The way the treatment or procedure will be administered
- The prognosis if the treatment or procedure is given
- Side effects
- Risks
- Possible consequences of refusing the treatment or procedure
- Other alternatives

All clients have the right to give informed consent before healthcare professionals perform interventions. Administration of

box
2.1 | Federal Bill of Rights for Mental Health Patients

1. The right to appropriate treatment and related services in a setting and under conditions that are the most supportive of such person's personal liberty, and restrict such liberty only to the extent necessary consistent with such person's treatment needs, applicable requirements of law, and applicable judicial orders.

2. The right to an individualized, written treatment or service plan (such plan to be developed promptly after admission of such person), the right to treatment based on such plan, the right to periodic review and reassessment of treatment and related service needs, and the right to appropriate revision of such plan, including any revision necessary to provide a description of mental health services that may be needed after such person is discharged from such program or facility.

3. The right to ongoing participation, in a manner appropriate to a person's capabilities, in the planning of mental health services to be provided (including the right to participate in the development and periodic revision of the plan).

4. The right to be provided with a reasonable explanation, in terms and language appropriate to a person's condition and ability to understand the person's general mental and physical (if appropriate) condition,

the objectives of treatment, the nature and significant possible adverse effects of recommended treatment, the reasons why a particular treatment is considered appropriate, the reasons why access to certain visitors may not be appropriate, and any appropriate and available alternative treatments, services, and types of providers of mental health services.

5. The right not to receive a mode or course of treatment in the absence of informed, voluntary, written consent to treatment except during an emergency situation or as permitted by law when the person is being treated as a result of a court order.

6. The right not to participate in experimentation in the absence of informed, voluntary, written consent (includes human subject protection).

7. The right to freedom from restraint or seclusion, other than as a mode or course of treatment or restraint or seclusion during an emergency situation with a written order by a responsible mental health professional.

8. The right to a humane treatment environment that affords reasonable protection from harm and appropriate privacy with regard to personal needs.

9. The right to access, on request, to such person's mental health care records.

continued on page 25

box
2.1 Federal Bill of Rights for Mental Health Patients *continued*

10. The right, in the case of a person admitted on a residential or inpatient care basis, to converse with others privately, to have convenient and reasonable access to the telephone and mails, and to see visitors during regularly scheduled hours. (For treatment purposes, specific individuals may be excluded.)

11. The right to be informed promptly and in writing at the time of admission of these rights.

12. The right to assert grievances with respect to infringement of these rights.

13. The right to exercise these rights without reprisal.

14. The right of referral to other providers upon discharge.

42 U.S.C.A. § 10841.

treatments or procedures without a client's informed consent can result in legal action against the primary provider and the healthcare agency.

A major problem with consent and clients who have psychiatric disorders involves their competence to agree to procedures. Many clients, such as those who are aware of their surroundings, understand others, can make decisions based on what they think is best, and can agree to treatments or procedures without coercion, can give informed consent. On the other hand, clients with psychiatric disorders, such as those whom the court has already determined to be incompetent or those who have not been so adjudicated but are so clearly impaired by their psychiatric illnesses that they cannot truly understand what healthcare professionals are communicating, are not able to give informed consent. Major considerations for informed consent in psychiatric-mental health nursing involve ongoing monitoring and observation of clients for the following:

- A state of legal capacity or competence when they are asked to give informed consent
- Continuing understanding of the information they have been given

- Power and opportunities to revoke consent at any time during treatment

Confidentiality

Nurses have a professional legal, and ethical duty to use knowledge gained about clients only to enhance their care and not for other purposes. Accordingly, nurses must strive to maintain the confidentiality of verbal and written information.

Preserving confidentiality is especially important for clients with mental illness. Despite some advances, society still attaches tremendous stigma to those with psychiatric diagnoses. Breaches of confidentiality about clients' diagnoses, symptoms, behaviors, and treatment outcomes can have negative consequences for clients' employment, promotion, marriage, insurance benefits, and so forth.

Health Insurance Portability and Accountability Act

The Health Insurance Portability and Accountability Act (HIPAA) of 1996 and Final Rule effective 2002 delineate specific guidelines and standards for the appropriate use and disclosure of the health information of clients, identifies privacy rights, requires certain privacy practices of healthcare providers, and requires the development and implementation of administrative, technical, and physical safeguards to ensure the security of health information. Protected health information under HIPAA is defined broadly as any individually identifiable health information and includes demographic data that either identifies or could reasonably be used to identify the person. Under the privacy rule, healthcare providers:

- Must guard against the misuse of any client's identifiable health information
- Limit the sharing of such information (affording significant new rights to enable clients to understand and to control the use and disclosure of their health information)
- May use and disclose protected health information without consent, authorization, or both when they are conducting treatment, payment, and healthcare operations

- May disclose information without consent or authorization
  if so mandated by state or federal reporting requirements, such
  as those related to public health, abuse, neglect, and domestic
  violence
- May disclose protected information to law enforcement officials
  under specific circumstances
- May disclose protected information without authorization to
  comply with laws related to workers' compensation, to a party
  responsible for paying the benefits, and to any agency responsible for handling the workers' compensation claim; special provi-
  sions for authorization apply to psychotherapy notes.

Privileged Communication

Each state has statutes regarding *privileged communication*, which
delineate which professionals have the legal privilege to withhold
conversations and communications. Although statutes vary, they cus-
tomarily provide this privilege to physicians, attorneys, and clergy.
Some states also extend privileged communication to psychologists,
nurses, and other healthcare providers.

Breach of Confidentiality

Courts have ruled that mandates protecting client confidentiality
end for therapists when confidences include threats against others.
Although courts recognize the duty to maintain confidentiality
between client and therapist, they have established that it is super-
seded by the duty to protect public safety. Healthcare professionals
must be aware that they cannot ignore or fail to attend to clients'
threats against others, especially when the opportunity for clients to
act on these threats is reasonable. Other legal situations that may
demand breaches of confidentiality include the following:

- Allegations of child abuse
- Threats of suicide
- Allegations of sexual misconduct against a therapist or other
  healthcare professional

Treatment in the Least Restrictive Environment

Courts have given guidance to the mental health system on many
matters, including standards for treatment settings. As early as 1969,

the court held that a person treated involuntarily should receive care in a setting least restrictive to liberty that still meets treatment needs. Least restrictive environments can be community resources instead of hospitalization, open units instead of locked units, or outpatient or home care instead of inpatient care. Continual assessment of the client's condition and status is necessary to ensure that more or less restrictive alternatives are consistent with the client's evolving needs.

Voluntary versus Involuntary Admission

When clients with psychiatric disorders are hospitalized, the type of admission determines the treatment plan. Civil commitment admissions include the following:

- Voluntary admissions
- Emergency admissions
- Involuntary commitments (indefinite duration)

Each state has specific statutory regulations pertaining to each status that mandate procedures for admission, discharge, and commitment for treatment (Table 2.1).

Cultural Perspectives of Mental Health and Mental Illness

Culture can influence perceptions of health and illness greatly, as well as how, when, and why people seek treatment for health problems. This factor becomes especially important in mental health. Many aspects of psychiatric care involve self-perception, roles and relationships, family dynamics and interactions, attitudes toward medications, values, and community supports.

Factors Affecting Use of Mental Health Services

Historically, many members of ethnically and racially diverse populations have avoided the mental healthcare delivery system. This avoidance arose from fear of being institutionalized, diagnosed incorrectly, or labeled "abnormal" because of culturally ingrained differences. Minority groups may display resistance to, and feel

table
2.1.
Types of Admission and Client Rights

Type of Admission	Description of Clients/Situation	Client's Rights
Voluntary	• Clients present themselves at psychiatric facilities and request hospitalization. • Clients are evaluated as being a danger to themselves or others or as so seriously mentally ill that they cannot adequately meet their own needs in the community but are willing to submit to treatment and competent to do so.	• Clients are considered competent (unless otherwise adjudicated) and therefore have the absolute right to refuse treatment, including psychotropic medications, unless they are dangerous to themselves or others. • Clients do not have an absolute right to discharge at any time but may be required to request discharge. The time delay gives healthcare personnel an opportunity to initiate a procedure to change a client's admission status to involuntary if he or she meets the necessary statutory requirements.
Emergency	• Client's behavior indicates that he or she is mentally ill and, consequently, likely to harm self or others (each state's statutes define the exact procedure for the initial evaluation, possible length of detainment, and attendant treatment available).	• Client's right to come and go is restricted. • Client's right to consult with an attorney to prepare for a hearing remains and must be protected. • Clients may be forced to take psychotropic medications, especially if they continue to be dangerous to themselves or others.

continued on page 30

table
2.1.

Types of Admission and Client Rights *continued*

Type of Admission	Description of Clients/Situation	Client's Rights
	• Diagnosis, evaluation, and emergency treatment are provided for all clients with emergency admission status.	• Invasive procedures, such as electroconvulsive therapy or psychosurgery, are not permitted unless they are ordered by the court or consented to by the client or his or her legal guardian.
	• At end of statutorily limited admission period, client discharge by facility, change in status to voluntary admission, or civil hearing via representative to determine the need for continuing involuntary treatment.	• No treatment should impair the client's ability to consult with an attorney at the time of a hearing.
Involuntary	• Individual refuses psychiatric hospitalization or treatment but poses a danger to self or others, is mentally ill, and is not judged suitable for less drastic options.	• Client is unable to leave facility when he or she wishes.

uncomfortable about, seeking mental health services for a variety of reasons, including:

- Stress experienced from forced migration, dislocation, or immigration
- Inability to speak or comprehend the dominant language and distrust of culturally inappropriate interpreter services
- Differences in religious beliefs and practices
- Environmental stress as a result of poverty or lack of equal access to education, employment, housing, or medical care
- Culture-specific beliefs about seeking help (eg, history, fear of being labeled or controlled by medications, shame, basic belief about illness)
- Use of traditional healers and alternative medicines for specific culture-bound situations
- Differing values and attitudes
- Misinterpretation of behaviors (eg, lateness, sense of bewilderment, codependence, assimilation, distrust, quietness)

Additionally, other factors may play a role:

- ***Variability and vulnerability:*** Variability in the incidence of mental illnesses among different cultural groups may be related to differences in genetic vulnerability (including variances among Native American tribes); biological variations that may be directly related to race include body structure, skin color, genetic code variations, susceptibility to disease, nutritional preferences and deficiencies, and psychological characteristics.
- ***Ethnopharmacology:*** Substantial racial and ethnic differences, which reflect both genetics and environment, influence responses to medications; racial and ethnic differences can affect metabolism of prescribed medications, which can influence a drug's safety and effectiveness with a particular client; clinical effectiveness and side effects also have been shown to vary among racial and ethnic groups.
- ***Traditional medicine:*** People from all parts of the world use traditional, complementary, or alternative medical practices; awareness of such "treatment" practices is crucial.

- *Accessibility:* The Americans with Disabilities Act of 1990 and Title VI of the Civil Rights Act of 1964 mandate accessibility to healthcare services and facilities for all U.S. citizens. Historically, however, mainstream mental health services have failed to meet the needs of the minority population adequately. Cultural barriers to treatment range from cultural insensitivity to obstacles such as difficulty understanding appointment procedures, lack of public transportation, signs written in a language not understood by the client, and formidable-looking buildings. Many services are inaccessible because of location or hours of service, and cultural barriers also may be related to historical circumstances that have led to a group's economic, social, and political status in the community

- *Racial bias:* Clients from nonwhite populations are institutionalized more frequently than are whites. This finding includes admissions to hospitals, involuntary commitments, and incarcerations. Racial bias affects such factors as definition of dangerousness, severity of diagnostic labels, and choice of treatments.

- *Religious and spiritual influences:* Many clients from minority populations interpret symptoms or signs of mental illness as spiritual. Consequently, they may choose to seek help from trusted spiritual leaders. Clients, families, and spiritual leaders may not identify signs or symptoms as indicating a mental health problem, or clients may be diagnosed with a mental health problem only after traditional healing methods have failed.

Culturally Competent and Congruent Care

To provide culturally congruent care, nurses must possess knowledge about cultural illnesses and healing practices as well as intercultural communication skills. They must develop self-awareness, flexibility, and working relationships that cross the lines of difference; they must become aware of their own cultural heritage and anticipate the culture shock of working outside their comfort zone.

When assessing and intervening with ethnic minorities, nurses must consider the following:

- Communication, including written and oral language, gestures, facial expressions, and body language

- Personal space, including both the space itself and the items sharing the designated space
- Social organization, including patterns of behavior during life events such as births, puberty, childbearing, illness, and death
- Time, both concrete and abstract
- Environment, including perceptions regarding control of the environment
- Biological variations among racial groups

Table 2.2 highlights four critical skills that nurses must acquire to provide culturally competent care.

table
2.2. **Critical Skills for Culturally Competent Care**

Skill	Strategies
Cross-cultural understanding (knowledge about how and why people of different cultures behave in certain ways)	• Study the relevant culture or identify a colleague from that culture and learn about the culture's values, norms, and mores. • Do not use this strategy in isolation because doing so may lead to over-generalization, ie, treating all members of a specific group exactly the same.
Intercultural communication (communication as the center of cross-cultural psychiatric-mental health nursing [some differences in communication are readily apparent; others are harder to discern, such as degree of openness, self-disclosure, emotional expression, insight, and even talkativeness])	• Develop listening skills, including learning to decipher nonverbal behavior and detect barriers that interfere with communication. • Gain expertise in this area; any unidentified intrapersonal stereotypes and biases would hinder their communicative skills. • Recognize if own communication style differs from that of a client; spend additional time with that client to improve understanding and ensure culturally competent care.

continued on page 34

table
2.2. Critical Skills for Culturally Competent Care *continued*

Skill	Strategies
	• Design strategies to minimize problems with language during interviews, such as using an interpreter to communicate effectively.
Facilitation skills	• Focus primarily on conflict resolution. • Gain the ability to negotiate interactions potentially inconsistent with the value and belief system of a client or family from a culture that differs from that of one's own.
Flexibility	• Learn to embrace change. • Modify expectations. • Adjust old operating norms and stereotypes. • Try new behaviors.

Assessment, Interviewing, and Communication

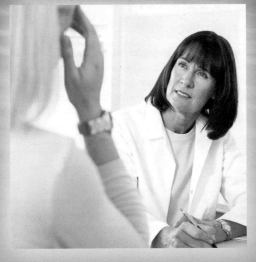

The Nurse–Client Relationship

The Nursing Process

The **nursing process** is an organized approach for providing quality psychiatric-mental health nursing care. The steps involved are the same as those used in other nursing specialties (eg, maternal-newborn, medical-surgical). Differences for psychiatric nursing, however, exist in terms of the manner and focus of the nurse's observations, the particulars of interviewing during data collection, and the types of interventions used for identified problems.

Assessment

Assessment, the first step of the nursing process, is the act of gathering, classifying, categorizing, analyzing, and documenting information about a client's health status. Nurses perform assessment with the understanding that all aspects of the client's life—spiritual, biological, psychological, social, cultural, cognitive, and behavioral—affect his or her well-being. Differences for psychiatric nursing, however, exist in terms of the manner and focus of the nurse's observations and the particulars of interviewing during data collection.

Assessment is the first standard of practice. Psychiatric mental health nurses obtain assessment data from several sources:

- Interviews with clients and their families
- Medical history and physical examination
- Mental status examination (MSE)
- Records from other healthcare facilities or prior treatments
- Laboratory and psychological tests
- Assessments by other professionals and paraprofessionals

Interviewing

The **psychiatric interview** is considered to be the primary assessment tool in clinical practice. The process of interview and assessment is a complex interaction between the nurse's communication and behavior styles and those of the client.

Nurses may conduct assessment interviews at different times during a client's treatment. When they encounter clients during a triage assessment (eg, in an emergency department), the nurses may obtain little background or historical information. In other circumstances, nurses conduct assessments of clients whom other healthcare professionals from various settings have already seen and treated. In these circumstances, nurses may have access (with the client's written consent) to a wealth of information about a client's medical history that they can use as a foundation for comparison and further assessment. Nurses need to be familiar with current laws as established in the Health Insurance Portability and Accountability Act (HIPAA) because these laws address legal parameters for sharing and receiving information from resources other than clients themselves (see Chapter 2).

In all circumstances, the nurse's understanding of the client's health history is helpful in preparing the interview setting, guiding the interview, and making recommendations for further care. Previous medical or surgical problems, psychiatric hospitalizations, psychotropic medications, and counseling interventions are just a few key components that can provide clues about which interventions have been successful or unsuccessful. Information about any family history of mental illness or suicidal tendencies can provide valuable information in assessing current risks. Historical data about the client's behavioral responses to intervention (eg, past verbal or physical aggression) can serve as important considerations when making decisions about where and how to conduct the interview in a way that minimizes risks for nurses and clients.

Communication

The quality of the interview and assessment depends on communication, the process of conveying information through various complex verbal and nonverbal behaviors. This process can be broken into several components:

- **Communicators**: people who simultaneously send and receive messages through words and nonverbal actions (eg, nodding, eye contact, facial expressions, posture)
- **Encoding**: the process by which a communicator puts into words or behaviors the ideas or feelings that he or she is trying to convey, such as shouting, crying, looking away, and choosing particular words
- **Decoding**: the process by which a communicator discerns or interprets what another is saying
- **Channel**: route or method a communicator chooses to convey a message, such as writing, talking, looking, e-mailing, and phoning
- **Feedback**: the discernible response, including all behaviors, that a receiver makes to a sender's message

Therapeutic Communication

Therapeutic communication occurs when the nurse demonstrates empathy, uses effective communication skills, and responds to the client's thoughts, needs, and concerns. This planned process allows nurse and client to build a trusting relationship in which the client is free to express thoughts, feelings, and options without fear of judgment (Table 3.1).

Nontherapeutic Communication

Nontherapeutic communication develops when nurses respond in ways that cause clients to feel defensive, misunderstood, controlled, minimized, alienated, or discouraged from expressing thoughts and feelings. Types include responding socially, using closed-ended questions, changing the subject, belittling, making stereotyped comments, giving false reassurance, moralizing, interpreting, advising, challenging, and defending. Although most people use nontherapeutic responses in everyday communication, it is important to be aware of how these responses deter open discussion and increase the likelihood of withdrawal by clients. Learning the labels for nontherapeutic approaches helps nurses to recognize and avoid them (Table 3.2).

Therapeutic Relationship

The **therapeutic relationship** is a close, helping relationship based on trust, which fosters collaboration. It is the foundation of all nursing care. The purpose of the therapeutic relationship in psychiatric-mental health nursing is to help clients solve problems, cope more effectively, and achieve developmental goals.

Elements of a Therapeutic Relationship

Certain key elements must exist, however, for a therapeutic relationship to develop:

- **Trust**: the foundation of all close relationships; involves taking the risk of sharing oneself with another, knowing that there is a chance of hurt, embarrassment, judgment, and disappointment; fostered by predictability, consistency, clear expectations, confidentiality, nonjudgmental acceptance
- **Professionalism**: application of a specific background of knowledge and skills with the purpose of promoting the client's mental health
- **Mutual respect**: sense of reverence for the human spirit and wonder at the uniqueness of each person without stigmatization
- **Caring**: demonstration of three primary behaviors: giving of the self, meeting the needs of clients in a timely manner, and providing comfort measures for clients and family; empathy, genuineness, and unconditional positive regard
- **Partnership**: role of clients and families as active partners in care with power sharing and negotiation

table
3.1. **Therapeutic Communication Techniques**

Technique	Description	Examples
Open-ended statements; broad openings	General questions to initiate conversation and encourage client to talk about any subject	"What would you like to talk about today?" "What brings you here?"
Validating	Reviewing and rephrasing key client statements	"Let me see if I understand." "It sounds like you are saying that you don't like having to take the medication. Is that correct?"
Clarifying	Questioning to better understand what client is saying; encourages the client to reconsider what was stated	I'm not sure what you mean by.…
Paraphrasing	Use of the nurse's words to reflect the meaning of the client's message; demonstrates to client that nurse has understood the client	"So you are saying that … helps you cope."
Reflection	Statement that indicates the underlying emotional basis of the message and redirects idea back to the client	Client: "Should I call my brother?" Nurse: "Should you call your brother?" "It sounds like you're unsure about.…?"

Focusing	Redirection of the client's attention toward something specific
	"Let's get back to talking about…." "You mentioned feeling…." Can you give me an example of when this occurs?"
Observation	Statement demonstrating what nurse has seen
	"Your lip quivers and you wring your hands when you talk about your wife. What are you feeling?"
Silence	No verbalization; remaining quiet
	Client: "I hate school" Nurse: <silence> Client: "I don't have any friends"
Confrontation; testing discrepancies	Cautious use of words nonjudgmentally to call attention to differences in client's statements
	"You said you're family never visits, but weren't they here earlier this afternoon?"
General leads	A means for elaborating via demonstration of interest in listening
	"I see." "Go on."

table
3.2. **Nontherapeutic Communication Techniques**

Technique	Description	Examples
False reassurance	Statement that trivializes client's feelings	"You're going to be just fine. Don't worry about anything."
Closed-ended questions	Questions that require a 'yes' or 'no' answer	"Do you understand everything I told you?" "Are you feeling sad today?"
Social responding	Superficial conversation that is not client-centered	Client: "I'm glad I'm being discharged today." Nurse: "Are you going to watch the game tonight?"
Clichés	Advice that has no meaning or worth to the client	"It's for your own good." "Just stay positive and everything will be okay." "Things get better with time."
Advising	Statements that offer the client specific suggestions	"I'd try the medication if I were you." "Why don't you try listening to music? That always helps me when I'm worried."

Belittling	Statement that discounts the client's feelings or makes the client's situation seem less than what the client feels it is	"There's nothing difficult about having to take medicine."
Patronizing	Statement that treats the client in a condescending manner	"Are we ready to go take our medicines?"
Changing the subject	Statement that ignores the current topic and introduces a new topic or a distantly related one	Client: "I'm worried about this therapy." Nurse: "What medications are you taking?" Client: "I think my wife is planning to divorce me." Nurse: "How long have you been married?"
Defending	Statement that argues or justifies a position rather than attempting to hear the client's concern	Client: "I can't get any help with this problem." Nurse: "We're doing the best we can to help, but we're really busy."
Interpreting	Intrusive comment in attempt to psychoanalyze the client	Client: "I don't want to take this medication." Nurse: "I think you're in denial about your illness."

43

table
3.3. **Social Versus Therapeutic Relationships**

Aspect	Social Relationships	Therapeutic Relationships
Purpose	Interactions provide companionship, recreation, and support for both parties.	The focus is health promotion, behavior change, and growth for the client.
Basis	Parties share equal give and take.	The nurse cares for the client; the client is not expected to respond to the nurse's personal needs.
Superficial discussions	Exploration of topics such as weather, sports, and television programs is normal.	Such talk blurs boundaries by introducing the nurse's background and personal preferences and distracting from the task of therapeutic change.
Self-disclosure	Both parties engage in increasingly free and revealing exchanges as the relationship develops.	The nurse facilitates the client's self-disclosure to promote change and growth. Nurses use self-disclosure only when it serves the client's needs.
Conflict	Both parties may argue freely, with relatively few constraints on words and emotions.	The nurse uses therapeutic communication skills to listen, confront, and set limits with clients while remaining calm, professional, and respectful. Even when clients are out of control, rude, or inappropriate, the nurse models appropriate communication.
Termination	Relationship may gradually fade or abruptly end if dissatisfaction or distance develops. Conversely, the relationship may be lifelong.	The nurse initiates and encourages discussion of any problems or behaviors that disrupt or inhibit the relationship. Termination is expected once the client resolves the presenting problem or moves to another therapeutic setting. Termination is planned and deliberate with therapeutic value.

Therapeutic versus Social Relationship

A therapeutic relationship is different from a social relationship. A social relationship is designed to meet the friendship needs of both parties (Table 3.3).

Phases of a Therapeutic Relationship

A therapeutic relationship a helping relationship based on trust, consists of three phases: the introductory phase; the middle or working phase; and termination. Each phase has predictable behaviors, dynamics, and challenges (Table 3.4).

table
3.4. **Phases of the Therapeutic Relationship**

Phase	Description
Introductory	The goal is to establish rapport and build a foundation for further work. Nurses focus on: • Introducing selves and greeting clients by name • Communicating interest in clients • Responding to any immediate concerns, such as questions, comfort needs, or emergency issues • Setting the parameters for nurse–client interactions; establishing contracts • Gathering data • Discerning the focal problem, setting goals, and beginning to plan interventions • Reducing client anxieties Client often tests nurse's commitment, eg, acting out, missing appointments. Goals must be met before moving on to next phase: • Trust is established, and both parties perceive the relationship as safe. • The client can verbalize thoughts and feelings. • Both the nurse and client have identified and agreed upon a focal problem or purpose for the relationship. • The client's strengths, weaknesses, and priorities for intervention are becoming clear. • The nurse has explained his or her role.
Middle or working phase	Clients are involved actively in achieving goals set during the initial phase. They make progress by testing new behaviors, identifying resources, and discovering avenues for change.

continued on page 46

table
3.4. **Phases of the Therapeutic Relationship** *continued*

Phase	Description
	As clients achieve goals, nurses provide feedback and support. Many clients go through periods of resisting change. Goals must be met before moving onto next phase:
	• The client has identified past behaviors that have been ineffective for coping with the focal problem.
	• The client has developed a plan of action, practiced implementing it, and evaluated its effectiveness.
	• The client has integrated a new self-concept, worldview, or attitude toward the illness as a result of changes in behavior and circumstances.
	• The client and family express increased hopefulness for the future and ability to function independently.
Termination	The relationship comes to a close.
	Clients often regress during the termination phase.
	The nurse's job is to remain consistent, caring, and hopeful about the client's progress.
	This is the time to review work, discuss any remaining questions, clear up misconceptions, and applaud the client's progress. On a more human level, it is a time to remember the high points in the relationship (moments of laughter or insight), acknowledge and let go of the low points, and appreciate the time that the nurse and client have spent together.
	During the termination phase, nurses should feel free to share their positive feelings and admiration for clients, as well as to express enjoyment of the relationship.
	Nurses educate families about the client's condition, advise them of the potential for symptom recurrence, and inform them about signs of relapse; make specific recommendations regarding how to help clients maintain their improved functioning.
	Before conclusion, the nurse and client evaluate whether they have met the following goals of the termination stage:
	• Contacts between nurse and client are spaced further apart or appointments are shorter to allow for increased independence.
	• Both parties have expressed feelings about the loss of the relationship.
	• Interactions are more relaxed, less intense, and focused on the future.
	• The nurse discourages cues that lead to new areas of exploration.
	• The nurse provides necessary referrals and links with community resources.

4

Common Psychiatric Assessment Tools

A ssessment tools are helpful in obtaining general information about a client or gathering specific information related to a condition or the client's current status or function. Various assessment tools are available for use when assessing clients with psychiatric mental health conditions.

General Assessment Tools
Brief Psychiatric Rating Scale

○ BOX 4.1 ○

DIRECTIONS: Place an X in the appropriate box to represent level of severity of each symptom.

	Not Present	Very Mild	Mild	Moderate	Moderate/Severe	Severe	Extremely Severe
SOMATIC CONCERN–preoccupation with physical health, fear of physical illness, hypochondriasis.	❏	❏	❏	❏	❏	❏	❏
ANXIETY–worry, fear, overconcern for present or future, uneasiness.	❏	❏	❏	❏	❏	❏	❏
EMOTIONAL WITHDRAWAL–lack of spontaneous interaction, isolation deficiency in relating to others.	❏	❏	❏	❏	❏	❏	❏
CONCEPTUAL DISORGANIZA-TION–thought processes confused, disconnected, disorganized, disrupted.	❏	❏	❏	❏	❏	❏	❏
GUILT FEELINGS–self-blame, shame, remorse for past behavior.	❏	❏	❏	❏	❏	❏	❏
TENSION–physical and motor mani-festations of nervousness, over-activation.							
MANNERISMS AND POSTURING–peculiar, bizarre unnatural motor behavior (not including tic).	❏	❏	❏	❏	❏	❏	❏
GRANDIOSITY–exaggerated self-opinion, arrogance, conviction of unusual power or abilities.	❏	❏	❏	❏	❏	❏	❏
DEPRESSIVE MOOD–sorrow, sad-ness, despondency, pessimism.	❏	❏	❏	❏	❏	❏	❏
HOSTILITY–animosity, contempt, belligerence, disdain for others.	❏	❏	❏	❏	❏	❏	❏
SUSPICIOUSNESS–mistrust, belief others harbour malicious or discrimi-natory intent.	❏	❏	❏	❏	❏	❏	❏
HALLUCINATORY BEHAVIOR–perceptions without normal external stimulus correspondence.	❏	❏	❏	❏	❏	❏	❏

BOX 4.1 *continued*

DIRECTIONS: Place an X in the appropriate box to represent level of severity of each symptom.

	Not Present	Very Mild	Mild	Moderate	Moderate/Severe	Severe	Extremely Severe
MOTOR RETARDATION–slowed weakened movements or speech, reduced body tone.	❏	❏	❏	❏	❏	❏	❏
UNCOOPERATIVENESS–resistance, guardedness, rejection of authority.	❏	❏	❏	❏	❏	❏	❏
UNUSUAL THOUGHT CONTENT–unusual, odd, strange, bizarre thought content.	❏	❏	❏	❏	❏	❏	❏
BLUNTED AFFECT–reduced emotional tone, reduction in formal intensity of feelings, flatness.	❏	❏	❏	❏	❏	❏	❏
EXCITEMENT–heightened emotional tone, agitation, increased reactivity.	❏	❏	❏	❏	❏	❏	❏
DISORIENTATION–confusion or lack of proper association for person, place, or time.	❏	❏	❏	❏	❏	❏	❏
Global Assessment Scale (Range 1–100)	❏	❏	❏	❏	❏	❏	❏

(Reprinted with permission from Overall, J. E. [1998]. The Brief Psychiatric Rating Scale [BPRS]: Recent developments in ascertainment and scaling. *Psychopharmacology Bulletin*, 24, 97–99.)

Brief Review of Sleep Patterns

BOX 4.2

1. Average hours/night _____

2. Routine times _____ Variable routine_____ No routine_____

3. Difficulty Falling Asleep _____ Staying Asleep _____ Early AM wakening _____

4. Nightmares _____ Night Terrors _____ Sleepwalking _____

5. Sleep Apnea _____ Snoring _____

6. Sedative/Hypnotic Medications (name, dose, duration of use, effectiveness):
_____
_____

FICA Spiritual Assessment Tool

BOX 4.3

F: Faith and Beliefs
I: Importance and influence
C: Community
A: Address

Detailed questions relating to acronym:

F: What is your faith or belief?
   Do you consider yourself spiritual or religious?
   What things do you believe in that give meaning to your life?
I: Is it important in your life?
   What influence does it have on how you take care of yourself?
   How have your beliefs influenced your behavior during this illness?
   What role do your beliefs play in regaining your health?
C: Are you part of a spiritual or religious community?
   Is this of support to you?
   Is there a person or group of people whom you really love or who are
   really important to you?
A: How would you like me, your [nurse], to address these issues in your
   healthcare?

General recommendations when taking a spiritual history:

1. Consider spirituality as a potentially important component of every client's
   physical well-being and mental health.
2. Address spirituality at each complete physical examination and continue
   addressing it at follow-up visits if appropriate. In patient care, spirituality
   is an ongoing issue.
3. Respect a client's privacy regarding spiritual beliefs; do not impose your
   beliefs on others.
4. Make referrals to chaplains, spiritual directors, or community resources as
   appropriate.
5. Be aware that your own spiritual beliefs will help you personally and will
   overflow in your encounters with those for whom you are to make the
   [nurse]–patient encounter a more humanistic one.

Adapted from Puchalski, C. (2001). Taking a spiritual history allows clinicians to understand
patients more M. Solomon, A. Romer, K. Heller, & D. Weissman (Eds.). *Innovations in end-of-life
care: Practical strategies and international perspectives* (Vol. II). Larchmont, NY: Mary
Ann Liebert.

Global Assessment of Functioning (GAF) Scale

BOX 4.4

Consider psychological, social, and occupational functioning on a hypothetical continuum of mental health-illness. Do not include impairment in functioning due to physical (or environmental) limitations.

CODE	(Note: Use intermediate codes when appropriate, eg, 45, 68, 72.)
100 – 91	**Superior functioning in a wide range of activities, life's problems never seem to get out of hand, is sought out by others because of his or her many positive qualities. No symptoms.**
90 – 81	**Absent or minimal symptoms** (eg, mild anxiety before an exam), **good functioning in all areas, interested and involved in a wide range of activities, socially effective, generally satisfied with life, no more than everyday problems or concerns** (eg, an occasional argument with family members).
80 – 71	**If symptoms are present, they are transient and expectable reactions to psychosocial stressors** (eg, difficulty concentrating after family argument); **no more than slight impairment in social, occupational, or school functioning** (eg, temporarily falling behind in schoolwork).
70 – 61	**Some mild symptoms** (eg, depressed mood and mild insomnia) **OR some difficulty in social, occupational, or school functioning** (eg, occasional truancy, or theft within the household), **but generally functioning pretty well, has some meaningful interpersonal relationships.**
60 – 51	**Moderate symptoms** (eg, flat affect and circumstantial speech, occasional panic attacks) **OR moderate difficulty in social, occupational, or school functioning** (eg, few friends, conflicts with peers or co-workers).

continued on page 52

○ BOX 4.4 *continued* ○

CODE	(Note: Use intermediate codes when appropriate, eg, 45, 68, 72.)
50 – 41	**Serious symptoms** (eg, suicidal ideation, severe obsessional rituals, frequent shoplifting) **OR any serious impairment in social, occupational, or school functioning** (eg, no friends, unable to keep a job).
40 – 31	**Some impairment in reality testing or communication** (eg, speech is at times illogical, obscure, or irrelevant) **OR major impairment in several areas, such as work or school, family relations, judgment, thinking, or mood** (eg, depressed man avoids friends, neglects family, and is unable to work; child frequently beats up younger children, is defiant at home, and is failing at school).
30 – 21	**Behavior is considerably influenced by delusions or hallucinations OR serious impairment in communication or judgment** (eg, sometimes incoherent, acts grossly inappropriately, suicidal preoccupation) **OR inability to function in almost all areas** (eg, stays in bed all day: no job, home, or friends).
20 – 11	**Some danger of hurting self or others** (eg, suicide attempts without clear expectation of death; frequently violent; manic excitement) **OR occasionally fails to maintain minimal personal hygiene** (eg, smears feces) **OR gross impairment in communication** (eg, largely incoherent or mute).
10 – 1	**Persistent danger of severely hurting self or others** (eg, recurrent violence) **OR persistent inability to maintain minimal personal hygiene OR serious suicidal act with clear expectation of death.**
0	Inadequate information.

From American Psychiatric Association. (2000). *Diagnostic and Statistical Manual of Mental Disorders* (4th ed. text rev.). Washington, DC: Author.

Mini-Mental State Examination

○ BOX 4.5 ○

MMSE Sample Items

Orientation to Time
"What is the date?"

Registration
"Listen carefully, I am going to say three words. You say them back after I stop. Ready? Here they are . . .
HOUSE (pause), CAR (pause), LAKE (pause). Now repeat those words back to me." [Repeat up to five times, but score only the first trial.]

Naming
"What is this?" [Point to a pencil or pen.]

Reading
"Please read this and do what it says." [Show examinee the words on the stimulus form.]
CLOSE YOUR EYES

PERSONS Acronym for Identifying Major Aspects of Psychiatric Mental Health Nursing Assessment

○ BOX 4.6 ○

P—Perceptions of the client, Presenting symptoms, Previous psychiatric treatment, Previous medication, Previous medical illness, Precipitating events, Physical assessment

E—Educational background, Employment background, Environment of home life

R—Relationships (with family, significant others, support systems), Review of systems

S—Substance use and abuse

O—Objective observations (of thought content, thought processes, mood/affect and behavior, physical examination)
Obstacles to treatment (including financial and environmental)

N—Needs that are specialized (language, hearing, reading/writing, cultural, spiritual)

S—Safety assessment (suicide potential, homicidal ideation, victimization issues such as abuse or neglect)

Psychosocial Assessment Guide with Questions

BOX 4.7

AREA OF FOCUS	INFORMATION TO CONSIDER
Client's complaint; present symptoms, focus of concern	• What caused the client to seek help at this time? • What symptoms is the client experiencing? • Is the client a danger to self or others?
Perceptions and expectations	• What are the client's perceptions about the problem? • Whose idea was it to seek help? • How does the client feel about receiving treatment? • When does the client anticipate no longer needing treatment in this setting? • If the client describes a cluster of problems, ask, "What would you say is the biggest problem you have now?"

Previous hospitalizations and mental health treatment (*The nurse should try not to spend too much time in this area at first. He or she can gather more data as the nurse–client relationship develops.*)	• How old was the client when he or she first saw a psychiatrist or counselor?
	• Has the client ever had any suicide attempts?
	  • If so, did the client want to die?
	  • Was the attempt impulsive or planned?
	  • Did the client write a note?
	  • Did the client tell anyone after the attempt?
	  • How did the client feel about surviving?

Family history	• Have the client's grandparents, parents, siblings, or children had any problems with mental illness or substance abuse? • What medical illnesses or addictions run in the client's family?
Developmental history (age related)	• Ask the adult client at the time of initial assessment. "Are you satisfied with the way your life has gone so far? Do you have any regrets?"
Health beliefs and practices	• What medications is the client taking? • What are they for? • Do they help? • Does the client experience side effects? • Is the client taking the medications exactly as prescribed? • Does the client ever forget them?

○ BOX 4.7 continued ○

AREA OF FOCUS	INFORMATION TO CONSIDER
	• What does the client know about his or her illness?
	• Does the client think that he or she can do things to help manage symptoms? If so, will he or she be able to do them?
Substance use	• Determine the last use of alcohol and illicit or abused drugs and the amount.
	• Ask, "At what point in your life did you start using more than you had intended?"
	• Has the client been addicted to drugs or alcohol in the past?
Sexual history	• Does the current problem affect sexual function?
	• Is the client satisfied with current sexual activity?
Abuse	• Has the client been physically, sexually, or verbally abused?
	• Was the client neglected as a child?
Spiritual	• What are the client's religious preferences, spiritual beliefs, and religious practices?
	• Does the client participate in church activities?
	• What does the client believe in?
	• How important are the client's religious beliefs to him or her?
Basic needs (diet, exercise, sleep, elimination)	• Ask the client to describe a typical day.
Sociocultural (occupation, education, race, culture, financial security, household members, satisfaction with living arrangements, leisure activities)	• Is the client spending as much time with other people as usual?
	• Are the other people responding to the client differently now?
	• Have the client's most significant or intimate relationships changed lately?
	• How do the client's friends feel about his or her situation now?
	• Who are the client's greatest supports?
	• Does the client get involved in community activities? Has that changed lately?
Coping patterns	• Have the client and family (or whomever the client lives with) been under any unusual stress in the past year? For example, has anyone in the family died or been very sick?
	• Have there been many changes in the client's life lately?

continued on page 56

○ BOX 4.7 *continued* ○

AREA OF FOCUS	INFORMATION TO CONSIDER
Self-esteem	• When under stress, what does the client usually do to help himself or herself? • How does this problem relate to other problems the client has had in the past? • Is there a pattern? • How does the client see himself or herself now? • Has this situation affected the client's self-esteem?
Medical concerns or assessment	• Ask the client to describe allergies, current medications, previous medical illness, and hospitalizations. • Conduct a review of systems.

Recent Life Changes Questionnaire

○ BOX 4.8 ○

SOCIAL AREA	LIFE CHANGES	LCU VALUES
Family	Death of spouse	105
	Marital separation	65
	Death of close family member	65
	Divorce	62
	Pregnancy	60
	Change in health of family member	52
	Marriage	50
	Gain of new family member	50
	Marital reconciliation	42
	Spouse begins or stops work	37
	Son or daughter leaving home	29
	In-law trouble	29
	Change in number of family get-togethers	26
Personal	Jail term	56
	Sex difficulties	49
	Death of a close friend	46
	Personal injury or illness	42
	Change in living conditions	39
	Outstanding personal achievement	33
	Change in residence	33
	Minor violations of the law	32
	Begin or end school	32

BOX 4.8 continued

SOCIAL AREA	LIFE CHANGES	LCU VALUES
	Change in sleeping habits	31
	Revision of personal habits	31
	Change in eating habits	29
	Change in church activities	29
	Vacation	29
	Change in school	28
	Change in recreation	28
	Christmas	26
Work	Fired at work	64
	Retirement from work	49
	Trouble with boss	39
	Business readjustment	38
	Change to different line of work	38
	Change in work responsibilities	33
	Change in work hours or conditions	30
Financial	Foreclosure of mortgage or loan	57
	Change in financial state	43
	Mortgage (eg, home, car)	39
	Mortgage or loan less than $10,000 (eg, stereo)	26

Directions: Sum the LCUs for your life change events during the past 12 months.
  250 and 400 LCUs per year: Minor life crisis
  Over 400 LCUs per year: Major life crisis
*LCU. Life change unit. The number of LCUs reflects the average degree or intensity of the life change.
(From Rahe. R. H. (2000). Recent Life Changes Questionnaire [RLCQ] (1997). Holmes. T. H. in American Psychiatric Association, Task Force for the Handbook of Psychiatric Measures. *Handbook of psychiatric measures.* Washington. DC: American Psychiatric Association, pp. 235–237.)

Sexual History

BOX 4.9

I. Identifying data
  A. Age
  B. Sex
  C. Occupation
  D. Relationship status—single, married, number of times previously married, separated, divorced, cohabiting, serious involvement, casual dating (difficulty forming or keeping relationships should be assessed throughout the interview)
  E. Sexual orientation—hetero-sexual, homosexual, or bisexual (this may also be ascertained later in the interview)
II. Current functioning
  A. Unsatisfactory to highly satisfactory

continued on page 58

BOX 4.9 continued

B. If unsatisfactory, why?
C. Feeling about partner satisfaction
D. Dysfunctions?—eg, lack of desire, erectile disorder, inhibited female arousal, anorgasmia, premature ejaculation, retarded ejaculation, pain associated with intercourse (dysfunction discussed later)
  1. Onset—lifelong or acquired
    a. If acquired, when?
    b. Did onset coincide with drug use (medications or illegal recreational drugs), life stresses (eg, loss of job, birth of child), interpersonal difficulties
  2. Generalized—occurs in most situations or with most partners
  3. Situational
    a. Only with current partner
    b. In any committed relationship
    c. Only with masturbation
    d. In socially proscribed circumstance (eg, affair)
    e. In definable circumstance (eg, very late at night, in parental home, when partner initiated sex play)
E. Frequency—partnered sex (coital and noncoital sex play)
F. Desire/libido—how often are sexual feelings, thoughts, fantasies, dreams, experienced? (per day, week, etc.)
G. Description of typical sexual interaction
  1. Manner of initiation or invitation (eg, verbal or physical? Does same person always initiate?)
  2. Presence, type, and extent of foreplay (eg, kissing, caressing, manual or oral genital stimulation)
  3. Coitus? positions used?
  4. Verbalization during sex? if so, what kind?
  5. Afterplay? (whether sex act is completed or disrupted by dysfunction); typical activities (eg, holding, talking, return to daily activities, sleeping)
  6. Feeling after sex: relaxed, tense, angry, loving
H. Sexual compulsivity?—intrusion of sexual thoughts or participation in sexual activities to a degree that interferes with relationships or work, requires deception, and may endanger the patient
III. Past sexual history
  A. Childhood sexuality
    1. Parental attitudes about sex—degree of openness or reserve (assess unusual prudery or seductiveness)
    2. Parents' attitudes about nudity and modesty
    3. Learning about sex
      a. From parents? (initiated by child's questions or parent volunteering information? which parent? what was child's age?); subjects covered (eg, pregnancy, birth, intercourse, menstruation, nocturnal emission, masturbation)
      b. From books, magazines, or friends at school or through religious group?

BOX 4.9 *continued*

c. Significant misinformation
d. Feeling about information
4. Viewing or hearing primal scene—reaction?
5. Viewing sex play or intercourse of person other than parent
6. Viewing sex between pets or other animals

B. Childhood sex activities
1. Genital self-stimulation before adolescence; age? reaction if apprehended?
2. Awareness of self as boy or girl; bathroom sensual activities? (regarding urine, feces, odor, enemas)
3. Sexual play or exploration with another child (playing doctor)—type of activity (eg, looking, manual touching, genital touching); reactions or consequences if apprehended (by whom?)

IV. Adolescence
A. Age of onset of puberty—development of secondary sex characteristics, age of menarche for girl, wet dreams or first ejaculation for boy (preparation for and reaction to)
B. Sense of self as feminine or masculine—body image, acceptance by peers (opposite sex and same sex), sense of sexual desirability, onset of coital fantasies
C. Sex activities
1. Masturbation—age begun; ever punished or prohibited? method used, accompanying fantasies, frequency (questions about masturbation and fantasies

are among the most sensitive for patients to answer)
2. Homosexual activities—ongoing or rare and experimental episodes, approached by others? If homosexual, has there been any heterosexual experimentation?
3. Dating—casual or steady, description of first crush, infatuation, or first love
4. Experiences of kissing, necking, petting ("making out" or "fooling around"), age begun, frequency, number of partners, circumstances, type(s) of activity
5. Orgasm—when first experienced? (may not be experienced during adolescence), with masturbation, during sleep, or with partner? with intercourse or other sex play? frequency?
6. First coitus—age, circumstances, partner, reactions (may not be experienced during adolescence); contraception and/or safe sex precautions used

V. Adult sexual activities (may be experienced by some adolescents)
A. Premarital sex
1. Types of sex play experiences—frequency of sexual interactions, types and number of partners
2. Contraception or safe sex precautions used
3. First coitus (if not

continued on page 60

BOX 4.9 continued

experienced in adolescence) age, circumstances, partner

4. Cohabitation—age begun, duration, description of partner, sexual fidelity, types of sexual activity, frequency, satisfaction, number of cohabiting relationships, reasons for breakup(s)

5. Engagement—age, activity during engagement period with fiancé(e), with others; length of engagement

B. Marriage (if multiple marriages have occurred, explore sexual activity, reasons for marriage, and reasons for divorce in each marriage)

1. Types and frequency of sexual interaction—describe typical sexual interaction (see above), satisfaction with sex life? view of partner's feeling

2. First sexual experience with spouse—when? what were the circumstances? was it satisfying? disappointing?

3. Honeymoon—setting, duration, pleasant or unpleasant, sexually active? frequency? problems? compatibility?

4. Effect of pregnancies and children on marital sex

5. Extramarital sex—number of incidents, partner; emotional attachment to

extramarital partners? feelings about extramarital sex

6. Postmarital masturbation—frequency? effect on marital sex?

7. Extramarital sex by partner—effect on interviewee

8. Ménage à trois or multiple sex (swinging)

9. Areas of conflict in marriage (eg, parenting, finances, division of responsibilities, priorities)

VI. Sex after widowhood, separation, divorce—celibacy, orgasms in sleep, masturbation, noncoital sex play, intercourse (number of and relationship to partners), other

VII. Special issues

A. History of rape, incest, sexual or physical abuse

B. Spousal abuse (current)

C. Chronic illness (physical or psychiatric)

D. History or presence of sexually transmitted diseases

E. Fertility problems

F. Abortions, miscarriages, or unwanted or illegitimate pregnancies

G. Gender identity conflict (eg, transsexualism, wearing clothes of opposite sex)

H. Paraphilias (eg, fetishes, voyeurism, sadomasochism)

Sleep Pattern Assessment

O BOX 4.10 O

Typical Sleep Pattern
- Bedtime
- Wakeup time
- Duration of sleep
- Frequency of nighttime awakenings
- Duration of time from lights out to sleep onset
- Daytime napping
- Perceived causes of nighttime awakenings
- Differences in sleep patterns between weekdays and weekends
- Events occurring during sleep: pain, parasomnias, snoring
- Limb movements or limb discomfort during sleep
- Recent changes in sleep pattern; perception of cause

Factors That May Influence Sleep
- Environment: noise, lighting
- Medical disorders
- Psychiatric disorders
- Stressors
- Medications

Consequences of Sleep
- Satisfaction with sleep
- Daytime sleepiness
- Cognitive function
- Memory
- Work performance
- Social relationships
- History of accidents/injury
- Mood
- Quality of life
- Unusual events occurring during sleep
- Snoring
- Parasomnias
- Sleep environment

Anxiety Assessment Tools
Hamilton Rating Scale for Anxiety

BOX 4.11

Instructions: This checklist is to assist the physician or psychiatrist in evaluating each patient as to his or her degree of anxiety and pathological condition. Please fill in the appropriate rating.

NONE = 0   MILD = 1   MODERATE = 2   SEVERE = 3   SEVERE, GROSSLY DISABLING = 4

ITEM		RATING	ITEM		RATING
Anxious mood	Worries, anticipation of the worst, fearful anticipation, irritability		Cardiovascular symptoms	Tachycardia, palpitations, pain in chest, throbbing of vessels, fainting feelings, missing beat	
Tension	Feelings of tension, fatigability, startle response, moved to tears easily, trembling, feelings of restlessness, inability to relax		Respiratory symptoms	Pressure or constriction in chest, choking feelings, sighing, dyspnea	
Fears	Of dark, of strangers, of being left alone, of animals, of traffic, of crowds		Gastrointestinal symptoms	Difficulty in swallowing, wind, abdominal pain, burning sensations, abdominal fullness, nausea, vomiting, borborygmi, looseness of bowels, loss of weight, constipation	
Insomnia	Difficulty in falling asleep, broken sleep, unsatisfying sleep and fatigue on				

	waking dreams, nightmares, night terrors	Genitourinary symptoms	Frequency of micturition, urgency of micturition, amenorrhea, menorrhagia, development of frigidity, premature ejaculation, loss of libido, impotence
Intellectual (cognitive)	Difficulty in concentration, poor memory		
Depressed mood	Loss of interest, lack of pleasure in hobbies, depression, early waking, diurnal swing	Autonomic symptoms	Dry mouth, flushing, pallor, tendency to sweat, giddiness, tension headache, raising of hair
Somatic (muscular)	Pains and aches, twitching, stiffness, myoclonic jerks, grinding of teeth, unsteady voice, increased muscular tone	Behavior at interview	Fidgeting, restlessness or pacing, tremor of hands, strained face, sighing or rapid respiration, furrowed brow, swallowing, belching, facial pallor, brisk tendon jerks, dilated pupils, exophthalmos
Somatic (sensory)	Tinnitus, blurring of vision, hot and cold flushes, feeling of weakness, picking sensation		

ADDITIONAL COMMENTS:

Investigator's signature:

Reprinted with permission from the British Journal of Medical Psychology *(1959), Vol. 32, 50–55. © British Psychological Society.*

Yale-Brown Obsessive Compulsive Scale

BOX 4.12

For each item circle the number identifying the response that best characterizes the patient.

1. Time occupied by obsessive thoughts
   How much of your time is occupied by obsessive thoughts? How frequently do the obsessive thoughts occur?
   0 None
   1 Mild (less than 1 h/day) or occasional (intrusion occurring no more than 8 times a day)
   2 Moderate (1–3 h/day) or frequent (intrusion occurring more than 8 times a day, but most of the hours of the day are free of obsessions)
   3 Severe (greater than 3 and up to 8 h/day) or very frequent (intrusion occurring more than 8 times a day and occurring during most of the hours of the day)
   4 Extreme (greater than 8 h/day) or near consistent intrusion (too numerous to count and an hour rarely passes without several obsessions occurring)

2. Interference due to obsessive thoughts
   How much do your obsessive thoughts interfere with your social or work (or role) functioning?
   Is there anything that you don't do because of them?
   0 None
   1 Mild, slight interference with social or occupational activities, but overall performance not impaired
   2 Moderate, definite interference with social

or occupational performance but still manageable
   3 Severe, causes substantial impairment in social or occupational performance
   4 Extreme, incapacitating

3. Distress associated with obsessive thoughts
   How much distress do your obsessive thoughts cause you?
   0 None
   1 Mild, infrequent, and not too disturbing
   2 Moderate, frequent, and disturbing but still manageable
   3 Severe, very frequent, and very disturbing
   4 Extreme, near constant, and disabling distress

4. Resistance against obsessions
   How much of an effort do you make to resist the obsessive thoughts?
   How often do you try to disregard or turn your attention away from these thoughts as they enter your mind?
   0 Makes an effort to always resist, or symptoms so minimal doesn't need to actively resist
   1 Tries to resist most of the time
   2 Makes some effort to resist
   3 Yields to all obsession without attempting to control them, but does so with some reluctance
   4 Completely and willingly yields to all obsessions

BOX 4.12 continued

5. Degree of control over obsessive thoughts

How much control do you have over your obsessive thoughts? How successful are you in stopping or diverting your obsessive thinking?

0 Complete control
1 Much control, usually able to stop or divert obsessions with some effort and concentration
2 Moderate control, sometimes able to stop or divert obsessions
3 Little control, rarely successful in stopping obsessions
4 No control, experienced as completely involuntary, rarely able to even momentarily divert thinking

6. Time spent performing compulsive behaviors

How much time do you spend performing compulsive behaviors? How frequently do you perform compulsions?

0 None
1 Mild (less than 1 h/day performing compulsions) or occasional (performance of compulsions occurring no more than 8 times a day)
2 Moderate (1–3 h/day performing compulsions) or frequent (performance of compulsions occurring more than 8 times a day, but most of the hours of the day are free of compulsive behaviors)
3 Severe (greater than 3 and up to 8 h/day performing

compulsions) or very frequent (performance of compulsions occurring more than 8 times a day and occurring during most of the hours of the day)
4 Extreme (greater than 8 h/day performing compulsions) or near consistent performance of compulsions (too numerous to count and an hour rarely passes without several compulsions being performed)

7. Interference due to compulsive behaviors

How much do your compulsive behaviors interfere with your social or work (or role) functioning? Is there anything that you don't do because of the compulsions

0 None
1 Mild, slight interference with social or occupational activities, but overall performance not impaired
2 Moderate, definite interference with social or occupational performance but still manageable
3 Severe, causes substantial impairment in social or occupational performance
4 Extreme, incapacitating

8. Distress associated with compulsive behavior

How would you feel if prevented from performing you compulsions? How anxious would you become? How anxious do you get while performing compulsions until you are satisfied they are completed?

continued on page 66

BOX 4.12 *continued*

0 None
1 Mild, only slightly anxious if compulsions prevented or only slightly anxious during performance of compulsions
2 Moderate, reports that anxiety would mount but remain manageable if compulsion prevented or that anxiety increases but remains manageable during performance of compulsions
3 Severe, prominent and very disturbing increase in anxiety if compulsions interrupted or prominent and very disturbing increases in anxiety during performance of compulsions
4 Extreme, incapacitating anxiety from any intervention aimed at modifying activity or incapacitating anxiety develops during performance of compulsions

9. Resistance against compulsions
How much of an effort do you make to resist the compulsions?
0 Makes an effort to always resist, or symptoms so minimal doesn't need to actively resist
1 Tries to resist most of the time
2 Makes some effort to resist
3 Yields to all compulsions without attempting to control them but does so with some reluctance
4 Completely and willingly yields to all compulsions

10. Degree of control over compulsive behavior
0 Complete control
1 Much control, experiences pressure to perform the behavior but usually able to exercise voluntary control over it
2 Moderate control, strong pressure to perform behavior, can control it only with difficulty
3 Little control, very strong drive to perform behavior, must be carried to completion, can only delay with difficulty
4 No control, drive to perform behavior experienced as completely involuntary

Reprinted with permission from Goodman, W. K., Price, L. H., Rasmussen, S. A., et al. (1989). The Yale-Brown Obsessive-Compulsive Scale, 1: Development, use and reliability. Arch Gen Psychiatry, 46, 1006.

Abuse and Violence Assessment Tools
Abuse Assessment Screen

BOX 4.13

1. Have you ever been emotionally or physically abused by your partner or someone important to you?
   YES _____
   NO _____

2. Within the past year have you been hit, stapped, kicked, or otherwise physically hurt by someone?
   YES _____
   NO _____
   If YES. By whom: _____
   Number of times: _____
   Mark the area of injury on body map

3. Within the past year has anyone forced you to have sexual activities?
   If YES. who: _____
   Number of times: _____

4. Are you afraid of your partner or anyone you listed above?
   YES _____
   NO _____

Burgess-Partner Abuse Scale for Teens

○ BOX 4.14 ○

Directions: During the past 12 months, you and one of your partners may have had a fight. Below is a list of things one of your partners may have done to you. Please circle the number of how often this partner did these things to you. This is not a test and there are no right or wrong answers. Remember, having a partner(s) does not mean you are having sex with the partner(s).

If you have not had a partner in the past 12 months, do not fill this form out

	NEVER	ONCE	A FEW TIMES	MORE THAN A FEW TIMES	ROUTINELY OR A LOT
1. My partner doesn't let me go out with my friends	0	1	2	3	4
2. My partner tells me what to wear	0	1	2	3	4
3. My partner says if I don't have sex with him/her then I don't love him/her	0	1	2	3	4
4. My partner says he/she will hurt me if I talk to another guy/girl	0	1	2	3	4
5. My partner calls me bad names like bitch	0	1	2	3	4
6. My partner says he/she will hurt me with a weapon	0	1	2	3	4
7. My partner forces me to have sex	0	1	2	3	4
8. My partner tells me I am stupid or dumb	0	1	2	3	4
9. My partner follows me when I do things with my friends or family	0	1	2	3	4
10. My partner hits or kicks something when he/she gets mad at me	0	1	2	3	4
11. My partner kicks me	0	1	2	3	4

12. My partner says he/she can have sex with other
    people even though he/she said I can't 0   1   2   3   4
13. My partner gives me sex infections 0   1   2   3   4
14. My partner hurts me using a weapon 0   1   2   3   4
15. My partner forces me to use drugs even though I don't
    want to 0   1   2   3   4
16. My partner beats me up so bad 0   1   2   3   4
17. My partner says he/she will hurt my family if I don't
    do what he/she says 0   1   2   3   4
18. My partner tells me what school activities I can and
    can't do 0   1   2   3   4
19. My partner tells me what friends I can hang out with . . 0   1   2   3   4
20. My partner chokes me if he/she gets mad at me 0   1   2   3   4
21. My partner yells at me if he/she doesn't know where
    I am 0   1   2   3   4
22. My partner says we can't break up even though I
    want to 0   1   2   3   4

How many partners have you had in the past 12 months? _____

SAFE Questions for Abuse

BOX 4.15

- **S**tress/**S**afety: What stress do you experience in your relationships? Do you feel safe in your relationships? Should I be concerned for your safety?
- **A**fraid/**A**bused: Have there been situations in your relationships where you have felt afraid? Has your partner ever threatened or abused you or your children? Have you ever been physically hurt or threatened by your partner? Are you in a relationship like that now? Has your partner ever forced you to engage in sexual intercourse that you did not want? People in relationships/ marriages often fight; what happens when you and your partner disagree?
- **F**riends/**F**amily: Are your friends aware that you have been hurt? Do your parents or siblings know about this abuse? Do you think you could tell them, and would they be able to give you support?
- **E**mergency plan: Do you have a safe place to go and the resources you (and your children) need in an emergency? If you are in danger now, would you like help in locating a shelter? Would you like to talk to a social worker/a counselor/me to develop an emergency plan?

Ashur M.L.C. (1993). Asking about domestic violence: SAFE questions. *JAMA 269*(18), 2367. © American Medical Association.

Violence Danger Assessment

BOX 4.16

Several risk factors have been associated with homicides (murders) of both batterers and battered women in research that has been conducted after the killings have taken place. We cannot predict what will happen in your case, but we would like you to be aware of the danger of homicide in situations of severe battering and to see how many of the risk factors apply to your situation. (The "he" in the questions refers to your husband, partner, ex-husband, ex-partner, or whoever is currently physically hurting you.)

1. Has the physical violence increased in frequency during the past year?
2. Has the physical violence increased in severity during the past year, or has a weapon or threat with a weapon been used?
3. Does he ever try to choke you?
4. Is there a gun in the house?
5. Has he ever forced you into sex when you did not wish to do so?

BOX 4.16 continued

6. Does he use drugs? By drugs, I mean "uppers" or amphetamines, speed, angel dust, cocaine, "crack," street drugs, heroin, or mixtures.

7. Does he threaten to kill you, or do you believe he is capable of killing you?

8. Is he drunk every day or almost every day? (In terms of quantity of alcohol.)

9. Does he control most or all of your daily activities? For instance, does he tell you whom you can be friends with, how much money you can take with you shopping, or when you can take the car? (If he tries, but you do not let him, check here—)

10. Has he ever beaten you while you were pregnant? (If never pregnant by him, check here—)

11. Is he violently and constantly jealous of you? (For instance, does he say, "If I can't have you, no one can.")

12. Have you ever threatened or tried to commit suicide?

13. Has he ever threatened or tried to commit suicide?

14. Is he violent toward the children?

15. Is he violent outside the home?

TOTAL YES ANSWERS:

THANK YOU. PLEASE TALK TO YOUR NURSE, ADVOCATE, OR COUNSELOR ABOUT WHAT THE DANGER ASSESSMENT MEANS IN TERMS OF YOUR SITUATION.

Adapted from Campbell. J., & Humphreys, J. (Eds.). (1993). *Nursing care of survivors of family violence* (p. 259). St. Louis: Mosby.

Dementia Assessment Tools

Questionnaire for Dementia

BOX 4.17

Subjective Data

Behavioral Changes (Often Asked of the Family)

Is there a change in behavior? If so,

a. How does the present behavior differ from former behavior?

b. When was this change in behavior first recognized?

Emotional Changes

- Are any of the following present: depression, anxiety, paranoia, agitation, grandiosity, confabulation?
- Does the client have insight into the fact that "things are not right?"
- Is the client complaining of many physical ailments for which there are no bases?
- Are certain previous personality traits becoming predominant or exaggerated?

Social Changes

- Is the client exhibiting embarrassingly loud and jocular behavior?
- Is there sexual acting-out beyond the bounds of propriety?
- Has the client shown signs of short temper, irritability, or aggressiveness?
- Is there an increasing inability to make social judgments?

Intellectual Behavior

- Has the ability to remember recent events decreased?
- Has the ability to problem-solve decreased? (This might be especially apparent in the work or job area.)
- Do new environments or even old environments result in the client's disorientation?

- Is it difficult for the client to carry out complex motor skills? Do his or her efforts result in many errors?
- Are any of the following language problems present:
  - Has the client's language changed?
  - Does the client's language ramble and wander from the point of the conversation?
  - Is the point of the conversation never clearly stated?
  - Is there difficulty comprehending complex material?
  - Does the client have trouble remembering names of people and objects?
  - Does the client have difficulty writing?

Functional Capacity

- Are there any changes in the client's ability to perform activities of daily living (ADLs)?
- Is there difficulty transferring or ambulating?
- Is there difficulty bathing, dressing, or grooming?
- Is there difficulty eating or toileting?
- Are there any changes in the client's ability to perform instrumental ADLs (IADLs)?
- Is the client able to make a grocery list, shop for food, and handle money?
- Is the client able to use the telephone?
- Can the client prepare a meal and complete housekeeping tasks?

○ BOX 4.17 continued ○

Objective Data

Level of Consciousness
Is the client confused, sleepy, withdrawn, adynamic, apathetic?

Appearance
Is there decreased personal hygiene?

Attention
- Does the client have decreased ability to repeat digits after the interviewer?
- Do other stimuli in the environment easily distract the client from the interviewer?
- Does the client focus on only one of the stimuli in the environment, and is he or she unable to turn attention from the one stimulus?

Language
- Outflow of words decreases.
- Patterns of repetitive, tangential, or concrete speech appear.
- Writing skills decrease more rapidly than the spoken word.

Memory
Test the client's ability to remember four unrelated words and recent events. (Confabulation and anger often will be used by the client to move the interviewer away from questions related to memory.)

Constructional Ability
The client is instructed to copy a series of line drawings; the client often is unable to do this, or the ability to do so declines dramatically over time.

Cortical Function
- The client's ability to perform arithmetic is faulty and reveals many errors.
- Proverb interpretation—Usually, the client gives only a concrete interpretation of the proverb.
- Similarities—The client often denies similarities between two objects and instead gives a concrete answer. For example, when asked, "What is the similarity between a tiger and a cat?" the client may reply, "One is small and one is large. There is no similarity."

Functional Dementia Scale

○ BOX 4.18 ○

Client _____
Observer _____
Position or relation to
patient _____
Facility _____
Date _____

Circle one rating for each item:
1. None or little of the time
2. Some of the time
3. Good part of the time
4. Most or all of the time

1	2	3	4	(1) Has difficulty in completing simple tasks on own (eg, dressing, bathing, doing arithmetic).
1	2	3	4	(2) Spends time either sitting or in apparently purposeless activity.
1	2	3	4	(3) Wanders at night or needs to be restrained to prevent wandering.
1	2	3	4	(4) Hears things that are not there.
1	2	3	4	(5) Requires supervision or assistance in eating.
1	2	3	4	(6) Loses things.
1	2	3	4	(7) Appearance is disorderly if left to own devices.
1	2	3	4	(8) Moans.
1	2	3	4	(9) Cannot control bowel function.
1	2	3	4	(10) Threatens to harm others.
1	2	3	4	(11) Cannot control bladder function.
1	2	3	4	(12) Needs to be watched so doesn't injure self (eg, by careless smoking, leaving the stove on, falling).

1	2	3	4	(13)	Destructive of materials around him/her (eg, breaks furniture, throws food trays, tears up magazines).
1	2	3	4	(14)	Shouts or yells.
1	2	3	4	(15)	Accuses others of doing him bodily harm or stealing his/her possessions—when you are sure the accusations are not true.
1	2	3	4	(16)	Is unaware of limitations imposed by illness.
1	2	3	4	(17)	Becomes confused and does not know where he/she is.
1	2	3	4	(18)	Has trouble remembering.
1	2	3	4	(19)	Has sudden changes of mood (eg, gets upset, angered, or cries easily).
1	2	3	4	(20)	If left alone, wanders aimlessly during the day or needs to be restrained to prevent wandering

Reprinted with permission from Moore, J.T., et al. (1983). A functional dementia scale. *Journal of Family Practice*, 16, 498. Copyright by Appleton and Lange.

Eating Disorder Assessment Tools
Criteria for Hospitalization: Eating Disorders

BOX 4.19

MEDICAL

- Weight loss, <75% below ideal
- Heart rate, <40 beats/min; children <20 beats/min
- Temperature, <36°C
- Blood pressure, <90/60 mm Hg; children, <80/50 mm Hg
- Glucose, <60 mg/dL
- Serum potassium, <3 mEq/L
- Severe dehydration
- Electrolyte imbalance

PSYCHIATRIC

- Risk for suicide
- Severe depression
- Failure to comply with treatment
- Inadequate response to treatment at another level of care (outpatient)

Adapted from Yoel, J. & Workgroup in Eating Disorders. (2000). Practice guidelines for the treatment of patients with eating disorder. *American Journal of Psychiatry, 157*(1), 1–35.

Disordered Eating Screening Questions

BOX 4.20

- How many diets have you been on in the past year?
- How often does your weight affect how you feel about yourself?
- How often do you feel you should be dieting?
- How often do you feel dissatisfied with your body size?

Reprinted with permission from Elsevier Science from "Rapid screening for disordered eating in college-aged females in the primary care setting" by Anstine, D. & Grinenko, D. *Journal of Adolescent Health, 26*(5), 338–342 © 2000 by the Society for Adolescent Medicine.

Eating Attitudes Test

BOX 4.21

Please place an (X) under the column that applies best to each of the numbered statements. All the results will be strictly confidential. Most of the questions relate to food or eating, although other types of questions have been included. Please answer each question carefully. Thank you.

	ALWAYS	VERY OFTEN	OFTEN	SOMETIMES	RARELY	NEVER
1. Like eating with other people.		—	—	—	—	—
2. Prepare foods for others but do not eat what I cook.	—		—	—	—	—
3. Become anxious prior to eating.	—	—	—	—	—	—
4. Am terrified about being overweight.	—	—	—	—	—	—
5. Avoid eating when I am hungry.	—	—	—	—	—	—
6. Find myself preoccupied with food.	—	—	—	—	—	—
7. Have gone on eating binges where I feel that I may not be able to stop.	—	—	—	—	—	—
8. Cut food into small pieces.	—	—	—	—	—	—
9. Aware of the calorie content of foods that I eat.	—		—	—	—	—
10. Particularly avoid foods with a high carbohydrate content (eg, bread, potatoes, rice, etc.).	—	—	—	—	—	—
11. Feel bloated after meals.	—	—	—	—	—	—

continued on page 78

BOX 4.2 | *continued*

	ALWAYS	VERY OFTEN	OFTEN	SOMETIMES	RARELY	NEVER
12. Feel that others would prefer I ate more.						
13. Vomit after I have eaten.						
14. Feel extremely guilty after eating.						
15. Am preoccupied with a desire to be thinner.						
16. Exercise strenuously to burn off calories.						
17. Weigh myself several times a day.						
18. Like my clothes to fit tightly.						
19. Enjoy eating meat.						
20. Wake up early in the morning.						
21. Eat the same foods day after day.						
22. Think about burning up calories when I exercise.						
23. Have regular menstrual periods.						
24. Other people think I am too thin.						
25. Am preoccupied with the thought of having fat on my body.						
26. Take longer than others to eat.						
27. Enjoy eating at restaurants.						
28. Take laxatives.						
29. Avoid foods with sugar in them.						

30. Eat diet foods.
31. Feel that food controls my life.
32. Display self-control around food.
33. Feel that others pressure me to eat.
34. Give too much time and thought to food.
35. Suffer from constipation.
36. Feel uncomfortable after eating sweets.
37. Engage in dieting behavior.
38. Like my stomach to be empty.
39. Enjoy trying new rich foods.
40. Have impulse to vomit after meals.

Scoring: The patient is given the questionnaire without the X's, just blank. Three points are assigned to endorsements that coincide with the X's; the adjacent alternatives are weighted as 2 points and 1 point, respectively. A total score of over 30 indicates significant concerns with eating behavior.

Inventory for Clients with Eating Problems

O BOX 4.22 O

Health Perception–Health Management

- How has your general health been?
- Do you have any health issues that need treatment?
- Have others been concerned about your health or your weight?
- Do you use laxatives or diuretics to control weight?

Nutrition–Metabolism

- Have you ever fasted to lose weight?
- Have you ever tried to vomit after eating?

Elimination

- Do you have to use laxatives to have a bowel movement?
- Do you have diarrhea often?

Activity–Exercise

- Do you feel weak or dizzy or have muscle cramping?
- Do you ever have palpitations?
- Do you follow a strict exercise regimen?
- Do you panic if you cannot exercise as much as you'd like?

Sleep–Rest

- Do you have difficulty sleeping?

Cognition–Perception

- Would you describe yourself as a perfectionist?
- Do you repeat things until you get them right?
- Have you ever been unable to get something out of your mind?
- Do you find yourself repeatedly thinking about the same things?

- How do you feel if you lose control, such as getting very angry or eating too much?
- What do you do when you feel you are losing control?
- Have you ever had times when you have eaten uncontrollably? What did you feel, and what did you do?

Self-perception–Self-concept

- What do you like the best about your body?
- What do you like the least about your body?
- If you could change how you look, how would you be different?
- What do you like the best about yourself?
- What do you like the least about yourself?
- How would you describe yourself to others?
- How would others (family, friends) describe you?
- What are your strengths?
- What are your weaknesses?

Roles–Relationships

- How is your relationship with your parents?
- How would you describe your family?
- Do you have many friends?
- Do you have a best friend?
- What do you like to do with your friends?
- What is school like?
- Do you study a lot?
- In what activities are you involved at school?
- Do you feel pressure to do well in school? If so, from whom?

◯ BOX 4.22 *continued* ◯

Sexuality–Reproduction

- Have your periods become irregular or stopped completely? (for female clients)
- How do you feel about the body changes that occur at adolescence (eg, in females, breast development, menstruation, broadening of hips)?
- Is dating something that you enjoy?
- Have you had any sexual experiences?
- How do you feel about your sexual experiences (or lack of them)?

Coping–Stress Tolerance

- How do you make decisions about everyday things?
- How do you spend your free time? (For example, do you usually ask someone for advice or think things out for yourself?)
- Is your life right now pretty much the way you want it? If not, what would you change? What can you do to make these changes?
- What do you do to feel better when you are sad or upset?

- Have you ever felt like hurting yourself when you are down?
- Have you ever thought about committing suicide?
- Have you ever used alcohol or drugs to feel better?
- Have you ever stolen anything (eg, food or money)? If so, how do you feel about that?
- Do you get along with your parents? What happens when you argue with them? What do you argue about? What happens when you talk to them about a problem or concern?
- How do you get along with your siblings? Can you talk to them about your feelings and problems?
- Do your friends help you if you have a problem?

Values–Beliefs

- What is important to you?
- What do you care about?
- What is the meaning of life for you?

Mood Disorder Assessment Tools
Beck Depression Inventory

BOX 4.23

Instructions: This questionnaire consists of 21 groups of statements. Please read each group of statements carefully, and then pick out the one statement in each group that best describes the way you have been feeling during the past two weeks, including today. Circle the number beside the statement you have picked. If several statements in the group seem to apply equally well, circle the highest number for that group. Be sure that you do not choose more than one statement for any group, including Item 16 (Changes in Sleeping Pattern) or Item 18 (Changes in Appetite).

1. Sadness
 0 I do not feel sad.
 1 I feel sad much of the time.
 2 I am sad all the time.
 3 I am so sad or unhappy that I can't stand it.

2. Pessimism
 0 I am not discouraged about my future.
 1 I feel more discouraged about my future than I used to be.
 2 I do not expect things to work out for me.
 3 I feel my future is hopeless and will only get worse.

3. Past Failure
 0 I do not feel like a failure.
 1 I have failed more than I should have.
 2 As I look back, I see a lot of failures.
 3 I feel I am a total failure as a person.

4. Loss of Pleasure
 0 I get as much pleasure as I ever did from the things I enjoy.
 1 I don't enjoy things as much as I used to.

 2 I get very little pleasure from the things I used to enjoy.
 3 I can't get any pleasure from the things I used to enjoy.

5. Guilty Feelings
 0 I don't feel particularly guilty.
 1 I feel guilty over many things I have done or should have done.
 2 I feel quite guilty most of the time.
 3 I feel guilty all of the time.

6. Punishment Feelings
 0 I don't feel I am being punished.
 1 I feel I may be punished.
 2 I expect to be punished.
 3 I feel I am being punished.

7. Self-Dislike
 0 I feel the same about myself as ever.
 1 I have lost confidence in myself.
 2 I am disappointed in myself.
 3 I dislike myself.

8. Self-Criticalness
 0 I don't criticize or blame myself more than usual.

○ BOX 4.23 continued ○

1 I am more critical of myself than I used to be.
2 I criticize myself for all of my faults.
3 I blame myself for everything bad that happens.

9. Suicidal Thoughts or Wishes
0 I don't have any thoughts of killing myself.
1 I have thoughts of killing myself, but I would not carry them out.
2 1 would like to kill myself.
3 I would kill myself if I had the chance.

10. Crying
0 I don't cry any more than I used to.
1 I cry more than I used to.
2 I cry over every little thing.
3 I feel like crying, but I can't.

11. Agitation
0 I am no more restless or wound up than usual.
1 I feel more restless or wound up than usual.
2 I am so restless or agitated that it's hard to stay still.
3 I am so restless or agitated that I have to keep moving or doing something.

12. Loss of Interest
0 I have not lost interest in other people or activities.
1 I am less interested in other people or things than before.
2 I have lost most of my interest in other people or things.
3 It's hard to get interested in anything.

13. Indecisiveness
0 I make decisions about as well as ever.

1 I find it more difficult than usual to make decisions.
2 I have much greater difficulty in making decisions than I used to.
3 I have trouble making any decisions.

14. Worthlessness
0 I do not feel I am worthless.
1 I don't consider myself as worthwhile and useful as I used to.
2 I feel more worthless as compared to other people.
3 I feel utterly worthless.

15. Loss of Energy
0 I have as much energy as ever.
1 I have less energy than I used to have.
2 I don't have enough energy to do very much.
3 I don't have enough energy to do anything.

16. Changes in Sleeping Pattern
0 I have not experienced any change in my sleeping pattern.
1a I sleep somewhat more than usual.
1b I sleep somewhat less than usual.
2a I sleep a lot more than usual.
2b I sleep a lot less than usual.
3a I sleep most of the day.
3b I wake up 1–2 hours early and can't get back to sleep.

17. Irritability
0 I am no more irritable than usual.
1 I am more irritable than usual.
2 I am much more irritable than usual.
3 I am irritable all the time.

continued on page 84

○ B O X 4.23 *continued* ○

18. Changes in Appetite

0 I have not experienced any change in my appetite.

1a My appetite is somewhat less than usual.

1b My appetite is somewhat greater than usual.

2a My appetite is much less than before.

2b My appetite is much greater than usual.

3a I have no appetite at all.

3b I crave food all the time.

19. Concentration Difficulty

0 I can concentrate as well as ever.

1 I can't concentrate as well as usual.

2 It's hard to keep my mind on anything for very long.

3 I find I can't concentrate on anything.

20. Tiredness or Fatigue

0 I am no more tired or fatigued than usual.

1 I get more tired or fatigued more easily than usual.

2 I am too tired or fatigued to do a lot of the things I used to do.

3 I am too tired or fatigued to do most of the things I used to do.

21. Loss of Interest in Sex

0 I have not noticed any recent change in my interest in sex.

1 I am less interested in sex than I used to be.

2 I am much less interested in sex now.

3 I have lost interest in sex completely.

Geriatric Depression Scale (short form)

BOX 4.24

1. Are you basically satisfied with your life?	Yes	No
2. Have you dropped many of your activities and interests?	Yes	No
3. Do you feel that your life is empty?	Yes	No
4. Do you often get bored?	Yes	No
5. Are you in good spirits most of the time?	Yes	No
6. Are you afraid that something bad is going to happen to you?	Yes	No
7. Do you feel happy most of the time?	Yes	No
8. Do you often feel helpless?	Yes	No
9. Do you prefer to stay at home rather than go out and do new things?	Yes	No
10. Do you feel you have more problems with memory than most?	Yes	No
11. Do you think it is wonderful to be alive now?	Yes	No
12. Do you feel pretty worthless the way you are now?	Yes	No
13. Do you feel full of energy?	Yes	No
14. Do you feel that your situation is hopeless?	Yes	No
15. Do you think that most people are better off than you are?	Yes	No

Score: /15 One point for "No" to questions 1, 5, 7, 11, 13

One point for "Yes" to other questions

Normal	3 ± 2
Mildly depressed	7 ± 3
Very depressed	12 ± 2

Adapted from Sheikh, J I., & Yesavage, J. A. (1986). Geriatric Depression Scale (GDS): Recent evidence and development of a shorter version. In T. L. Brink (Ed.). *Clinical gerontology: a guide to assessment and intervention* (pp. 165–173). Binghamton, NY: Haworh Press. © By the Haworth Press, Inc. All rights reserved. Reprinted with permission.

Hamilton Rating Scale for Depression

○ B O X 4.25 ○

For each item select the "cue" that best characterizes the patient.

1. Depressed mood (sadness, hopeless, helpless, worthless)
   0 Absent
   1 These feeling states indicated only on questioning
   2 These feeling states spontaneously reported verbally
   3 Communicates feeling states nonverbally— ie, through facial expression, posture, voice, and tendency to weep
   4 Patient reports VIRTUALLY ONLY these feeling states in his spontaneous verbal and nonverbal communication

2. Feelings of Guilt
   0 Absent
   1 Self-reproach, feels he has let people down
   2 Ideas of guilt or rumination over past errors or sinful deeds
   3 Present illness is a punishment; delusions of guilt
   4 Hears accusatory or denunciatory voices and/or experiences threatening visual hallucinations

3. Suicide
   0 Absent
   1 Feels life is not worth living
   2 Wishes he were dead or any thoughts of possible death to self
   3 Suicide ideas or gesture
   4 Attempts at suicide (any serious attempt rates 4)

4. Insomnia early
   0 No difficulty falling asleep
   1 Complains of occasional difficulty falling asleep— ie, more than 1/4 hour

   2 Complains of nightly difficulty falling asleep

5. Insomnia middle
   0 No difficulty
   1 Patient complains of being restless and disturbed during the night
   2 Waking during the night— any getting out of bed rates 2 (except for purpose of voiding).

6. Insomnia late
   0 No difficulty
   1 Waking in early hours of the morning but goes back to sleep
   2 Unable to fall asleep again if gets out of bed

7. Work and activities
   0 No difficulty
   1 Thoughts and feelings of incapacity, fatigue or weakness related to activities, work, or hobbies
   2 Loss of interest in activities, hobbies, or work—either directly reported by patient, or indirect in listlessness, indecision, and vacillation (feels he has to push self to work or activities)
   3 Decrease in actual time spent in activities or decrease in productivity. In hospital, rate 3 if patient does not spend at least 3 hours a day in activities (hospital job or hobbies) exclusive of ward chores
   4 Stopped working because of present illness. In hospital, rate 4 if patient engages in no activities except ward chores or if patient fails to perform ward chores unassisted.

○ BOX 4.25 *continued* ○

8. Retardation (slowness of thought and speech; impaired ability to concentrate; decreased motor activity)
  0 Normal speech and thought
  1 Slight retardation at interview
  2 Obvious retardation at interview
  3 Interview difficult
  4 Complete stupor
9. Agitation
  0 None
  1 Playing with" hands, hair, etc.
  2 Hand wringing, nail biting, hair pulling, biting of lips
10. Anxiety psychic
  0 No difficulty
  1 Subjective tension and irritability
  2 Worrying about minor matters
  3 Apprehensive attitude apparent in face or speech
  4 Fears expressed without questioning
11. Anxiety somatic
  0 Absent
     Physiological concomitants of anxiety, such as:
  1 Mild
     Gastrointestinal—dry mouth, wind, indigestion, diarrhea, cramps, belching
  2 Moderate
     Cardiovascular—palpitations, headaches
  3 Severe
     Respiratory—hyperventilation, sighing
  4 Incapacitating   Urinary frequency Sweating
12. Somatic symptoms gastrointestinal
  0 None
  1 Loss of appetite but eating without staff encouragement. Heavy feelings in abdomen.

  2 Difficulty eating without staff urging. Requests or requires laxatives or medication for bowels or medication for GI symptoms.
13. Somatic symptoms general
  0 None
  1 Heaviness in limbs, back or head. Backaches, headache, muscle aches. Loss of energy and fatigability.
  2 Any clearcut symptom rates 2
14. Genital symptoms
  0 Absent   Symptoms such as:
  1 Mild   Loss of libido
  2 Severe   Menstrual disturbances
15. Hypochondriasis
  0 Not present
  1 Self-absorption (bodily)
  2 Preoccupation with health
  3 Frequent complaints, requests for help, etc.
  4 Hypochondriacal delusions
16. Loss of weight
  A: When rating by history
  0 No weight loss
  1 Probable weight loss associated with present illness
  2 Definite (according to patient) weight loss
  B: On weekly ratings by ward psychiatrist, when actual weight changes are measured
  0 Less than 1 lb weight loss in week
  1 Greater than 1 lb weight loss in week
  2 Greater than 2 lb weight loss in week
17. Insight
  0 Acknowledges being depressed and ill
  1 Acknowledges illness but attributes cause to bad food,

continued on page 88

○ B O X 4 . 2 5 *continued* ○

climate, overwork, virus, need for rest, etc.
2 Denies being ill at all

18. Diurnal variation

AM	PM		If symptoms are worse in the morning or evening, note which it is and rate severity of variation
0	0	Absent	
1	1	Mild	
2	2	Severe	

19. Depersonalization and derealization
   0 Absent
   1 Mild   Such as:
   2 Moderate   Feeling of unreality
   3 Severe   Nihilistic ideas
   4 Incapacitating

20. Paranoid symptoms
   0 None
   1
     Suspiciousness
   2
   3 Ideas of reference
   4 Delusions of reference and persecution

21. Obsessional and compulsive symptoms
   0 Absent
   1 Mild
   2 Severe

22. Helplessness
   0 Not present
   1 Subjective feelings that are elicited only by inquiry
   2 Patient volunteers his helpless feelings

   3 Requires urging, guidance, and reassurance to accomplish ward chores or personal hygiene
   4 Requires physical assistance for dress, grooming, eating, bedside tasks, or personal hygiene

23. Hopelessness
   0 Not present
   1 Intermittently doubts that "things will improve" but can be reassured
   2 Consistently feels "hopeless" but accepts reassurances
   3 Expresses feelings of discouragement, despair, pessimism about future, which cannot be dispelled
   4 Spontaneously and inappropriately perseveres "I'll never get well" or its equivalent

24. Worthlessness (ranges from mild loss of esteem, feelings of inferiority, self-depreciation to delusional notions of worthlessness)
   0 Not present
   1 Indicates feelings of worthlessness (loss of self-esteem) only on questioning
   2 Spontaneously indicates feelings of worthlessness (loss of self-esteem)
   3 Different from 2 by degree. Patient volunteers that he is "no good," "inferior," etc.
   4 Delusional notions of worthlessness—ie, "I am a heap of garbage" or its equivalent

Reprint with permission from Hamiler, M. (1960). A rating scale for depression. *J Neurol Neurosurg Psychiatry, 23,* 56.

Mood Disorder Questionnaire

continued on page 90

BOX 4.26

The following questionnaire can be used as a starting point to help you recognize the signs/symptoms of bipolar disorder but is not meant to be a substitute for a full medical evaluation. Bipolar disorder is complex and **an accurate, thorough diagnosis can be made through a personal evaluation by your doctor.** However, a positive screening may suggest that you might benefit from seeking an evaluation from your doctor. Regardless of the questionnaire results, if you or your family has concerns about your mental health, please contact your physician and/or other healthcare professional.

When completed, you may want to print out your responses.

Instructions: Please answer each question as best you can.

	YES	NO
1. Has there ever been a period of time when you were not your usual self and …		
… you felt so good or so hyper that other people thought you were not your normal self or you were so hyper that you got into trouble?	☐	☐
… you were so irritable that you shouted at people or started fights or arguments?	☐	☐
… you felt much more self-confident than usual?	☐	☐
… you got much less sleep than usual and found you didn't really miss it?	☐	☐
… you were much more talkative or spoke much faster than usual?	☐	☐
… thoughts raced through your head or you couldn't slow your mind down?	☐	☐
… you were so easily distracted by things around you that you had trouble concentrating or staying on track?	☐	☐
… you had much more energy than usual?	☐	☐

BOX 4.26 *continued*

... you were much more active or did many more things than usual? ☐ ☐

... you were much more social or outgoing than usual, for example, you telephoned friends in the middle of the night? ☐ ☐

... you were much more interested in sex than usual? ☐ ☐

... you did things that were unusual for you or that other people might have thought were excessive, foolish, or risky? ☐ ☐

... spending money got you or your family into trouble? ☐ ☐

2. If you checked YES to more than one of the above, have several of these ever happened during the same period of time? ☐ ☐

3. How much of a problem did any of these cause you—like being unable to work; having family, money, or legal troubles; getting into arguments or fights? Please select one response only.

[☐] No Problem   [☐] Minor Problem   [☐] Moderate Problem   [☐] Serious Problem

4. Have any of your blood relatives (children, siblings, parents, grandparents, aunts, uncles) had manic-depressive illness or bipolar disorder? ☐ ☐

5. Has a healthcare professional ever told you that you have manic-depressive illness or bipolar disorder? ☐ ☐

Hirschfeld, R. M. A., Williams, J. B., Spitzer, R. L., et al. (2000). Development and validation of a screening instrument for bipolar spectrum disorder: The Mood Disorder Questionnaire. *American Journal of Psychiatry* 157(11), 1873–1875.

Suicide Assessment

BOX 4.27

Questions to Ask for a Comprehensive Suicide Assessment

- Ask the client directly if he or she has thoughts of suicide:
  - "Have you had thoughts about death or about killing yourself?"
  - "Are the thoughts pervasive or do they come and go (intermittent)?"
  - "Do these thoughts stay with you for a while, or do they tend to come and go?"
  - "Have you heard voices telling you to hurt or kill yourself?"
  - "Do thoughts tend to have some connection to certain situations?"
  - "Has anything happened lately that has prompted you to think about suicide more?"
  - "Are there situations or ideas that always seem to be present when you are thinking about suicide?"
- Ask the client if he or she has a plan; ask for details about how extensive the plan is and identify means or method and lethality:
  - "Do you have a plan for how you would kill yourself?"
  - "Are there means available (eg, pills, a gun and bullets, or poison)?"
  - "Have you actually rehearsed or practiced how you would kill yourself?"
  - '"How strong is your intent to do this?"
- Can the client resist the impulse to commit suicide?
  - "Are you an impulsive person?"

- "Can you resist the impulse to do this?"
- "What would keep you from committing suicide?"
- "Tell me about your hopes for the future."
- Has the client ever had ideas about or attempted suicide?
  - "Have you ever thought about hurting or killing yourself?"
  - "Have you tried to hurt or kill yourself in the past? When?"
- Has anyone in the client's immediate or extended family or a significant other ever committed suicide?
  - "What was that person's relationship to you?"
  - "What were the circumstances of his or her death?"
  - "What was your experience of this event?"

Questions to Ask if Assessing a Recent Suicide Attempt

- What were the means; how did you try to commit suicide?
- Where was the attempt made?
- Did anyone know about the attempt beforehand or during the attempt?
- Who found you?
- How many attempts have you made in the past?
- Did you have a plan that you had thought out and prepared, or was the attempt done more on an impulsive feeling?
- Did you have any physical harm or impairment from the attempt?
- How did you get treated, and what was required?

Adapted from Bobo, W. V., et al. 2001. *VHA/DOD clinical practice guideline for the management of major depressive disorder in adults.* Washington, DC: Department of Veterans Affairs.

Schizophrenia and Related Assessment Tools

Abnormal Involuntary Movement Scale (AIMS)

○ BOX 4.28 ○

	NONE	MINIMAL	MILD	MODERATE	SEVERE
Facial and Oral Movements					
1. Muscles of facial expression, eg, movements of forehead, eyebrows, periorbital area, cheeks: include frowning, blinking, smiling, grimacing	0	1	2	3	4
2. Lips and perioral area, eg, puckering, pouting, smacking	0	1	2	3	4
3. Jaw, eg, biting, clenching, chewing, mouth opening, lateral movement	0	1	2	3	4
4. Tongue, rate only increase in movement both in and out of mouth. NOT inability to sustain movement	0	1	2	3	4
Extremity Movements					
5. Upper (arms, wrists, hands, fingers) Include choreic movements (ie, rapid, objectively purposeless, irregular, spontaneous). Athetoid movements (ie, slow, irregular, complex, serpentine). Do NOT include tremor (ie, respective, regular, rhythmic)	0	1	2	3	4

		0	1	2	3	4
Trunk Movements	6. Lower (legs, knees, ankles, toes), eg, lateral knee movement, foot lapping, heel dropping, foot squinning, inversion and eversion of foot	0	1	2	3	4
	7. Neck, shoulders hips, eg, rocking, twisting, squirming. pelvic gyrations	0	1	2	3	4
	8. Severity of abnormal movements	0	1	2	3	4
Global Judgment	9. Incapacitation due to abnormal movements	0	1	2	3	4
	10. Patient's awareness of abnormal movements Rate only patient's report	No awareness	Aware, no distress	Aware, mid distress	Aware, moderate distress	Aware, severe distress
		0	1	2	3	4

Reprinted from Guy. W. [1976]. *ECDEU: Assessment manual for psychopharmacology* [DHEW publication no. 76-338). Washington. DC: Department of Health. Education, and Welfare. Psychopharmacology Research Branch.

Simplified Diagnoses for Tardive Dyskinesia (SD-TD)

BOX 4.29

PREREQUISITES—The three prerequisites are as follows. Exceptions may occur.

1. A history of at least 3 months' total cumulative neuroleptic exposure. Include amoxapine and metoclopramide in all categories below as well.
2. **SCORING/INTENSITY LEVEL.** The presence of a **TOTAL SCORE OF FIVE (5) OR ABOVE.** Also be alert for any change from baseline or scores below five that have at least a "moderate" (3) or "severe" (4) movement on any item or atleast two "mild" (2) movements on two items located in different body areas.
3. Other conditions are not responsible for the abnormal involuntary movements.

DIAGNOSES—The diagnosis is based upon the current exam and its relation to the last exam. The diagnosis can shift depending upon: (a) whether movements are present or not, (b) whether movements are present for 3 months or more (6 months if on a semiannual assessment schedule), and (c) whether neuroleptic dosage changes occur and affect movements.

- **NO TD**—Movements **are not** present on this exam or movements are present, but some other condition is responsible for them. The last diagnosis must be NO TD, PROBABLE TD, or WITHDRAWAL TD.
- **PROBABLE TD**—Movements **are** present on this exam. This is the first time they are present **or** they have never been present for 3 months or more. The last diagnosis must be NO TD or PROBABLE TD.
- **PERSISTENT TD**—Movements **are** present on this exam **and** they have been present for 3 months or more with this exam or at some point in the past. The last diagnosis can be any except NO TD.
- **MASKED TD**—Movements **are not** present on this exam **but** this is due to a neuroleptic dosage increase or reinstitution after a prior exam when movements were present. Also use this conclusion if movements are not present due to the addition of a non-neuroleptic medication to treat TD. The last diagnosis must be PROBABLE TD, PERSISTENT TD, WITHDRAWAL TD, or MASKED TD.
- **REMITTED TD**—Movements **are not** present on this exam **but** PERSISTENT TD has been diagnosed **and** no neuroleptic dosage increase or reinstitution has occurred. The last diagnosis must be PERSISTENT TD or REMITTED TD. If movements re-emerge, the diagnosis shifts back to PERSISTENT TD.
- **WITHDRAWAL TD**—Movements **are not seen while** receiving neuroleptics or at the last dosage level **but are seen within** 8 weeks following a neuroleptic reduction or discontinuation. The last diagnosis must be NO TD or WITHDRAWAL TD. If movements continue for 3 months or more

○ B O X 4 . 2 9 *continued* ○

after the neuroleptic dosage reduction or discontinuation, the diagnosis shifts to PERSISTENT TD. If movements do not continue for 3 months or more after the reduction or discontinuation, the diagnosis shifts to NO TD.

INSTRUCTIONS

1. The rater completes the Assessment according to the standardized exam procedure. If the rater also completes Evaluation items 1–4 he/she must also sign the preparer box. The form is given to the physician. Alternatively, the physician may perform the assessment.
2. The physician completes the Evaluation section. The physician is responsible for the entire Evaluation section and its accuracy.
3. IT IS RECOMMENDED THAT THE PHYSICIAN EXAMINE ANY INDIVIDUAL WHO MEETS THE THREE PREREQUISITES OR WHO HAS MOVEMENTS NOT EXPLAINED BY OTHER FACTORS. NEUROLOGICAL ASSESSMENTS OR DIFFERENTIAL DIAGNOSTIC TESTS THAT MAY BE NECESSARY SHOULD BE OBTAINED.
4. File form according to policy or procedure.

OTHER CONDITIONS
(partial list)

1. Age
2. Blind
3. Cerebral Palsy
4. Contact Lenses
5. Dentures/No Teeth
6. Down Syndrome
7. Drug Intoxication (specify)
8. Encephalitis
9. Extrapyramidal Side Effects (specify)
10. Fahr's Syndrome
11. Heavy Metal Intoxication (specify)
12. Huntington's Chorea
13. Hyperthyroidism
14. Hypoglycemia
15. Hypoparathyroidism
16. Idiopathic Torsion Dystonia
17. Meige syndrome
18. Parkinson's Disease
19. Stereotypies
20. Syndenham's Chorea
21. Tourette's Syndrome
22. Wilson's Disease
23. Other (specify)

Sprague, R. L. & Kalachnik, J. E. (1991). Reliability, validity, and a total score cutoff for the Dyskinesia Identification System, Condensed User Scale (DISCUS) with mentally ill and mentally retarded populations. *Psychopharmacology Bulletin, 27*(1), 51–58.

Simpson-Angus Rating Scale

○ BOX 4.30 ○

1. GAIT: The patient is examined as he walks into the examining room; his gait, the swing of his arms, his general posture, all form the basis for an overall score for this item. This is rated as follows:

0 Normal
1 Diminution in swing while the patient is walking.
2 Marked diminution in swing with obvious rigidity in the arm.
3 Stiff gait with arms held rigidly before the abdomen.
4 Stooped shuffling gait with propulsion and retropulsion.

2. ARM DROPPING: The patient and the examiner both raise their arms to shoulder height and let them fall to other sides. In a normal subject, a stout slap is heard as the arms hit the sides. In the patient with extreme Parkinson's syndrome, the arms fall very slowly.

0 Normal, free fall with loud slap and rebound.
1 Fall slowed slightly with less audible contact and little rebound.
2 Fall slowed, no rebound.
3 Marked slowing, no slap at all.
4 Arms fall as though against resistance; as though through glue.

3. SHOULDER SHAKING: The subject's arms are bent at a right angle at the elbow and are taken one at a time by the examiner who grasps one hand and also clasps the other around the patient's elbow. The subject's upper arm is pushed to and fro, and the humerus is externally rotated. The degree of resistance from normal to extreme rigidity is scored as follows:

0 Normal
1 Slight stiffness and resistance.
2 Moderate stiffness and resistance.
3 Marked rigidity with difficulty in passive movement.
4 Extreme stiffness and rigidity with almost a frozen shoulder.

4. ELBOW RIGIDITY: The elbow joints are separately bent at right angles and passively extended and flexed, with the subject's biceps observed and simultaneously palpated. The resistance to this procedure is rated. (The presence of cog-wheel rigidity is noted separately.) Scoring is from 0 to 4, as in the Shoulder Shaking test.

0 Normal
1 Slight stiffness and resistance.
2 Moderate stiffness and resistance.

3 Marked rigidity with difficulty in passive movement.

4 Extreme stiffness and rigidity with almost a frozen shoulder.

5. FIXATION OF POSITION OR WRIST RIGIDITY: The wrist is held in one hand and the fingers held by the examiner's other hand, with the wrist moved to extension flexion and both ulnar and radial deviation. The resistance to this procedure is rated as in Items 3 and 4.

0 Normal

1 Slight stiffness and resistance.

2 Moderate stiffness and resistance.

3 Marked rigidity with difficulty in passive movement.

4 Extreme stiffness and rigidity with almost a frozen shoulder.

6. LEG PENDULOUSNESS: The patient sits on a table with his legs hanging down and swinging free. The ankle is grasped by the examiner and raised until the knee is partially extended. It is then allowed to fall. The resistance to falling and the lack of swinging form the basis for the score on this item.

0 The legs swing freely.

1 Slight diminution in the swing of the legs.

2 Moderate resistance to swing.

3 Marked resistance and damping of swing.

4 Complete absence of swing.

7. HEAD DROPPING: The patient lies on a well-padded examining table and his head is raised by the examiner's hand. The hand is then withdrawn, and the head allowed to drop. In the normal subject, the head will fall upon the table. The movement is delayed in extrapyramidal system disorder, and in extreme parkinsonism it is absent. The neck muscles are rigid and the head does not reach the examining table. Scoring is as follows:

0 The head falls completely, with a good thump as it hits the table.

1 Slight slowing in fall, mainly noted by lack of slap as head meets the table.

2 Moderate slowing in the fall, quite noticeable to the eye.

3 Head falls stiffly and slowly.

4 Head does not reach examining table.

8. GLABELLA TAP: Subject is told to open his eyes wide and not to blink. The glabella region is tapped at a steady, rapid speed. The number of times patient blinks in succession is noted:

0 0 to 5 blinks

1 6 to 10 blinks

2 11 to 15 blinks

3 16 to 20 blinks

4 21 or more blinks

9. TREMOR: Patient is observed walking into examining room and then is re-examined for this item:

0 Normal

1 Mild finger tremor, obvious sight and touch.

2 Tremor of hand or arm occurring spasmodically.

continued on page 98

BOX 4.30 *continued*

3 Persistent tremor of one or more limbs.

4 Whole body tremor.

10. SALIVATION: Patient is observed while talking and then asked to open his mouth and elevate his tongue. The following ratings are given:

0 Normal

1 Excess salivation to the extent that pooling takes place if the mouth is open and the tongue raised.

2 When excess salivation is present and might occasionally result in difficulty in speaking.

3 Speaking with difficulty because of excess salivation.

4 Frank drooling.

Scoring: Each item is rated on a 5-point scale, with 0 meaning the complete absence of the condition and 4 meaning the presence of the condition in extreme form. The score is obtained by adding the items and dividing by 10.

Reprinted with permission from Simpson G. M., Angus, J. W. S. (1970). A rating scale for extrapyramidal side effects. *Acta Psychiatrica Scandinavica, 212* (Suppl.). 11–19. Copyright 1970, Munksgaard International Publishers, Ltd.

Substance Disorder Assessment Tools

Addiction Research Foundation Clinical Institute Withdrawal Assessment for Alcohol Revised (CIWA-AR)

BOX 4.31

NAUSEA AND VOMITING—Ask "Do you feel sick to your stomach? Have you vomited?" Observation.
0 no nausea and no vomiting
1 mild nausea with no vomiting
2
3
4 intermittent nausea with dry heaves
5
6
7 constant nausea, frequent dry heaves and vomiting

TREMOR—Arms extended and fingers spread apart. Observation.
0 no tremor
1 not visible, but can be felt fingertip to fingertip
2
3
4 moderate, with patient's arms extended
5
6
7 severe, flapping tremors

PAROXYSMAL SWEATS—Observation.
0 no sweat visible
1 barely perceptible sweating, palms moist
2
3
4 beads of sweat obvious on forehead
5
6
7 drenching sweats

ANXIETY—Ask, " Do you feel nervous?" Observation.
0 no anxiety, at ease
1 mildly anxious
2
3
4 moderately anxious, or guarded, so anxiety is inferred
5
6
7 equivalent to acute panic states as seen in severe delirium or acute psychotic reactions

AGITATION—Observation.
0 normal activity
1 somewhat more than normal activity
2
3
4 moderately fidgety and restless
5
6
7 paces back and forth during most of the interview, or constantly thrashes about

TACTILE DISTURBANCES—Ask, "Have you any itching, pins and needles sensations, any burning, any numbness or do you feel bugs crawling on or under your skin?" Observation.
0 none
1 very mild itching, pins and needles, burning or numbness
2 mild itching, pins and needles, burning or numbness
3 moderate itching, pins and needles, burning or numbness

continued on page 100

○ B O X 4.31 | continued ○

AUDITORY DISTURBANCES—
Ask, "Are you more aware of
sounds around you? Are they
harsh? Do they frighten you? Are
you hearing anything that is disturbing to you? Are you hearing
things you know are not there?"
Observation.
0 not present
1 very mild harshness or ability to
   frighten
2 mild harshness or ability to frighten
3 moderate harshness or ability to
   frighten
4 moderately severe hallucinations
5 severe hallucinations
6 extremely severe hallucinations
7 continuous hallucinations

VISUAL DISTURBANCES—Ask,
"Does the light appear too bright? Is
its color different? Does it hurt your
eyes? Are you seeing anything that
is disturbing to you? Are you seeing
things you know are not there?"
Observation.
0 not present
1 very mild sensitivity
2 mild sensitivity
3 moderate sensitivity
4 moderately severe hallucinations
5 severe hallucinations
6 extremely severe hallucinations
7 continuous hallucinations

HEADACHE, FULLNESS IN
HEAD—Ask, "Does your head feel
different? Does it feel like there is a
band around your head?" Do not
rate for dizziness or lightheaded-
ness. Otherwise, rate severity.
Observation.
0 not present
1 very mild
2 mild
3 moderate
4 moderately severe
5 severe
6 very severe
7 extremely severe

ORIENTATION AND CLOUDING
OF SENSORIUM—Ask, "What day
is this? Where are you? Who am I?"
Observation.
0 oriented and can do serial
   additions
1 cannot do serial additions or is
   uncertain about date
2 disoriented for date by no more
   than 2 calendar days
3 disoriented for date by more than
   2 calendar days
4 disoriented for place and/or person

Maximum Possible Score 67

A score of less than 10 usually indicates no need for additional withdrawal medication.

Alcohol Use Disorder Identification Test (AUDIT)

◯ BOX 4.32 ◯

The following questionnaire will give you an indication of the level of risk associated with your current drinking pattern. To accurately assess your situation, you will need to be honest in your answers. This questionnaire was developed by the World Health Organization and is used in many countries to assist people to better understand their current level of risk in relation to alcohol consumption.

1. How often do you have a drink containing alcohol? (0) Never, (1) Monthly or less, (2) 2 to 4 times a month, (3) 2 to 3 times a week, (4) 4 or more times a week.
2. How many standard drinks do you have on a typical day when you are drinking? (0) 1 or 2, (1) 3 or 4, (2) 5 or 6, (3) 7 to 9, (4) 10 or more.
3. How often do you have six or more drinks on one occasion? (0) Never, (1) Less than monthly, (2) Monthly, (3) Weekly, (4) Daily or almost daily.
4. How often during the last year have you found that you were not able to stop drinking once you had started? (0) Never, (1) Less than monthly, (2) Weekly, (3) Weekly, (4) Daily or almost daily.
5. How often during the past year have you failed to do what was normally expected of you because of drinking? (0) Never, (1) Less than monthly, (2) Monthly, (3) Weekly, (4) Daily or almost daily.
6. How often during the last year have you needed a drink in the morning to get yourself going after a heavy drinking session? (0) Never, (1) Less than monthly, (2) Monthly, (3) Weekly, (4) Daily or almost daily.
7. How often during the last year have you had a feeling of guilt or remorse after drinking? (0) Never, (1) Less than monthly, (2) Monthly, (3) Weekly, (4) Daily or almost daily.
8. How often during the last year have you been unable to remember what happened the night before because you had been drinking? (0) Never, (1) Less than monthly, (2) Monthly, (3) Weekly, (4) Daily or almost daily.
9. Have you or someone else been injured as a result of your drinking? (0) Never, (1) Less than monthly, (2) Monthly, (3) Weekly, (4) Daily or almost daily.
10. Has a relative, a doctor, or other health worker been concerned about your drinking or suggested that you cut down? (0) No, (2) Yes, but not in the last year, (4) Yes, during the last year.

Adapted from Babor, T., de la Fuente, J. R., Saurders, J., et al., (1992). *Alcohol Use Disorders Identification Test (AUDIT). Guidelines for Use in Primary Health Care.* World Health Organization, Geneva. Used with permission. Bohn, Babor, & Kranziev (1995).

CAGE Questionnaire

BOX 4.33

- Have you ever felt you should Cut down on your drinking?
- Have people Annoyed you by criticizing your drinking?
- Have you ever felt bad or Guilty about your drinking?
- Have you ever had a drink (or Eye-opener) first thing in the morning to steady your nerves or to get rid of a hangover?

From Ewing, J. A. (1984). Detecting alcoholism: The CAGE questionnaire. Journal of the American Medical Association, 252. *1902–1907.*

Michigan Alcoholism Screening Test (MAST)

BOX 4.34

Scoring Yes to 3 or more indicates alcoholism.

1. Do you feel you are a normal drinker?
2. Do friends or relatives think you are a normal drinker?
3. Have you ever attended a meeting of Alcoholics Anonymous?
4. Have you ever gotten in trouble at work because of drinking?
5. Have you ever lost friends or girlfriends/boyfriends because of drinking?
6. Have you ever neglected your obligations, your family, or your work for 2 or more days in a row because of your drinking?
7. Have you ever had delirium tremens (DTs), severe shaking, or heard voices or seen things that were not there after heavy drinking?
8. Have you ever gone to anyone for help about your drinking?
9. Have you ever been in a hospital because of your drinking?
10. Have you ever been arrested for drunken driving or other drunken behavior?

From Pokormy, A.D., Miller, B.A., & Kaplan, H.B. (1972). The brief MAST: A shortened version of the Michigan Alcohol Screening Test. American Journal of Psychiatry, *129, 342–345; reprinted by permission. Copyright © by 1972 American Psychiatric Association; http://ajp. psychiatry online.org.*

Substance Use Inventory

◯ BOX 4.35 ◯

Health History Questions

Demographic Data

- Name:
- Age:
- Sex:
- Ethnic group:
- Marital status:
- Religious affiliation:
- Significant other:
- Reason for seeking care/motivation for treatment:

Current Substance Information

- What types of substances do you currently use?
  - Alcohol (specify beer, wine, whiskey)
  - Cocaine
  - Heroin
  - Marijuana
  - Sedative–hypnotics
  - Hallucinogens
- Which of the above drugs do you use in combination?
- What is the predominant substance of choice?
- Do you use any prescription drugs?
- What is the approximate amount of alcohol or drugs that you use?
  - How many six packs, quarts, fifths?
  - How many bags?
  - How many pills or hits daily?
- How do you take any drugs that you use?
- How frequently do you use substances? Daily, several times a week?

- Does use increase on weekends or other times?
- Do you engage in binge drinking?
- Have you ever tried to control or cut down drinking or substance use? How?
- When was your last drink or use of drugs?
- Have you developed tolerance? (explain)
  - When did it begin?
  - Has there been a change in tolerance?
- Are withdrawal symptoms present (explain)
  - Is there a history of withdrawal?
  - Is there a history of seizures?
  - Is there a history of hallucinations? (explain)

Past Medical History

- Are there any present medical problems?
- Are there any chronic medical problems?
- Is there a history of any of the following: liver disease, hepatitis, diabetes, heart disease, anemia, drug overdose?
- Have there been any recent falls, injuries, accidents?
- Are you taking any prescribed medications?
- Do you have any known allergies?

Past Substance History

- Have you ever stopped drinking or using drugs?
- How long was the period of abstinence?

continued on page 104

○ BOX 4.35 *continued* ○

- Why did you abstain; what was the motivation?
- When did you start using substances?
- When did you first begin having difficulty in life circumstances because of substances?
- Have you ever been in treatment for substance abuse or dependency?
- What type of treatment did you have for substance abuse or dependency?
- How many times were you in treatment for the above?
- Is there a family history of alcohol abuse or dependency?
- Is there a family history of drug abuse or dependency?

Psychosocial History

- What is your spouse's, partner's, family's reaction to your use of substances?
- Do family members also abuse substances?
- Is substance use causing marital conflicts?
- Do you have children? How many, ages, and sex?
- Have children had school problems, health problems, or physical, emotional, sleeping problems?
- Is the family suffering from housing or nutritional problems because of substances?

- What are your present living conditions?
- Do you live alone?
- What are your leisure activities or hobbies?
- Has your participation in these activities changed because of substance use?
- Have your friends changed or been lost because of substance use?
- Do social activities center on the substance use?
- What is your occupation and present place of employment?
- How long have your been with your present employer?
- Have you ever missed work from substance use?
- Have you abused substances while working?
- Is substance use jeopardizing work or business?
- How much time do you spend on substances?
- Do substances provide you with a source of income?
- Have you had any violations while intoxicated?
- Are any present legal offenses pending from substance abuse or dependency?
- Is present treatment court recommended?

○ BOX 4.36 ○

Physical Examination

Area of Focus	Common positive findings/indicators of drug problems
Vital Signs	
Blood pressure	Hypotension or hypertension
Pulse	Rapid, regular, irregular
Temperature	Elevated
Respirations	Rapid, shallow, depressed
Appearance	
Gait	Unsteady, normal, weaving, shuffling
Eyes	Conjunctival injection; bloodshot; dilated, pin-point pupils; lacrimation (tearing); vacant stare; poor eye contact; intense eye contact
Skin	Perspiration, cool, clammy, dry, bruises, needle tracks, scars, abrasions, gooseflesh, excoriations, reddened palms
Nose	Running (rhinorrhea), congested, red
Tremors	Fine or coarse, slight–moderate or severe
Grooming	Unkempt, unshaven, odor (alcohol, foul)
Mental Status/Behavior	
Speech	Slurred, incoherent, loud, monotone, hesitant, pressured, distracted
Attitude	Quiet, calm, demanding, agitated, irritable, impatient, vague, withdrawn, suspicious, anxious, tearful, happy, silly
Dominant mood—affect	Euphoric, depressed, angry, sad
Sensorium	Lack of orientation to time, person, place; changes in memory
Perception	Illusions, hallucinations, delusions, hallucinosis

Therapeutic Modalities

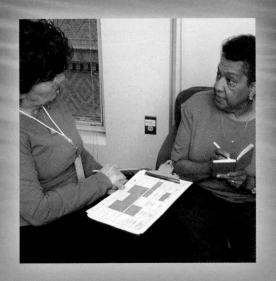

SECTION
three

5

Individual, Group, and Family Therapies and Interventions

Behavioral Therapy

Description

- Fundamental assumption that human responses are learned and therefore may be unlearned
- Based on the work of B. F. Skinner (1904–1990)
  - Conceptualized several principles to explain how behaviors can be developed and altered
  - Theory of operant conditioning
- No attempts to explain how the mind works or causes of mental disorders

Focus

- Observable behaviors and efforts on measures to bring about changes in them
- Reinforcement or promotion of desirable behaviors
- Alteration of undesirable behaviors
- Belief that change in behaviors are accompanied by changes in thoughts and feelings

Uses/Indications

- Anorexia nervosa (see Chapter 17)
- Attention deficit hyperactivity disorder (ADHD) (see Chapter 31)
- Anxiety disorders (see Chapter 14)
- Borderline personality disorder (BPD) (see Chapter 20)
- Major depressive disorder (see Chapter 19)
- Obsessive-compulsive disorder (OCD) (see Chapter 14)
- Phobias
- Sleep disorders (see Chapter 22)

Components

- All behavior learned
- Behavior modification through a system of rewards and punishments
  - Rewards or positive reinforcement as motivation for continued behavior, increasing likelihood that behavior will be repeated
  - Punishment or negative reinforcement to change undesirable behavior
  - Continuous reinforcement as the quickest method to improve behavior, but behavior returns after reinforcement ends
  - Random intermittent reinforcement as a slower method to improve behavior, but behavior lasts longer after reinforcement ends
- Examples: token economy and psychoeducation
  - Token economy: tokens used as rewards for client behavior; clients can use tokens for special purchases, items, or privileges
  - Psychoeducation: information provided via educational strategies to result in a change in knowledge and behavior

Nurse's Role

- Remaining consistent when implementing the plan of care
- Maintaining good communication both verbally and in writing among all healthcare personnel to ensure appropriate reinforcement for clients

- Emphasizing what clients will do instead of what they will not do
- Assisting clients with exploration of thoughts and feelings

Client-Centered Therapy
Description

- Humanistic theoretical approach
- Developed by Carl Rogers (1902–1987)
- Strong belief that quality of client–therapist relationship alone has healing potential
- Individual as a "client" rather than a "patient"

Focus

- Emphasis on therapeutic relationship and empathetic responses to clients
- View of clients as capable of learning about and accepting themselves, and exploring their personal abilities
- Learning to view self as a person of worth and achieving self-actualization
- Repeated conflicts with others or involvement in unsupportive relationships leading to loss of self-esteem, defensiveness, and interference with self-actualization

Uses/Indications

- Depressive disorders (see Chapter 19)
- Anxiety disorders (see Chapter 14)
- Personality disorders (see Chapter 20)
- Alcohol-related disorders (see Chapter 24)
- Panic disorder (see Chapter 14)

Components

- Three major concepts essential to therapeutic relationship:
  - **Empathy**: emotionally knowing another person; involves listening carefully, being in tune with what clients are saying, and

having insight into the meaning of their thoughts, feelings, and behavior
- **Genuineness**: true engagement in knowing and interacting with clients in open, human exchanges; comes through as an attitude that arises from deep concern; also being able to relax and resist trying to impress others
- **Unconditional positive regard**: being able to give to clients with "no strings attached"; clients worthy of respect and attention regardless of their behavior and despite their flaws and setbacks
- Clients regarded as the experts on their lives; therapists acting in a supportive role
- Clients doing the work; supportive and nurturing client–therapist relationship key to progress

Nurse's Role

- Using empathy with clients, such that nurses can feel for them while also maintaining an emotional boundary
- Carefully listening and attending to clients
- Using therapeutic communication skills
  - Direct eye contact
  - Concerned expression
  - Forward leaning position
  - Reflection
  - Clarifying
  - Paraphrasing
- Accepting clients for who they are without evaluation
- Ensuring that clients feel accepted to promote:
  - Increased capacity for honesty and openness
  - Willingness to self-explore
  - Greater likelihood of thriving in the therapeutic environment

Cognitive Therapy
Description

- Psychoeducational and copying model of therapy
- Active, directive, time-limited, structured approach
- Person's beliefs determine feelings and behavior

Focus

- Client's thinking about self and world
- Examination of beliefs and influence on behavior and feelings
- Identification and alteration of dysfunctional beliefs that distort experiences
- Emphasis on process (how) rather than content (what)
- Goal of increased self-efficacy or proficiency and sense of self-control

Uses/Indications

- Anxiety (see Chapter 14)
- Eating disorders (see Chapter 17)
- Personality disorders (see Chapter 20)
- Suicidal ideation (see Chapter 28)
- Sexual disorder (see Chapter 21)

Components

- Three issues underlying psychological disorders:
  - Cognitive triad (client's perception of self, world, and future)
  - Cognitive distortion (positive or negative) (Table 5.1)
  - Schema (core beliefs; basic rules of life; accumulation of learning and experiences from family, religion, ethnicity, gender, regional subgroups, and society)
- Client's perception of event rather than event itself as determining relevance and emotional response
- Treatment approach
  - Trust-building, active listening, empathy
  - Development of working problem list
  - Homework assignments and review of successes
  - Session agenda setting
  - Work on agenda
  - Review of session

Nurse's Role

- Listening actively and empathetically
- Assisting clients to identify situations and possible triggers

table
5.1. Cognitive Distortions

Distortion	Example	Commonly Associated Psychiatric Diagnoses
All-or-nothing thinking	"I'm either a success or a failure." "The world is either black or white."	Borderline personality disorder Obsessive-compulsive personality disorder
Mind reading	"They probably think that I'm incompetent." "I just know that he disapproves."	Avoidant personality disorder Paranoid personality disorder
Emotional reasoning	"Because I feel inadequate, I am inadequate." "Because I feel uncomfortable, the world is dangerous."	Anxiety disorders
Overgeneralization	"Everything I do turns out wrong." "My choices are always wrong."	Depression
Catastrophizing	"If I _____, there will be terrible consequences." "If I _____, it always fails."	Social anxiety Social phobia Panic disorders
Control fallacies	"If I'm not in complete control all the time, I will go out of control." "I must control all things in my life."	Obsessive-compulsive disorder Obsessive-compulsive personality disorder
Disqualifying the positive	"This success was only a fluke."	Depression

continued on page 114

table
5.1. **Cognitive Distortions** *continued*

Distortion	Example	Commonly Associated Psychiatric Diagnoses
Perfectionism	"I must do everything perfectly or I will be criticized and a failure."	Anxiety disorders
Selective abstraction	"The rest of the information doesn't matter." "I must focus on negative details and ignore all the positive aspects of this."	Depression
Externalization of self-worth	"My worth depends on what others think of me." "They think/believe _____, therefore I am _____."	Depression
Should/shouldn't/must/ought statements	"I should visit my family every time they want me to." "You/They should do whatever I say because it is right."	Obsessive-compulsive disorders
Jumping to conclusions	"I know they will not let me join."	Depression
Fallacy of change	"You should change your behavior because I want you to." "They should act differently because I expect it."	Narcissistic personality disorder

Fallacy of worrying	"If I worry about it enough, it will be resolved." "One cannot be too concerned."	Anxiety disorders
Fallacy of ignoring	"If I ignore it maybe it'll go away." "If I don't pay attention, I won't be responsible."	Depression Anxiety disorders
Fallacy of fairness	"Life should be fair." "People should be fair."	Avoidant personality disorder Social anxiety disorder
Fallacy of attachment	"I can't live without a man." "If I were in a relationship, all my problems would be gone."	Depression Anxiety disorders
Being right	"I must prove that I am right, as being wrong is unthinkable." "To be wrong is to be a bad person."	Obsessive-compulsive personality disorder Narcissistic personality disorder

- Supporting client–therapist interaction
- Reinforcing use of new skills to respond to negative distortions (Table 5.2)

Cognitive-Behavioral Therapy
Description
- Type of cognitive therapy that involves cognitive and behavioral techniques
- Highly structured psychotherapeutic method
- Examination of thoughts, feelings, and behavior together

Focus
- Emphasis on changing current thinking and behavior in clients
- No exploration of how clients became a certain way
- Results-oriented and specifically defined goals for monitoring progress toward them
- Goal of restructuring perceptions of events to promote behavioral and emotional change in clients

Uses/Indications
- Anorexia nervosa (see Chapter 17)
- Antisocial personality disorder (see Chapter 20)
- Anxiety disorders (see Chapter 14)
- Bipolar disorder (see Chapter 19)
- Body dysmorphic disorder (see Chapter 23)
- Bulimia nervosa (see Chapter 17)
- Hypochondriasis
- Impulse-control disorders (see Chapter 18)
- Obsessive-compulsive personality disorder (see Chapter 20)
- Somatization disorder (see Chapter 23)
- Substance-related disorder (see Chapter 24)

Components
- Involvement of three cognitive processes: cognitive triad, cognitive distortions, and schema (see Cognitive-Behavioral Therapy above)

table
5.2. Therapeutic Techniques of Cognitive Therapy

Technique	Description	Examples
Look for idiosyncratic meaning	Ask the client directly about what words and thoughts mean to him or her.	"What does that mean to you?" "Give me an example."
Question the evidence	Examine the source of data and recognize that the client may be overlooking parts.	"That sounds like what your mother would say." "It also might mean ___." "What evidence do you have that that is true?"
Reattribute	Distribute responsibility among all relevant parties, not just the client.	"Your brother and sister were also part of that." "As a child you could not know ___."
Decatastrophize	Recognize that the client is overestimating the catastrophic nature of the situation.	"What is the worst that can happen?" "If it does occur, what would be so terrible?"
Fantasize consequences	Ask the client to describe the situation. Often, he or she can see the irrationality of his or her ideas. If the problem remains real, then help the client develop coping strategies.	"What might be the effects in 10 years?"

continued on page 118

117

table
5.2. **Therapeutic Techniques of Cognitive Therapy** *continued*

Technique	Description	Examples
Weigh advantages and disadvantages	Ask the client to look at all sides of the issue before defining a reasonable course of action. Writing helps concretize thoughts.	"What are the pros and cons?"
Examine options and alternatives	Ask the client to generate additional options. This is especially difficult for the suicidal client. Don't discount his or her feelings.	"You may be right, something may be wrong with you. What other conclusion might there be?"
Turn adversity to advantage	Present opportunities that stem from challenges.	"Losing this job may be an entry point to a new career."
Use thought stopping	Stopping dysfunctional thoughts is best at the beginning, not the middle. Dysfunctional thoughts can have a snowball effect. Encourage the client to use devices to stop negative thoughts as they arise.	Examples include snapping fingers, popping a rubber band around the wrist, or tapping on the knee.
Use distraction	Distraction is especially helpful with anxiety problems because it is difficult to maintain two thoughts at the same time. Anxious thoughts generally preclude more adaptive thinking. A focused thought distracts the anxiogenic thought.	Have the client count to 200 by 13s (not by 2, 5, 10, or 11); count people wearing yellow or count only small trucks. Have the client do physical activity such as walking, focusing on the in and out of breathing, or counting every other step; it works best when using a complex activity.

- Belief that clients have innate ability to solve their own problems
- Goals developed in partnership with therapist; focus on future rather than on past
- First step: engagement and assessment
  - Development of rapport and identification that problems can be managed
  - Exploration of problem
  - Development of prioritized problem list that forms focus for follow-up sessions
  - Establishment of contract for specified number of sessions
- Second step: interventions
  - Homework assignments
  - Identification of underlying beliefs
  - Challenging of negative beliefs and self-talk
  - Testing of validity of automatic thoughts
  - Bibliotherapy, journaling, diary
- Third step: evaluation and termination
  - Continual determination of progress to goals
  - Encouragement for continued increase in self-awareness and self-reliance
  - Preparation for possible setbacks, including ways to deal with them

Nurse's Role

- Listening actively and empathetically
- Encouraging completion of homework assignments
- Supporting client–therapist interaction
- Reinforcing positive thoughts and effective coping responses

Dialectical Behavior Therapy (DBT)
Description

- Specific form of behavioral therapy
- Developed by Marsha Linehan (1993) specifically for treatment of BPD

Focus

- Emphasis on emotion regulation system
- Invalidating environment as one in which clients receive a message felt invalidating their participation, and that if they were more effective, feelings wouldn't occur
- Continued exposure to invalidating environment, which leads to pervasive dysfunction in regulating emotions
- Sole focus on change without validation of emotions in clients
- Achievement of a balance between acceptance and change of emotions

Uses/Indications

BPD (see Chapter 20)

Components

- Five functions of treatment:
  - Enhancement of client's capabilities
  - Generalization of treatment skills to client's environment
  - Improvement in motivation and decrease in dysfunctional behavior
  - Maintenance of therapist's capabilities and motivation
  - Structuring of the environment
- Use of mindfulness to help clients accept and attend to what is currently happening; encouragement of clients to embrace feeling while attending to one thing at a time, thereby focusing on behavior
- Self-monitoring form (eg, diary card) to track treatment targets (self-harm, emotional distress); used for prioritizing sessions
- Therapist consultation team meetings on a weekly basis for support, problem-solving, and fostering of compassionate attitude
- Use of individual therapy, group therapy, and consultation with therapist

Nurse's Role

- Maintaining a positive approach with clients
- Reinforcing skills learned

- Assisting clients with coping
- Promoting client safety
- Modeling self-respect by being assertive, observing personal limits
- Communicating expectations clearly

Exposure Therapy
Description

- Type of conditioning technique
- Exposure to real or simulated feared object or situation

Focus

- Exposure to fear without relaxation
- Clients given some control over duration of exposure to the fear-causing object
- Forms: graduated, implosive, and flooding

Uses/Indications

- Anxiety disorders (see Chapter 14)
- Agoraphobia

Components

- Graduated exposure
  - Clients control time and frequency of exposure to fear-causing stimulus
  - Over time, stimulus eventually losing its effect
- Implosive therapy:
  - Identification of fear-causing stimuli by therapists
  - Intense, anxiety-provoking image presented to clients
  - Dramatic and vivid description of image to clients
- Flooding
  - Identification of a specific fear associated with client's anxiety
  - Repeated and constant exposure of clients to fear without interruption until anxiety lessens

Nurse's Role

- Assisting clients in identifying fear(s)
- Offering support when confronting fear-causing situations or stimuli
- Educating about ways to handle stress in the future
- Promoting the use of positive coping strategies

Family Therapy

Description

- View of family as the unit of care
- Type of group therapy involving client and family members
- Often involves incorporation of M. Bowen's Family System Therapy Model or S. Minuchin's Family Structure Model

Focus

- Understanding of family dynamics and influence/effect on client's status
- Discovery of others within the family who also have emotional difficulties
- Maintenance of family integrity

Uses/Indication

Applicable for any mental health condition or disorder

Components

- Mobilization of client's and family's strengths and resources
- Restructuring of dysfunctional family behaviors
- Enhancement of family's problem-solving skills and capabilities
- Bowen's Family System Therapy Model:
  - Differentiation of self
  - Triangles
  - Family projection process
  - Nuclear family emotional process
  - Multigenerational transmission process

- Sibling position
- Emotional cutoff
- Minuchin's Family Structure Model
  - Family structure
  - Family rules
  - Subsystems
  - Boundaries

Nurse's Role

- Promoting family health
- Assisting family to adapt to stressors
- Observing family interactions and family relationships
- Assisting in helping family members improve family function
- Helping family build on strengths and perceive crises with hope
- Connecting family to appropriate resources

Group Therapy
Description

- Group therapy as a means to offer multiple stimuli to reveal, examine, and resolve distortions in interpersonal relationships
- Different types of therapy groups
  - Psychotherapeutic groups: use of many different theoretical approaches, including psychoanalysis, transactional analysis, cognitive, rational-emotive, humanistic, gestalt, interpersonal, and psychodrama (to explore the truth through dramatic methods)
  - Growth groups: self-help, encounter, training, community support
- Purpose of each group related to its goals and expected outcomes

Focus

- Interventions for mentally disordered behavior, thinking, and feeling
- Development of intellectual understanding and insight
- Certain level of insight necessary for change

- Maximal therapeutic benefit of psychotherapy or group growth dependent on factors for each member:
  - Extent of personality disorganization and its effects on interpersonal functioning as a family member, provider, and productive citizen
  - Degree of functional ability and role success or failure
  - Ability to harness impulses in stressful group situations
  - Purpose in joining a group, including both articulated and hidden agendas
  - Ability to share and support others in problem-solving tasks
  - Ability to use the material produced in a group to solve unique problems

Uses/Indications

Applicable for any mental health condition or disorder (Table 5.3)

Components

- Interdependent therapeutic factors in group therapy; different factors more functional and helpful to group process at different stages
- Emphasis and importance of therapeutic factors variable on the basis of group type
- Twelve curative factors that relate to different parts of the change process and are necessary for change:
  - Interpersonal learning
  - Catharsis
  - Group cohesiveness
  - Self-understanding
  - Development of socializing techniques
  - Existential factors
  - Universality
  - Instillation of hope
  - Altruism
  - Corrective family reenactment
  - Guidance
  - Identification/imitative behavior

table
5.3. **Advantages and Disadvantages of Group Therapy**

Advantages	Disadvantages
• More clients can be treated at once, fostering cost effectiveness. • Members benefit by hearing others discuss similar problems; feelings of isolation, alienation, and uniqueness often decrease, encouraging members to share problems. • Group therapy allows clients to explore their specific styles of communication in a safe atmosphere where they can receive feedback and undergo change. • Members learn from others multiple ways to solve problems, and group exploration may help them discover new ways. • Members learn about the functional roles of individuals in a group. Sometimes, a member shares the responsibility as the co-therapist. Members become culture carriers. • The group provides for its members' understanding, confrontation, and identification with more than one person. The member gains a reference group.	• A member's privacy may be violated, such as when a conversation is shared outside the group. This behavior obstructs confidentiality and hampers complete and honest participation. • Clients from various diagnostic groups may differ on the basis of neurobiological functioning. For example, a client with schizophrenia may have multiple deficits in information processing such as attention, learning, and memory. Because of these possible deficits, the group leader must be cognizant of the limitations and adjust the group process accordingly. • Clients may experience difficulty exposing themselves to a group or believe that they lack the skills to communicate effectively. Some clients may use these factors as resistance; others may be reluctant to expose themselves because they do not want to change. • Group therapy is not helpful if the therapist conducts the group as if it is individual therapy. Such a therapist may see dynamics and group processes as incidental or antagonistic to the therapeutic process. An effective group leader is skilled in techniques and interventions that foster group interaction and shape group behavior and growth.

Nurse's Role

- Using appropriate therapeutic communication techniques
- Establishing therapeutic relationship
- Accepting the feelings of group members
- Assisting in facilitating group process
- Helping with development of goals and group roles
- Participating as a member of the group as appropriate
- Encouraging the development of the group

Individual Psychotherapy

Description

- Process involving application of principles for establishing a professional relationship by a trained professional with a client seeking help for psychological problems
- Learning or human development as the result
- People providing psychotherapy: psychiatrists (MD), clinical psychologists (PhD), social workers (LMSW), licensed professional counselors (LPC), and psychiatric-mental health advanced practice registered nurses (APRN-PMH)

Focus

- Relationship between client and therapist as the common element
- Overall goals:
  - Decreased psychological distress
  - Increased client self-awareness and self-esteem
  - Learning of new, more functional coping methods

Uses/Indications

Applicable for any mental health condition or disorder

Components

- Purposeful one-to-one client–therapist relationship
- Therapist as trained professional with a knowledge base of guiding principles

- Therapeutic verbal and nonverbal communication techniques
- Numerous theories, therapies, and styles of practice varying with discipline (Table 5.4)

Nurse's Role

- Using therapeutic communication techniques
- Assisting with using newly learned coping strategies and suggested changes
- Promoting the use of positive coping strategies
- Educating about ways to reduce stress
- Encouraging continued participation with therapy

Limit Setting
Description

- Establishment of boundaries by someone in authority
- A framework for functioning in an acceptable manner

Focus

- Acceptable functioning to promote feelings of security, self-awareness, and self-esteem
- Boundaries set in response to client's need for control without being punitive

Uses/Indications

- Anger, aggression, violence (directed at self or others) (see Chapter 26)
- Suicidal intent
- Impulse-control disorders (see Chapter 18)
- Mood disorders (see Chapter 19)
- BPD (see Chapter 20)

Components

- Description of unacceptable client behavior
- Communication of expected behavior

table
5.4.

Selected Approaches to Psychotherapy

Approach	Focus	Key Points for Nurses	Desired Outcome
Psychoanalysis Psychodynamic psychotherapy	Client's conscious and unconscious conflicts	Transference Countertransference Defense mechanisms (see Chap. 1)	Insight into repressed conflicts Restructuring of the personality
Cognitive–behavioral therapy	Changing distorted thoughts, with the result being positive behavioral change	Identification of situations involving undesirable thoughts and actions Homework assignments	New skills
• Cognitive therapy	*Client's perception of self, world, and future (cognitive triad) Exploration of client's thought processes*	*Development of problem lists Session agendas Homework Evaluation of successes and failures*	*Recognition of self-defeating thought patterns Release of self-blame Enhancement of functional responses*
• Rational emotive behavior therapy	*Exploration of irrational thinking*	*Identification of activating situations and negative emotions, leading to irrational beliefs*	*Client control of behavior and thinking Change in thinking leading to positive change in behavior*

• Dialectical behavior therapy	Acceptance of emotions fused with acknowledgment of need for behavior change	Empathy Reflection of feelings Exploration of perceptual distortions and dysfunctional behaviors	*Client's embracing of intense emotions (living in the moment)* *Self-acceptance* *Change in cognitions leading to more functional coping patterns*
Behavior therapy	Promoting desirable behaviors Extinguishing undesirable behaviors	Token economies Reinforcements	Reshaping of behavior with elimination of negative behaviors
Client-centered therapy	Relationship with therapist Self-acceptance leading to insight	Unconditional positive regard Empathy Reflection of feelings	Increased self-esteem Positive foundation so that client sees self and situations more clearly
Solution-focused therapy	Problems result from mishandling life's events	Joint partnership between therapist and client Client development of alternate views of situation based on identification of past successes and factors maintaining the problem	Satisfactory life adjustments and ability to change, interact, and reach goals through solutions

- Provision of acceptable alternatives to the behavior
- Explanation of rationale for limits
- Description of consequences for violating limits

Nurse's Role

- Stating limits in a matter-of-fact manner
- Assisting clients to understand the reasons for limits
- Explaining the consequences for testing or violating limits
- Enforcing the limits consistently
- Ensuring that all healthcare team members are aware of limits and respond uniformly to testing or violation of them

Milieu Therapy
Description

- Also known as "therapeutic environment"
- Use of a stable, logical, organized social atmosphere
- Collaboration of client and all healthcare providers

Focus

- Facilitation of client interactions
- Promotion of personal client growth
- Emphasis on client involvement in treatment decisions and unit/setting operation
- Maintenance of family as part of client's life

Uses/Indications

- Antisocial personality disorder (see Chapter 20)
- Depressive disorders (see Chapter 19)
- Schizophrenia (see Chapter 25)
- Dissociative disorders (see Chapter 16)

Components

- **Containment**: provision of safety and security (physical and psychological) with freedom of movement within this environment

- **Validation**: affirmation of the client's individuality with focus on respect for clients and their rights
- **Structured interaction**: client interaction and active participation with others that is purposeful
- **Open communication**: sharing of information willingly by clients and team members
  - Encouragement of client self-disclosure as part of nurse–client relationship
  - Modeling of appropriate therapeutic communication techniques
  - Environmental arrangement to facilitate interaction
  - Client education

Nurse's Role

- Working collaboratively with clients and other healthcare team members
- Ensuring appropriate structure and safety of the environment
- Using appropriate therapeutic communication techniques in all interactions
- Encouraging and maintaining family involvement
- Demonstrating respect for clients during any interaction
- Offering support, praise, and reassurance to promote client's self-esteem
- Providing client education

Psychoanalysis
Description

- Form of therapy developed by Sigmund Freud (1856–1939)
- Exploration of the client's conscious and unconscious conflicts with past coping patterns
- Long-term treatment approach

Focus

- Belief that adult behaviors and problems resulted from faulty relationships and client's early mother–child experiences

- Conflicts among three personality parts (id, ego, and superego) cause mental illness
- Promotion of insight and integration of repressed conflicts into the personality
- Improved functioning and happiness as goal of therapy

Use/Indications

Applicable for any mental health condition or disorder

Components

- **Transference**: unconscious reenactment of patterns and feelings of past relationships; client distorts therapist's behaviors and unconsciously places positive or negative feeling about the past situation or person on the therapist
  - Current relationship ignited something in the client's past from an old relationship, usually one involving an authority figure, such as a parent
  - Need to identify and resolve transference for client change and growth
- **Countertransference**: extreme emotional responses (positive or negative) to clients
- Defense mechanisms (see Chapter 1)

Nurse's Role

- Being alert to any extreme emotional response that clients direct toward nurse
- Remaining compassionate and avoiding defensiveness if clients develop transference
- Assisting clients to identify the feelings and possible past reasons for them
- Understanding and closely monitoring countertransference; seeking assistance from a mental health colleague or the treatment team if it occurs

Rational-Emotive Behavior Therapy (REBT)
Description

- Initially developed in 1955 by Albert Ellis after he became dissatisfied with psychoanalysis

- Renamed rational-emotive behavior therapy to encompass a behavioral component
- Form of cognitive-behavioral therapy

Focus

- Clients disturbed not by things or events but by their view of them
- Rational beliefs viewed as evaluative and non-absolute cognitions; expressed as wishes, likes, and dislikes that may or may not be attained
- Irrational beliefs viewed as dogmatic and expressed in the form of rigid "musts," "shoulds," "oughts," or "have-tos," leading to negative emotions that interfere with goal pursuit and attainment
- Realization by clients that they are the creator of the psychological disturbance and that they can change it
  - Client understanding that such disturbance primarily results from irrational beliefs as crucial
  - Once identified, beliefs disputed and philosophically restructured, ultimately leading to change
  - Change as moving from absolutes to "preferences" (ie, what clients would like to happen)

Uses/Indications

- Antisocial personality disorder (see Chapter 20)
- Anxiety disorders (see Chapter 14)
- Bipolar disorder (see Chapter 19)
- Body dysmorphic disorder (see Chapter 23)
- Eating disorders (see Chapter 17)
- Obsessive-compulsive personality disorder (see Chapter 20)
- Somatization disorder (see Chapter 23)

Components

- Replacement of irrational beliefs with rational ones
- ABC approach to resolving irrational beliefs
  - Client's realization that the activating event (A) does not directly cause emotional and behavioral consequences (C)
  - Client's beliefs (B) about the activating event (A) as contributing primarily to the consequences (C) (irrational beliefs about events leading to inappropriate consequences)

- Unconditional self-acceptance regardless of professional or personal failings
- Acceptance of others as people, not necessarily on the basis of their behaviors
- Acceptance of life and a high tolerance of frustration helping clients live a functional life

Nurse's Role

- Listening actively and empathetically
- Supporting client–therapist interaction
- Assisting clients with challenging irrational beliefs
- Reinforcing positive thoughts and effective coping responses

Seclusion/Restraints
Description

- **Seclusion**: the involuntary confinement of clients in a hazard-free room or area that is locked and where clients can be directly observed
- **Restraint**: any manual method or physical or mechanical device, material, or equipment attached to a person's body that restricts freedom of movement or normal access to one's body
- Use of seclusion, restraint, or both as a source of controversy

Focus

- Use limited to emergencies involving imminent risk of a client physically harming self, staff, or others
- Application only when other less restrictive methods to ensure client safety have failed; nonphysical interventions as the first choice
- Discontinuation as soon as possible

Uses/Indications

- Aggression
- Violence (directed at self or others)
- Impulse-control disorders (see Chapter 18)

Components

- Ordered by physician with specialized training and experience in diagnosis and treatment of mental disorders or by a licensed independent practitioner with specialized training and experience in use of emergency safety interventions; as permitted by the state and facility
- Order limited to 4 hours for clients 18 years or older; 2 hours for children 9 to 17 years old; 1 hour for children less than 9 years old
- New order necessary if additional time needed
- Face-to-face evaluation of client within 1 hour of initiating restraint/seclusion to assess need for ongoing use
- Collaboration with client and staff on ways to help client regain control
- Ongoing assessment of client by staff when initiating restraint/seclusion and every 15 minutes afterward, including direct eye contact
- Debriefing within 24 hours after episode involving client, staff, and client's family if appropriate to discuss circumstances and factors resulting in use of seclusion/restraint and ways to prevent future episodes
- Accurate documentation

Nurse's Role

- Using all available means of nonphysical interventions
- Utilizing seclusion/restraint only as a last resort
- Continually assessing client during seclusion/restraint
- Ensuring client and staff safety during episode
- Adhering to appropriate standards of care for use of seclusion/restraint
- Documenting all aspects of situation before, during, and after use of seclusion/restraint
- Participating in debriefing sessions

Solution-Focused Therapy
Description

- Developed over the past 50 years through the collaboration of numerous therapists.
- Emphasis on helping clients find solutions to their problems

Focus

- No use of predetermined solutions
- Joint collaboration of therapist and client
- Problems best understood on the basis of solutions
- View of client as individual with strengths and achievements
- Client in state of constant change

Uses/Indications

- Thought disorders (see Chapter 25)
- Delusions, hallucinations

Components

- Some initial discussion of problem, then a focus on change
- Determination of central issue with concentration on resolution
- Use of goal-oriented questions to facilitate movement toward effective solution
- Step-wise process:
  - Setting the agenda
  - Understanding the effects of the problem
  - Identifying the exceptions
  - Making sense of the exceptions
  - Using future orientation
  - Asking the "miracle question"
  - Asking for a "video description"
  - Reinforcing small steps
  - Using scale questions
  - Continuing to work toward solutions

Nurse's Role

- Encouraging clients to focus on solution rather than on problem
- Viewing the client as an individual
- Emphasizing strengths and resources
- Assisting with development of realistic achievable goals

Systematic Desensitization

Description

- Classic conditioning technique
- Type of exposure therapy (see page 121)

Focus

- Replacement of anxiety or panic response with relaxation response
- Education involving the use of muscle relaxation

Uses/Indications

- Specific phobias
- Social phobias
- Agoraphobia
- Post-traumatic stress disorder (see Chapter 14)

Components

- Progressive, gradual confrontation of an object of fear in very small, controlled steps while in a deeply relaxed state
- Increasing degree of complexity and intensity with each progressive exposure or confrontation to decrease anxiety
- Another form involving creation of list in which client rates anxiety-inducing situations by degree of fear, using a scale of 0 to 10
  - Confrontation initiated with situations rated as 1 or 2 and practicing relaxation techniques
  - Gradual progression to higher-rated situations

Nurse's Role

- Assisting client in identifying fear(s)
- Offering support when confronting fear-causing situations or stimuli
- Educating about ways to handle stress in the future
- Promoting the use of positive coping strategies

6

Integrative and Somatic Therapies

Complimentary and Alternative Medicine (CAM) Therapies

Description

- Many are based on Eastern philosophies.
- **Alternative therapies**: those used in place of Western therapies.
- **Complementary therapies**: those used in conjunction with Western therapies.
- **CAM therapies**: practices generally not considered "conventional" in Western medical practice (ie, not taught widely in medical schools, not typically used in hospitals, and not usually reimbursed by medical insurance companies).
- More comprehensive use of the term "integrative therapies" to imply the use of practices in conjunction with traditional health-care modalities in the care of clients.

Focus

- Holistic, integrative approach in unifying physical, mental, and spiritual well-being

- Four domains:
  - **Mind–body medicine**: use mindful stress-reduction techniques to restore bodily functions
  - **Biologically based practices**: rely on natural substances such as herbs, diet and nutrition supplements, light modalities, and aromatherapy to restore health
  - **Manipulative and body-based practices**: focus on the manipulation or movement of one or more body parts
  - **Energy medicine**: energy fields that originate from inside (biofields) or outside (electromagnetic fields) the body (Table 6.1)

Uses/Indications

Will vary with the type of therapy
- Anxiety disorders (see Chapter 14)
- Mood disorders (see Chapter 19)
- Substance-related disorders (see Chapter 24)
- Cognitive disorders (see Chapter 15)

Components

- Focus on the person rather than on the illness
- Wide variety of methods
- Many herbal remedies with soothing effects on the nervous system (Table 6.2)

Nurse's Role

- Being knowledgeable about the basic CAM therapies
- Providing clients with appropriate resources for information
- Assisting clients in selecting the most appropriate therapy
- Educating clients about therapy
- Advocating in decision-making and providing support for decision
- Respecting client's wishes and beliefs in pursuing therapies

table
6.1. **Selected Review of Common Integrative Modalities**

Mind–body medicine: Approaches use mindful stress-reduction techniques to restore physiologic functions. Additional approaches to those covered include art therapy, dance therapy, guided imagery, humor, hypnotherapy, prayer and spirituality, and support groups.

Meditation	Clients try to achieve awareness without thought and positively alter physiology. Moment-to-moment attention leads to perceptual and cognitive changes. Focus on breathing diverts concentration from stressors. Meditation is done at prescribed frequencies and durations.
Music therapy	Use of music can alter behavior, emotions, or physiology. Musical vibrations and artistic expressions can help restore or enhance regulatory function. Such modalities may help clients develop self-awareness and creativity, improve learning, clarify values, and cope with various illnesses.
Pet therapy	Pet therapy programs are found nationwide. Studies support the benefits of interaction with pets, which include decreased blood pressure, enhanced mood and socialization, and improved cardiovascular symptoms. Pets can be helpful companions for depressed clients, as well as those with cognitive challenges.

Biologically based practices: These methods use natural substances to restore health and healing. Additional approaches to those covered include apitherapy, macrobiotics, nutritional supplements, and vitamin therapy.

Herbal therapy	Herbal therapy uses plants or their parts to manage illness. Most herbs act by correcting underlying causes of disease. Each herb has a complex mixture of active ingredients, often making it difficult to identify the effective agent. Use of herbs requires knowledgeable practitioners and reliable products because the strength and purity of preparations vary.
Aromatherapy	Aromatherapy uses essential oils for health benefits. It is not known if aromatherapy achieves its efficacy from placebo response, effects of touch and smell on the nervous system, learned memory of aromas, pharmacokinetic potentiation of drugs by essential oils, or pharmacologically active ingredients that have analgesic effects.

table
6.1. **Selected Review of Common Integrative Modalities** *continued*

Manipulative and body-based practices: These modalities involve the manipulation or movement of one or more body parts. Additional approaches to those covered include chiropractic, massage (more than 80 forms), osteopathy, and reflexology.

Yoga	Yoga is used to relieve anxiety, stress, and pain; treat addictions and migraines; enhance spatial memory; and increase auditory and visual perceptions. There are many styles of yoga; each is a unique combination of physical postures and exercises (*asanas*), breathing techniques (*pranayamas*), relaxation, diet, and proper thinking.
Reflexology	Reflexology involves massaging specific areas of the hands or feet to relieve stress or pain in corresponding related body areas. Use of reflexology is reported to improve pain, digestion, insomnia, premenstrual syndrome, menopausal symptoms, fertility, respiratory conditions, asthma, and cardiovascular problems.
Tai chi	Tai chi consists of a series of choreographed, continuous slow movements performed with mental concentration and coordinated breathing. Clients learn to connect with energies, balance energies within the body, and maintain equilibrium with the opposing forces of nature (yin and yang). This powerful centering activity may precede meditation, prayer, or other exercises.

Energy medicine: Energy therapies focus on energy fields that originate from inside (biofields) or outside (electromagnetic fields) of the body. Additional approaches to those covered include acupressure, Reiki, shiatsu, and therapeutic touch.

Acupuncture	Acupuncture involves the placement of needles on specific points of the body to treat specific illnesses. Needle placement helps correct and rebalance energy flow and consequently relieve pain and restore health. It redirects energy to organs with health deficiencies.
Bioelectromagnetic therapy	Clients use magnetic fields to prevent and treat disease and as first aid. Natural mineral magnets are used for insomnia, chronic pain, broken bones, stress, and musculoskeletal disorders.

table
6.2. **Selected Herbs, Minerals, and Vitamins for Mental Health Use**

Herbs, Minerals, and Vitamins	Uses	Actions and Precautions	Dose
California poppy, yellow and orange	Relieves pain Acts as sedative Relieves mild anxiety	Poppy contains mild alkaloids similar to codeine and morphine. Do not use with monoamine oxidase inhibitors (MAOIs).	1 tsp/cup tea 2–3 times a day
Ginkgo biloba	Reduces senility Reduces short-term memory loss in normal older adults Improves peripheral circulation	Use as a circulatory aid and antioxidant. Fruit or seed should not be handled or eaten. May enhance papaverine. Possible side effects include gastrointestinal (GI) distress, headache, and allergic reaction. Cautious use is recommended if taking aspirin or other blood-thinning drugs.	60 mg BID Alzheimer's—240 mg divided 2–3 times a day
Ginseng (Asian and American)	Reduces stress and fatigue Improves physical and mental function, especially with elderly clients Assists smoking cessation efforts	Use the root. Use may raise blood pressure and serum glucose levels and can increase the growth of estrogen-dependent cancer.	American—0.03% ginsenoside, 1–2 g fresh root Asian—1.5% ginseng, 1–2 g fresh root For both, 200–600 mg liquid extract daily

Guarana	Enhances cognition Reduces combat fatigue Acts as a "cerebral stimulant"	It is a food additive/dietary supplement. It contains an extremely high caffeine level: 2.6–7%, compared to coffee beans with 1–2% and dried tea leaves with 1–4%.	Not recommended for use Range for use: 250–1200 mg/day
Hops	Has a sedative effect Reduces anxiety	Forms include tea, extract, or capsule. The active ingredient is in glandular hairs on its scaly, conelike fruits.	1 tsp/cup tea 2–3 times a day or 30–40 drops tincture
Passion flower	Causes mild hypnosis Reduces insomnia Reduces nervousness, restlessness, and agitation	Depresses the central nervous system (CNS) for mild sedative effect. Forms include tea, capsules, and extracts.	Infusion of 2–5 g (1 tsp) dried herb TID
Rosemary and other mints	Normalizes nerve impulses Acts as an antioxidant Relieves headache Acts as a sedative Helps improve memory and prevent dementia	Slows/inhibits action of acetylcholinesterase to acetylcholine, which stays in synapse longer. Antioxidant is carnosic acid that is concentrated in young growing leaves, peaks in the summer, lessens in older leaves, and is hardly present in old wood stems. Forms include whole essential oils for external use (see Aromatherapy section in text)	Tincture (1:5) 2–4 mL TID

continued on page 144

143

table
6.2. **Selected Herbs, Minerals, and Vitamins for Mental Health Use** *continued*

Herbs, Minerals, and Vitamins	Uses	Actions and Precautions	Dose
St. John's wort	Treats mild to moderate depression, loss of interest, anorexia, fatigue, chronic fatigue immune dysfunction syndrome, and anxiety	Leaves or flowering tips can be used; hypericin is the active ingredient. May interfere with HIV drugs. Use may cause light sensitivity. Use with other drugs can be dangerous; do not take with other psychoactive medications (ie, selective serotonin reuptake inhibitors [SSRIs], tricyclics, and MAOIs). Has fewer side effects compared with antidepressants. May lower activity of nonsedating antihistamines, oral contraceptives, anti-epileptics, calcium channel blockers, cyclosporins, macrolides, and some antifungals.	300–500 mg TID with meals for 4–6 weeks 0.5 mg hypericin per capsule
SAMe (S-adenosylmethionine)	Treats mild to moderate depression and arthritis, protects the liver, eases fibromyalgia	SAMe is a naturally occurring compound that regulates action of serotonin and dopamine. Approved as prescription drug in Italy, Germany, Spain, and Russia.	200–800 or 1600 mg BID 1 hour before breakfast and lunch For arthritis 400–800 mg a day For fibromyalgia, 800 mg a day

		Takes effect in 10 days, faster than prescription drugs. Use enteric-coated tablets with 96% pure product. Do not use for bipolar disorder. Must take 800 µg folic acid and 1000 µg vitamin B_{12} daily; the herb will not work if these vitamin levels are low.	
Valerian	Relieves anxiety and insomnia	Forms include a tea (2–3 g dried root several times a day) or capsules. Herb is nonaddictive. Do not take with tranquilizers, sedatives, or alcohol. Possible side effects include blurred vision, excitability, and changes in heartbeat if taken in large doses or for more than 2 weeks.	300–400 mg 1–2 times a day
5-Hydroxytryptophan (5-HTP)	Treats bipolar disorder in conjunction with lithium Reduces depression Relieves insomnia	This amino acid is a precursor of serotonin. Taken from *Griffonia simplicifolia* seed.	Bipolar disorder—200 mg, Depression—150–300 mg, Insomnia—200–600 mg

Electroconvulsive Therapy (ECT)

Description

- Application of a small dose of electricity to the brain to induce a seizure
- Exact mechanism unclear
- Belief that ECT alters neurotransmitter receptors and thereby the chemistry of the brain

Focus

- Somatic therapy
- Belief that electrically induced seizure most likely modifies the neurochemical environment
- Therapy for clients for whom all other therapeutic interventions have failed and whose lives are at risk
- Usually given twice weekly on nonconsecutive days
- Treatments ranging from a few to 15 sessions, depending on client response
- Procedures lasting less than 1 hour, although each client's recovery time varies
- Graduated schedule, usually once a week for 1 month, once every 2 weeks for 2 months, once every 3 weeks for 2 months, and once every month for 2 to 4 months

Uses/Indications

- Major depression (see Chapter 19)
- Schizoaffective disorders
- Mania (see Chapter 19)
- Schizophrenia (see Chapter 25)

Components

- Brief general anesthesia with succinylcholine prior to the procedure to prevent severe muscle contractions that might result in muscle or bone injuries
- Anticholinergic agents used, possibly to dry secretions that might interfere with respiration
- Ultra-brief anesthetic agents to induce unconsciousness

- Electrode placement on the temple to induce a grand mal seizure via an electric current passed through the electrode for 0.10 to 1.0 second
- Induced convulsion lasting approximately 1 minute
- Oxygen administered to the client; oxygen saturation and cardiac functioning monitored

Nurse's Role

- Before the procedure:
  - Ensuring that client has fasted after midnight on the day of the procedure
  - Carefully assessing clients about to undergo ECT, including completion of appropriate history, physical examination, and laboratory testing
  - Informing client and family what to expect both immediately before and after the procedure
  - Reassuring client and family that the procedure is safe and that most side effects are transitory
- After the procedure:
  - Closely observing client's cardiovascular status and airway patency
  - Assessing carefully for postictal confusion
  - Reorienting the client as necessary; recording the duration and severity of any disorientation
  - Assessing for possible side effects such as headache, muscle aches, or nausea; administering prescribed agents for side effects
  - Providing gentle but firm direction to clients so that they remain in bed during disorientation
  - Promoting comfort by giving small sips of water, ice chips, or juice

Phototherapy
Description

- Use of artificial light to aid in regulating the cycle of darkness and daylight

- Light considered one of the most powerful regulators of human circadian rhythms

Focus

- Levels of melatonin and serotonin depend on the exposure of the pineal gland to sunlight
- Light acting as a trigger to reset the client's circadian rhythm

Uses/Indications

- Seasonal affective disorder (SAD)
- Circadian rhythm sleep disorder

Components

- Artificial light source (fluorescent light box with a filter to screen out ultraviolet rays) as the gold standard (usually 2500 lux [approximately 200 times brighter than normal indoor lighting])
- Exposure to the light from 30 to 120 minutes per day in the morning to mimic the natural circadian rhythm
- Antidepressant effect usually beginning in 1 to 4 days, with full effect occurring in approximately 2 weeks

Nurse's Role

- Teaching clients about using phototherapy
- Emphasizing the need to continue treatment even if feeling better
- Monitoring for possible side effects (rare), including complaints of headaches, eyestrain, nausea, sweating, visual disturbances, and sedation
- Instructing clients to consult an ophthalmologist before commencing treatment and to avoid looking directly into the light

Psychopharmacology

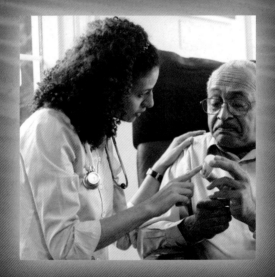

Anxiolytics/ Sedative-Hypnotics

Overview

Primary Indications

Generalized anxiety disorder (*see Chapter 14, p. 300*), acute anxiety states (*see p. 319*), social phobias, performance anxiety, and simple phobias

Other Indications

Insomnia (*see Chapter 22, p. 437*), alcohol withdrawal, agitation, mania, and acute psychoses (when safe and rapid sedation with relatively few side effects is desired)

Signs and Symptoms

Symptoms that indicate a possible need for anxiolytics and sedative-hypnotics include chronic and excessive worrying, motor tension, autonomic hyperactivity, apprehensive expectation, chronic hyper-vigilance for potential threats, impatience, irritability, feelings of being "on edge," intense fear or terror.

Major Categories

- **Benzodiazepines:** act directly on gamma-aminobutyric acid (GABA) receptors, possibly increasing available GABA to dampen neural overstimulation

- alprazolam (*see p. 151*)
- chlordiazepoxide (*see p. 159*)
- clonazepam (*see p. 160*)
- diazepam (*see p. 162*)
- estazolam (*see p. 164*)
- flurazepam (*see p. 166*)
- lorazepam (*see p. 169*)
- midazolam
- quazepam (*see p. 175*)
- temazepam (*see p. 178*)
- triazolam (*see p. 179*)
- **Barbiturates**: Depress the central nervous system (CNS), inhibiting impulse conduction, depressing cerebral cortex, altering cerebellar function, depressing motor output
  - amobarbital (*see p. 153*)
  - butabarbital (*see p. 156*)
  - mephobarbital (*see p. 170*)
  - pentobarbital (*see p. 171*)
  - phenobarbital (*see p. 173*)
  - secobarbital (*see p. 177*)
- Other agents
  - buspirone (*see p. 155*)
  - chloral hydrate (*see p. 157*)
  - eszopiclone (*see p. 165*)
  - hydroxyzine (*see p. 168*)
  - ramelteon (*see p. 176*)
  - zaleplon (*see p. 180*)
  - zolpidem (*see p. 182*)

Key Drug Monographs
alprazolam (Xanax, Xanax XR)
Drug Class
Benzodiazepine, anxiolytic

Indications and Dosage

Anxiety (*see p. 300*)	*Adults*: Initially, 0.25 to 0.5 mg PO three times daily (tid), to a maximum of 4 mg daily in divided doses. *Elderly clients*: Initially, 0.25 mg PO two times daily (bid) or tid to a maximum of 4 mg daily in divided doses.
Panic disorders (*see p. 311*)	*Adults*: 0.5 mg PO tid, increasing in 1-mg increments at intervals of 3 to 4 days, up to a maximum of 10 mg daily in divided doses. If using extended-release form, 0.5 to 1 mg PO once daily, increasing by no more than 1 mg every 3 to 4 days to a maximum daily dose of 10 mg.

Half-life

Immediate release: 12 to 15 hours
Extended release: 11 to 16 hours

Common Adverse Reactions

Central nervous system (CNS): Insomnia, irritability, dizziness, headache, anxiety, confusion, drowsiness, light-headedness, sedation, somnolence, difficulty speaking, impaired coordination, impaired memory, fatigue, depression, suicide
Gastrointestinal (GI): Diarrhea, dry mouth, constipation
Other: Emergence of anxiety between doses, dependence

Key Interactions

Increased CNS depression with: Anticonvulsants, antidepressants, antihistamines, barbiturates, benzodiazepines, general anesthetics, narcotics, phenothiazines, kava, valerian root, alcohol
Increased drug level with: Azole antifungals (including fluconazole, itraconazole, ketoconazole, miconazole), cimetidine, fluoxetine, fluvoxamine, hormonal contraceptives, nefazodone, grapefruit juice

Decreased drug effectiveness with: Carbamazepine, propoxyphene, smoking

Decreased drug level with: St. John's wort

Increased level of co-administered drug with: Tricyclic antidepressants (TCAs)

Nursing Considerations

- Administer extended-release form once daily in the morning.
- Alert: Avoid abrupt withdrawal of the drug, which can induce withdrawal symptoms, including seizures.
- Alert: Abuse, addiction, or both are possible.
- Monitor hepatic, renal, and hematopoietic function periodically in clients receiving repeated or prolonged therapy.
- Alert: Do not confuse alprazolam with alprostadil or Xanax with Zantac.
- Warn client to avoid hazardous activities that require alertness and physical coordination until effects of drug are known.
- Tell clients to avoid alcohol while taking the drug; advise that smoking may decrease the drug's effectiveness.
- Warn client not to take the drug with grapefruit juice.
- Tell client to swallow extended-release tablets whole; if using an orally disintegrating tablet, tell client to remove it from the bottle with dry hands and to immediately place it on his or her tongue, where it will dissolve and can be swallowed with saliva.
- If client is taking half of a scored, orally disintegrating tablet, instruct him or her to discard the unused half.
- Advise client to discard the cotton from the bottle of orally disintegrating tablets and to keep the bottle tightly sealed to prevent moisture from dissolving the tablets.

amobarbital sodium (Amytal Sodium)

Drug Class

Barbiturate, sedative-hypnotic

Indications and Dosage

Insomnia (short-term therapy; *see p. 437*)	*Adults*: 30 to 50 mg intramuscularly (IM) or intravenously (IV) (not to exceed 50 mg/min) bid to tid for sedation; 65 to 200 mg IM or IV (not to exceed 50 mg/min) for hypnotic effect.

Half-life
16 to 40 hours

Common Adverse Reactions
CNS: Somnolence, agitation, confusion, hyperkinesias, ataxia, vertigo, CNS depression, nightmares, lethargy, residual sedation
GI: Nausea, vomiting, constipation, diarrhea
Skin: Pain at the injection site
Other: Hypoventilation, tolerance, dependence

Key Interactions
Increased CNS depression with: CNS depressants, phenothiazines, alcohol, antihistamines
Increased drug level with: Monoamine-oxidase inhibitors (MAOIs)
Decreased effect of co-administered drug with: Oral anticoagulants, TCAs, corticosteroids, hormonal contraceptives, estrogen, acetaminophen, metronidazole, carbamazepine, β-blockers, phenylbutazones, theophyllines, quinidine, doxycycline

Nursing Considerations
- Assess mental status of clients before starting therapy.
- Administer drug via deep IM injection into a large muscle mass.
- If using IV administration, monitor IV insertion site for infiltration or extravasation.
- Assess vital signs closely during IV administration.
- Alert: Watch for signs of barbiturate toxicity: coma, pupillary constriction, cyanosis, clammy skin, and hypotension. Overdose can be fatal.

- Do not stop drug abruptly; withdraw gradually.
- Inform clients that morning hangover is common after hypnotic dose.
- Caution clients to avoid activities that require mental alertness or physical coordination while using the drug.
- Warn clients to avoid alcohol use while using the drug.

buspirone hydrochloride (BuSpar)

Drug Class
Anxiolytic

Indications and Dosage

Anxiety disorders (*see p. 300*)	*Adults*: Initially, 7.5 mg PO bid, increasing by 5-mg increments daily at intervals of 2 to 3 days; usual maintenance dose of 20 to 30 mg daily in divided doses, not to exceed 60 mg daily.

Half-life
2 to 3 hours

Common Adverse Reactions
CNS: Dizziness, drowsiness, headache
GI: Dry mouth, nausea, diarrhea, abdominal distress

Key Interactions
Increased risk for adverse effects with: Azole antifungals
Increased CNS depression with: CNS depressants, alcohol
Increased drug level with: Drugs metabolized by CYP3A4 (erythromycin, nefazodone), grapefruit juice
Increased risk for hypertension with: MAOIs

Nursing Considerations
- Monitor client closely for adverse CNS effects. Although buspirone is less sedating than other anxiolytics, its CNS effects can be unpredictable.

- Alert: Before client begins therapy with buspirone, do not stop a previous regimen with a benzodiazepine abruptly. Doing so can lead to a withdrawal reaction.
- Alert: Do not confuse buspirone with bupropion.
- Warn client to avoid hazardous activities that require alertness and physical coordination until effects of drug are known.
- Remind client that drug effects may not be noticeable for several weeks.
- Tell client to avoid alcohol during therapy.

butabarbital sodium (Butisol sodium)

Drug Class
Barbiturate, sedative-hypnotic

Indications and Dosage

Sedation (short-term use)	*Adults*: 15 to 30 mg PO three (tid) to four times daily (qid) for daytime sedation; 50 to 100 mg PO at bedtime for use as hypnotic.

Half-life
50 to 100 hours

Common Adverse Reactions
CNS: Somnolence, agitation, confusion, hyperkinesias, ataxia, vertigo, CNS depression, nightmares, residual sedation, paradoxical excitement, nervousness, psychiatric disturbances, hallucinations, insomnia, anxiety, dizziness, abnormal thinking
CV: Bradycardia, hypotension, syncope
GI: Nausea, vomiting, constipation, diarrhea, epigastric pain
Respiratory: Hypoventilation, apnea, respiratory depression
Other: Tolerance, dependence, withdrawal syndrome

Key Interactions
Increased CNS depression with: Alcohol

Decreased effectiveness of co-administered drug with: Oral anti-coagulants, TCAs, corticosteroids, hormonal contraceptives, estrogen, metronidazole, carbamazepine, β-blockers, phenylbutazones, theophyllines, quinidine, doxycycline

Nursing Considerations

- Monitor respiratory status of client closely during administration.
- Alert: Do not administer this drug for more than 2 weeks; it is habit-forming, and its effectiveness disappears after a short time.
- Alert: Watch for signs of barbiturate toxicity: coma, pupillary constriction, cyanosis, clammy skin, and hypotension. Overdose can be fatal.
- Do not stop drug abruptly; taper dose gradually.
- Inform client that morning hangover is common after a hypnotic dose.
- Caution client to avoid activities that require mental alertness or physical coordination until effects of drug are known.
- Warn client to avoid alcohol use while using the drug.

chloral hydrate (Aquachloral Supprettes, Somnote)

Drug Class

CNS depressant, sedative-hypnotic

Indications and Dosage

Sedation	*Adults*: 250 mg PO or PR tid after meals up to a maximum single or daily dose of 2 g. *Children*: 8 mg/kg PO tid to a maximum dose of 500 mg tid.
Insomnia (*see p. 437*)	*Adults*: 500 mg to 1 g PO or PR 15 to 30 minutes before bedtime to a maximum daily dose of 2 g. *Children*: 50 mg/kg PO or PR 15 to 30 minutes before bedtime to a maximum single dose of 1 g.

Half-life

7 to 10 hours

Common Adverse Reactions

CNS: Drowsiness, hangover, somnolence, disorientation, confusion, paranoid behavior
GI: Nausea, vomiting, diarrhea
Hematologic: Leukopenia, eosinophilia
Skin: Irritation
Other: Tolerance, dependence

Key Interactions

Increased CNS effects with: CNS depressants including opioid analgesics, alcohol
Increased risk of bleeding with: Oral anticoagulants
Decreased level of co-administered drug with: Phenytoin

Nursing Considerations

- Alert: Double-check dose carefully when giving oral liquid form, which is available in two strengths. To minimize unpleasant taste and stomach irritation, dilute or administer with liquid. Tell client to take drug after meals.
- Instruct client to swallow capsule whole with a full glass of water or juice.
- Take precautions to prevent hoarding or overdosing by clients who are depressed, suicidal, or drug-dependent, or who have history of drug abuse.
- Be aware that the drug loses its effectiveness in promoting sleep after 14 days of continued use. Long-term use may cause drug dependence, and client may experience withdrawal symptoms if the drug is stopped suddenly.
- Monitor blood urea nitrogen level because large doses of chloral hydrate may raise it.
- Warn client to avoid alcohol during drug therapy.
- Caution client to avoid activities that require mental alertness or physical coordination.

chlordiazepoxide (Librium)

Drug Class

Benzodiazepine, anxiolytic

Indications and Dosage

Mild to moderate anxiety	*Adults*: 5 to 10 mg PO, tid or qid. *Children 6 years and older*: 5 mg PO, bid to qid to a maximum of 10 mg PO bid or tid.
Severe anxiety	*Adults*: 20 to 25 mg PO tid or qid. *Elderly clients*: 5 mg PO bid to qid.
Withdrawal symptoms of acute alcoholism	*Adults*: 50 to 100 mg PO, IV or IM, repeating in 2 to 4 hours, as needed (p.r.n.), up to a maximum dose of 300 mg daily.

Half-life

5 to 30 hours

Common Adverse Reactions

CNS: Drowsiness, lethargy
GI: Nausea, constipation
Hematologic: Agranulocytosis
Skin: Swelling and pain at injection site

Key Interactions

Increased risk for adverse effects with: Cimetidine, disulfiram
Increased CNS depression with: CNS depressants, alcohol
Increased CNS sedation with: Kava
Increased level of co-administered drug with: Digoxin
Increased drug level with: Fluconazole, itraconazole, ketoconazole, miconazole

Decreased drug effectiveness with: Smoking
Decreased effectiveness of co-administered drug with: Levodopa

Nursing Considerations

- Administer IV doses carefully over 1 minute; ensure that necessary equipment and staff for emergency airway management are available. Monitor respirations every 5 to 15 minutes and before each IV dose.
- Keep powder refrigerated and away from light; mix just before use and discard remainder.
- Alert: 5-mg and 25-mg capsules may look similar in color through packaging. Verify contents and read label carefully.
- For IM administration, add 2 mL of diluent to powder; agitate gently until clear. Do not use supplied diluent for IV use. Use reconstituted solution immediately. Be aware that IM form may be absorbed erratically.
- If client is receiving repeated or prolonged therapy, monitor hepatic, renal, and hematopoietic function periodically.
- Alert: Use of this drug may lead to abuse and addiction. Do not withdraw the drug abruptly after long-term use because withdrawal symptoms may occur.
- Warn client to avoid hazardous activities that require alertness and physical coordination until effects of drug are known.
- Tell client to avoid alcohol while using the drug.
- Notify client that smoking may decrease drug's effectiveness.

clonazepam (Klonopin)

Drug Class
Benzodiazepine, anxiolytic, anticonvulsant

Indications and Dosage

Panic disorder (*see p. 311*)	*Adults*: Initially, 0.25 mg PO bid, increasing to a target dose of 1 mg after 3 days; if necessary increase dosage to a maximum of 4 mg daily by increasing dosage every 3 days in increments of 0.125 to 0.25 mg bid as tolerated until control achieved; then taper the dose, decreasing 0.125 mg bid every 3 days until drug is stopped.
Acute mania associated with bipolar disorders (*see p. 388*)	*Adults*: 0.5 to 16 mg PO daily.
Schizophrenia (adjunct therapy; *see p. 488*)	*Adults*: 0.5 to 2 mg PO daily.
Periodic leg movements during sleep	*Adults*: 0.5 to 2 mg PO daily.

Half-life
18 to 50 hours

Common Adverse Reactions
CNS: Drowsiness, sedation, depression, lethargy, apathy, fatigue, light-headedness, disorientation, confusion, headache
GI: Nausea, vomiting, constipation, diarrhea, dry mouth
Hematologic: Leukopenia, thrombocytopenia
Respiratory: Respiratory depression

Key Interactions
Decreased drug level with: Phenytoin, carbamazepine, phenobarbital, smoking
Increased CNS depression with: CNS depressants, alcohol

Nursing Considerations
- Watch for behavioral disturbances; monitor client for oversedation.
- Do not stop drug abruptly; gradually taper dosage.

- Administer drug as prescribed; for panic disorder, possibly give one dose at bedtime to decrease risk of somnolence.
- Caution client to avoid activities that require mental alertness or coordination until the effects of the drug are known.
- Advise clients to avoid alcohol.
- If client experiences GI distress, encourage them to take drug with food.

diazepam (Diastat, Valium)

Drug Class
Benzodiazepine, anxiolytic

Indications and Dosage

Anxiety	*Adults*: Depending on severity, 2 to 10 mg PO bid to qid; alternatively, 2 to 10 mg IM or IV every 3 to 4 hours, p.r.n. *Children 6 months and older*: 1 to 2.5 mg PO tid or qid, increasing gradually, as needed and tolerated. *Elderly clients*: Initially, 2 to 2.5 mg once daily or bid, increasing gradually.
Acute alcohol withdrawal	*Adults*: 10 mg PO tid or qid for the first 24 hours, reducing dosage to 5 mg PO tid or qid, p.r.n.; alternatively, 10 mg IV or IM, then 5 to 10 mg IV or IM every 3 to 4 hours, p.r.n.

Half-life
Approximately 1 to 12 days

Common Adverse Reactions
CNS: Drowsiness, dysarthria, slurred speech, tremor, transient amnesia, fatigue, ataxia, headache, insomnia, paradoxical anxiety, disorientation
Cardiovascular (CV): Bradycardia, tachycardia
GI: Constipation, diarrhea (with rectal form)
Genitourinary (GU): Incontinence, urine retention, changes in libido
Hematologic: Neutropenia

Respiratory: Respiratory depression, apnea
Other: Pain, phlebitis at injection site, dependence

Key Interactions

Increased risk of adverse reactions with: Cimetidine, disulfiram, fluoxetine, fluvoxamine, hormonal contraceptives, isoniazid, metoprolol, propoxyphene, propranolol, valproic acid
Increased CNS depression with: CNS depressants, alcohol, diltiazem
Increased sedation with: Kava
Increased drug level with: Fluconazole, itraconazole, ketoconazole, miconazole
Increased risk of toxicity of co-administered drug with: Digoxin
Increased drug level and level of co-administered drug with: Phenobarbital

Nursing Considerations

- Be aware that the IV route is the more reliable parenteral route; the IM route isn't recommended because absorption is variable and injection is painful.
- Alert: Keep emergency resuscitation equipment and oxygen at bedside, especially with IV administration.
- If possible, inject directly into a large vein. Otherwise, inject slowly through infusion tubing as close to the insertion site as possible. Give at no more than 5 mg/min. Watch closely for phlebitis at injection site. Change from IV to oral form as soon as possible.
- Monitor respirations every 5 to 15 minutes when administering IV and before each dose.
- When using oral solution, dilute dose just before giving.
- Monitor periodic hepatic, renal, and hematopoietic function studies in clients receiving repeated or prolonged therapy.
- Monitor elderly clients for dizziness, ataxia, and mental status changes. Clients are at an increased risk for falls.
- Alert: Use of this drug may lead to abuse and addiction. Do not withdraw the drug abruptly after long-term use; withdrawal symptoms may occur.
- Alert: Do not confuse diazepam with diazoxide.
- Warn client to avoid activities that require alertness and physical coordination until effects of drug are known.

- Advise client not to discontinue the drug abruptly; taper dose gradually after long-term therapy.

estazolam (ProSom)

Drug Class
Benzodiazepine, sedative-hypnotic

Indications and Dosage

Insomnia (*see p. 437*)	*Adults*: 1 mg PO before bedtime; possibly 2 mg necessary for some clients. *Elderly clients*: 1 mg PO before bedtime.

Half-life
10 to 24 hours

Common Adverse Reactions
CNS: Fatigue, dizziness, daytime drowsiness, somnolence, asthenia
GI: Dyspepsia, abdominal pain

Key Interactions
Increased CNS depression with: Cimetidine; disulfiram; hormonal contraceptives; isoniazid; CNS depressants, including antihistamines; opioid analgesics; other benzodiazepines; calendula; hops; kava; lemon balm; passion flower; skullcap; valerian; alcohol
Increased level of co-administered drug with: Digoxin, phenytoin
Increased drug level with: Fluconazole, itraconazole, ketoconazole, miconazole
Decreased drug effectiveness with: Rifampin, theophylline, smoking

Nursing Considerations
- Check liver and renal function and complete blood count (CBC) before and periodically during long-term therapy.
- Take precautions to prevent clients who are depressed, suicidal, or drug-dependent with a history of drug abuse from hoarding drug.

- Clients who receive prolonged treatment with benzodiazepines may experience withdrawal symptoms if they suddenly stop the drug (possibly after 6 weeks of continuous therapy).
- Alert: Do not confuse ProSom with Proscar, Prozac, or Psorcon E.
- Tell client not to increase dosage if he or she thinks that the drug is no longer effective, but instead to tell the prescriber.
- Caution client to avoid activities that require mental alertness or physical coordination.
- Warn client that drinking alcohol while or within 24 hours after taking drug can increase depressant effects.
- Caution client not to abruptly stop use after taking drug for 1 month or longer.

eszopiclone (Lunesta)

Drug Class
Sedative-hypnotic

Indications and Dosage

Insomnia (*see p. 437*)	*Adults*: 2 mg PO immediately before bedtime, increasing to 3 mg, p.r.n. *Elderly clients having trouble falling asleep*: 1 mg PO immediately before bedtime, increasing to 2 mg, p.r.n. *Elderly clients having trouble staying asleep*: 2 mg PO immediately before bedtime.

Half-life
6 hours

Common Adverse Reactions
CNS: Somnolence, headache
Ear, eye, nose, and throat (EENT): Unpleasant taste
GI: Diarrhea, dry mouth
Respiratory: Respiratory tract infection

Key Interactions

Increased CNS depression with: CNS depressants, alcohol

Increased risk of drug toxicity with: CYP3A4 inhibitors (clarithromycin, itraconazole, ketoconazole, nefazodone, nelfinavir, ritonavir, troleandomycin)

Risk for impaired cognition or memory with: Olanzapine

Decreased drug activity with: Rifampin

Decreased drug absorption with: High-fat meals

Nursing Considerations

- Evaluate client for physical and psychiatric disorders before treatment.
- Use the lowest effective dose.
- Alert: Give drug immediately before client goes to bed or after he or she has gone to bed and had trouble falling asleep.
- Use only for short periods (eg, 7 to 10 days). If client still has trouble sleeping, check for other psychological disorders.
- Monitor client for changes in behavior, including those that suggest depression or suicidal thinking.
- Caution client not to take drug unless he or she can get a full night's sleep.
- Advise client to avoid taking drug after a high-fat meal.
- Caution client to avoid activities that require mental alertness until drug's effects are known.
- Urge client to avoid alcohol while using the drug.
- Instruct client to immediately report changes in behavior and thinking.
- Warn client not to stop drug abruptly or change dose without consulting the prescriber.
- Inform client that he or she may develop tolerance or dependence if the drug is taken for a prolonged period.

flurazepam (Dalmane)

Drug Class

Benzodiazepine, sedative-hypnotic

Indications and Dosage

Insomnia (*see p. 437*)	*Adults*: 15 to 30 mg PO at bedtime, repeating dose once, p.r.n. *Elderly clients*: 15 mg PO at bedtime initially, until response is determined.

Half-life

2 to 4 days

Common Adverse Reactions

CNS: Daytime sedation, dizziness, drowsiness, disturbed coordination, lethargy, confusion, disorientation
GI: Nausea, vomiting

Key Interactions

Increased CNS depression with: Cimetidine; CNS depressants, including opioid analgesics; calendula; hops; kava; lemon balm; passion flower; skullcap; valerian; alcohol
Risk for co-administered drug toxicity with: Digoxin
Increased risk of drug toxicity with: Disulfiram, hormonal contraceptives, isoniazid
Increased drug level with: Fluconazole, itraconazole, ketoconazole, miconazole
Increased level of co-administered drug with: Phenytoin
Decreased drug effectiveness with: Rifampin, smoking

Nursing Considerations

- Check hepatic and renal function and CBC before and periodically during long-term therapy.
- Alert: Assess mental status before client starts. Elderly clients are more sensitive to drug's adverse CNS reactions.
- Take precautions to prevent hoarding or self-overdosing by clients who are depressed, suicidal, or drug-dependent, or those with a history of drug abuse.
- Be aware that long-term use may lead to physical and psychological dependence.

- Inform client that drug is more effective on second, third, and fourth nights of treatment, because the drug accumulates in the body.
- Warn client not to abruptly stop drug after taking it for 1 month or longer.
- Tell client to avoid alcohol while using the drug.
- Caution client to avoid activities that require mental alertness or physical coordination.

hydroxyzine hydrochloride (Atarax, Vistaril)

Drug Class
Anxiolytic

Indications and Dosage

Anxiety	*Adults*: 50 to 100 mg PO qid. *Children 6 years and older*: 50 to 100 mg PO daily in divided doses. *Children younger than 6 years*: 50 mg PO daily in divided doses.

Half-life
3 hours

Common Adverse Reactions
CNS: Drowsiness
GI: Dry mouth

Key Interactions
Increased anticholinergic effects with: Anticholinergics
Increased CNS depression with: CNS depressants, alcohol
Inhibition of co-administered drug with: Epinephrine

Nursing Considerations

- Observe for oversedation if client takes other CNS drugs.
- Be aware that elderly clients may be more sensitive to adverse anticholinergic effects; monitor these clients for dizziness, excessive sedation, confusion, hypotension, and syncope.
- Alert: Do not confuse hydroxyzine with hydroxyurea or hydralazine.
- Warn client to avoid hazardous activities that require alertness and physical coordination until effects of drug are known.
- Urge client to avoid alcohol while using the drug.
- Advise client to use sugarless hard candy or gum to relieve dry mouth.

lorazepam (Ativan)

Drug Class

Benzodiazepine, anxiolytic

Indications and Dosage

| Anxiety (*see p. 300*) | *Adults*: 2 to 6 mg PO daily in divided doses to a maximum of 10 mg daily.
Elderly clients: 1 to 2 mg PO daily in divided doses to a maximum of 10 mg daily. |
| Insomnia secondary to anxiety | *Adults*: 2 to 4 mg PO at bedtime. |

Half-life

10 to 20 hours

Common Adverse Reactions

CNS: Drowsiness, sedation, amnesia
CV: Hypotension
EENT: Visual disturbances
GI: Abdominal discomfort, nausea

Key Interactions

Increased CNS depression with: CNS depressants, kava, alcohol
Increased risk of co-administered drug toxicity with: Digoxin

Nursing Considerations

- Monitor hepatic, renal, and hematopoietic function periodically in clients receiving repeated or prolonged therapy.
- Alert: Use of this drug may lead to abuse and addiction. Do not stop drug abruptly after long-term use because withdrawal symptoms may occur.
- Alert: Do not confuse lorazepam with alprazolam.
- Warn client to avoid hazardous activities that require alertness or physical coordination until effects of drug are known.
- Tell client to avoid alcohol while using the drug.
- Notify client that smoking may decrease drug's effectiveness.
- Warn client not to stop drug abruptly because withdrawal symptoms may occur.

mephobarbital (Mebaral)

Drug Class

Barbiturate, sedative-hypnotic

Indications and Dosage

Anxiety	*Adults*: 32 to 100 mg PO tid to qid, with an optimal dose of 50 mg tid to qid PO. *Children*: 16 to 32 mg tid to qid PO.

Half-life

11 to 67 hours

Common Adverse Reactions

CNS: Somnolence, confusion, lethargy, residual sedation
GI: Nausea, vomiting, constipation, diarrhea, epigastric pain
Other: Tolerance, dependence

Key Interactions

Increased CNS depression with: CNS depressants, alcohol

Decreased effectiveness of co-administered drug with: Theophylline, oral anticoagulants, β blockers, doxycycline, corticosteroids, hormonal contraceptives and estrogen, metronidazole, phenylbutazones, quinidine, carbamazepine

Nursing Considerations

- Assess mental status before client starts therapy.
- Alert: Watch for signs of barbiturate toxicity: coma, pupillary constriction, cyanosis, clammy skin, and hypotension. Overdose can be fatal.
- Instruct client to take the drug exactly as prescribed.
- Do not stop drug abruptly; withdraw gradually.
- Inform client that morning hangover may occur.
- Advise client to take the drug with food if GI upset occurs.
- Caution client to avoid activities that require mental alertness or physical coordination.
- Warn client to avoid alcohol use while using the drug.

pentobarbital sodium (Nembutal sodium)

Drug Class

Barbiturate, sedative-hypnotic

Indications and Dosage

Sedation	*Adults*: 20 mg PO tid or qid. *Children*: 2 to 6 mg/kg PO daily in three divided doses up to a maximum daily dose of 100 mg.
Insomnia (*see p. 437*)	*Adults*: 100 to 200 mg PO at bedtime; alternatively, 150 to 200 mg deep IM, or 100 mg IV initially, with further small doses up to total of 500 mg; or 120 or 200 mg rectally. *Children*: 2 to 6 mg/kg or 125 mg/m^2 IM to a maximum dose of 100 mg. *Children 12 to 14 years*: 60 or 120 mg rectally. *Children 5 to 11 years*: 60 mg rectally. *Children 1 to 4 years*: 30 or 60 mg rectally. *Children 2 months to 1 year*: 30 mg rectally.

Half-life

35 to 50 hours

Common Adverse Reactions

CNS: Drowsiness, lethargy, hangover, paradoxical excitement in elderly clients, somnolence
GI: Nausea, vomiting
Respiratory: Respiratory depression
Skin: Reactions at tissue site
Other: Dependence

Key Interactions

Increased CNS depression with: CNS depressants including opioid analgesics, alcohol
Prolonged CNS depression with: MAOIs, valproic acid
Decreased effectiveness of co-administered drug with:
Corticosteroids, doxycycline, estrogens and hormonal contraceptives, oral anticoagulants, theophylline, verapamil, metoprolol, propranolol
Decreased absorption of co-administered drug with: Griseofulvin
Decreased drug effect with: Rifampin

Nursing Considerations

- Alert: IV barbiturates may cause severe respiratory depression, laryngospasm, or hypotension. Reserve their use for emergencies, under close supervision, with resuscitation equipment nearby.
- Do not mix in syringe, solutions, or lines with other drugs; give slowly at a rate no greater than 50 mg/min.
- Assess patency of site before and during parenteral administration. Parenteral solution is alkaline. Local tissue reactions and injection site pain may occur. Monitor site for extravasation.
- Assess mental status before clients start therapy.
- Reduce doses in elderly clients, who may be more sensitive to adverse CNS effects.
- Alert: Give IM injection deep into a large muscle mass with no more than 5 ml of drug at any one site. Superficial injection may cause pain, sterile abscess, and sloughing.
- Do not divide suppositories to ensure accurate dosage.

- Take precautions to prevent hoarding by clients who are depressed, suicidal, or drug-dependent, or who have a history of drug abuse.
- Watch for signs of barbiturate toxicity: coma, pupillary constriction, cyanosis, clammy skin, and hypotension. Overdose can be fatal.
- Inspect skin. Skin eruptions may precede fatal reactions. If skin reactions occur, stop drug and call prescriber. In some clients, high temperature, stomatitis, headache, or rhinitis may precede skin reactions.
- Be aware that the drug has no analgesic effect and may cause restlessness or delirium in clients with pain.
- Know that long-term use for insomnia isn't recommended; drug loses its effectiveness in promoting sleep after 14 days of continuous use. Long-term high dosage may cause drug dependence, and clients may experience withdrawal symptoms if they suddenly stop drug. Withdraw barbiturates gradually.
- Alert: Do not confuse pentobarbital with phenobarbital.
- Inform client that morning hangover is common after hypnotic dose, which suppresses REM sleep. Client may experience increased dreaming after stopping drug.
- Caution client to avoid activities that require mental alertness or physical coordination.
- Urge client to avoid alcohol use while using the drug.

phenobarbital sodium (Luminal)

Drug Class

Barbiturate, sedative-hypnotic

Indications and Dosage

Sedation	*Adults*: 30 to 120 mg PO, IV, or IM daily in divided doses bid or tid to a maximum dose of 400 mg daily. *Children*: 8 to 32 mg PO.
Insomnia (short term therapy; *see p. 437*)	*Adults*: 100 to 200 mg PO or 100 to 320 mg IM or IV at bedtime.

Half-life
5 to 7 days

Common Adverse Reactions
CNS: Drowsiness, lethargy, hangover, paradoxical excitement in elderly clients
CV: Bradycardia
GI: Nausea, vomiting
Respiratory: Respiratory depression, apnea
Skin: Erythema multiforme, angioedema, pain at injection site

Key Interactions
Increased CNS depression with: Chloramphenicol, MAOIs, CNS depressants including opioid analgesics, alcohol
Decreased effectiveness of co-administered drug with: Corticosteroids, doxycycline, estrogens and hormonal contraceptives, oral anticoagulants, TCAs, metoprolol, propranolol
Increased drug level with: Valproic acid, mephobarbital, primidone
Decreased drug level with: Rifampin
Increased drug effect and effect of co-administered drug with: Diazepam

Nursing Considerations
- Alert: Give IV dose slowly under close supervision at a rate of no more than 60 mg/min; have emergency equipment readily available.
- Administer IM injection deep into large muscle mass; superficial injection may cause pain, sterile abscess, and tissue sloughing.
- Assess mental status before client starts therapy.
- Reduce doses in elderly clients, who may be more sensitive to adverse CNS effects.
- Watch for signs of barbiturate toxicity: coma, pupillary constriction, cyanosis, clammy skin, and hypotension. Overdose can be fatal.
- Inspect skin. Skin eruptions may precede fatal reactions. If skin reactions occur, stop drug and call prescriber. In some clients, high temperature, stomatitis, headache, or rhinitis may precede skin reactions.
- Know that long-term use for insomnia isn't recommended; drug loses its effectiveness in promoting sleep after 14 days of

continuous use. Long-term high dosage may cause drug
dependence, and clients may experience withdrawal symptoms
if they suddenly stop the drug. Withdraw barbiturates
gradually.
- Alert: Do not confuse phenobarbital with pentobarbital.
- Caution client to avoid activities that require mental alertness or
physical coordination.
- Urge client to avoid alcohol use while using the drug.

quazepam (Doral)

Drug Class
Benzodiazepine, sedative-hypnotic

Indications and Dosage

Insomnia (*see p. 437*)	*Adults*: Initially, 15 mg PO at bedtime, possibly reducing dosage to 7.5 mg in some clients.

Half-life
41 hours

Common Adverse Reactions
CNS: Drowsiness, sedation, depression, lethargy, apathy, fatigue,
light-headedness, disorientation, restlessness, confusion
CV: Bradycardia, tachycardia
GI: Constipation, diarrhea
GU: Incontinence, urinary retention, changes in libido
Other: Dependence, withdrawal

Key Interactions
Increased CNS depression with: CNS depressants, alcohol
Increased drug effects with: Cimetidine, disulfiram, hormonal contraceptives
Decreased sedative effects with: Theophylline, aminophylline, smoking

Nursing Considerations

- **Alert:** Don't stop drug abruptly after long-term use, which may induce withdrawal symptoms.
- Warn client to avoid hazardous activities that require alertness or physical coordination until effects of drug are known.
- Tell client to avoid alcohol while using the drug.
- Notify client that smoking may decrease drug's effectiveness.
- Warn client not to stop the drug abruptly because withdrawal symptoms may occur.

ramelteon (Rozerem)

Drug Class

Sedative-hypnotic, melatonin-receptor agonist

Indications and Dosage

Insomnia (characterized by difficulty falling asleep; *see p. 437*)	*Adults*: 8 mg PO within 30 minutes of bedtime.

Half-life

Parent Drug: 1 to 2.5 hours
Metabolite: 2 to 5 hours

Common Adverse Reactions

CNS: Depression, dizziness, fatigue, headache, somnolence, worsened insomnia
GI: Diarrhea, nausea
Other: Flu-like symptoms

Key Interactions

Increased CNS depression with: CNS depressants, alcohol
Increased drug level with: Fluconazole (strong CYP2C9 inhibitor), ketoconazole (strong CYP3A4 inhibitor), weak CYPIA2 inhibitors, fluvoxamine (strong CYPIA2 inhibitor)
Decreased drug level with: Rifampin (strong CYP enzyme inducer)
Delayed time to peak effect with: High-fat meal

Nursing Considerations

- Thoroughly evaluate the cause of insomnia before starting drug.
- Assess client for behavioral or cognitive disorders.
- Administer drug within 30 minutes of bedtime.
- Be aware that drug does not cause physical dependence.
- Advise client not to take drug with or after a heavy meal.
- Caution against performing activities that require mental alertness or physical coordination after taking drug.
- Urge client to avoid alcohol while using the drug.
- Tell client to consult prescriber if insomnia worsens or behavior changes.
- Urge female clients to consult prescriber if menses stops, libido decreases, or galactorrhea or fertility problems develop.

secobarbital sodium (Seconal Sodium)

Drug Class

Barbiturate, sedative-hypnotic

Indications and Dosage

Sedation (bedtime; short-term use)	*Adults*: 100 mg PO at bedtime for less than a 2-week period.

Half-life

15 to 40 hours

Common Adverse Reactions

CNS: Somnolence, agitation, confusion, ataxia, vertigo, nightmares, residual sedation, paradoxical excitement, nervousness, psychiatric disturbance, insomnia, anxiety, dizziness
CV: Bradycardia, hypotension, syncope
GI: Nausea, vomiting, constipation, diarrhea, epigastric pain
Respiratory: Respiratory depression, hypoventilation, apnea
Other: Tolerance, dependence, withdrawal

Key Interactions

Increased CNS depression with: CNS depressants, alcohol

Decreased effect of co-administered drug with: Oral anticoagulants, corticosteroids, hormonal contraceptives and estrogen, metronidazole, metoprolol, propranolol, doxycycline, oxyphenbutazone, phenylbutazone, quinidine, theophylline

Nursing Considerations

- Alert: Do not administer this drug as a bedtime sedative for longer than 2 weeks.
- Assess mental status before client starts therapy
- Reduce doses in elderly clients, who may be more sensitive to drug's adverse CNS effects.
- Watch for signs of barbiturate toxicity: coma, pupillary constriction, cyanosis, clammy skin, and hypotension. Overdose can be fatal.
- Taper dose gradually.
- Inform client that morning hangover is possible.
- Caution client to avoid activities that require mental alertness or physical coordination.
- Advise client to change positions slowly.
- Urge client to avoid alcohol use while using the drug.

temazepam (Restoril)

Drug Class

Benzodiazepine, sedative-hypnotic

Indications and Dosage

Insomnia (*see p. 437*)	*Adults*: 15 to 30 mg PO at bedtime. *Elderly clients*: 15 mg PO at bedtime, individualizing dose as necessary.

Half-life

10 to 17 hours

Common Adverse Reactions

CNS: Drowsiness, dizziness, lethargy, disturbed coordination, daytime sedation, confusion

EENT: Blurred vision
GI: Diarrhea, nausea, dry mouth
Other: Dependence

Key Interactions

Increased CNS depression with: CNS depressants, alcohol
Increased sedation with: Calendula, hops, kava, lemon balm, passion flower, skullcap, valerian

Nursing Considerations

- Reduce doses in elderly clients, who may be more sensitive to drug's adverse CNS effects.
- Take precautions to prevent hoarding by clients who are depressed, suicidal, or drug-dependent, or who have history of drug abuse.
- Alert: Do not confuse Restoril with Vistaril.
- Tell client to avoid alcohol while using the drug.
- Caution client to avoid activities that require mental alertness or physical coordination.
- Warn client not to stop drug abruptly.
- Tell client that onset of drug's effects may take as long as 2 to 2.25 hours.

triazolam (Halcion)

Drug Class

Benzodiazepine, sedative-hypnotic

Indications and Dosage

Insomnia (*see p. 437*)	*Adults*: 0.125 to 0.5 mg PO at bedtime. *Elderly or debilitated clients*: 0.125 mg PO at bedtime, increasing p.r.n. to 0.25 mg PO at bedtime.

Half-life

1.5 to 5.5 hours

Common Adverse Reactions

CNS: Drowsiness, amnesia, ataxia, dizziness, rebound insomnia
GI: Nausea, vomiting
Other: Dependence

Key Interactions

Increased drug level with: Cimetidine, erythromycin, fluoxetine, fluvoxamine, isoniazid, nefazodone, ranitidine, itraconazole, ketoconazole, miconazole
Increased CNS depression with: CNS depressants, alcohol, diltiazem
Increased risk of sedation with: Calendula, hops, kava, lemon balm, passion flower, skullcap, valerian
Increased drug effect with: Grapefruit
Decreased drug effect with: Smoking

Nursing Considerations

- Assess mental status before clients start therapy.
- Reduce doses in elderly clients, who may be more sensitive to drug's adverse CNS effects.
- Monitor CBC, chemistry, and urinalysis.
- Take precautions to prevent hoarding or overdosing by clients who are depressed, suicidal, or drug dependent, or who have history of drug abuse.
- Alert: Do not confuse Halcion with Haldol or halcinonide.
- Warn clients not to take more than prescribed amount; overdose can occur at total daily dose of 2 mg (or four times the highest recommended amount).
- Tell clients to avoid alcohol use while using the drug.

zaleplon (Sonata)

Drug Class

Sedative-hypnotic

Indications and Dosage

Insomnia (*see p. 437*)	*Adults*: 10 mg PO daily at bedtime, possibly increasing to 20 mg p.r.n.; alternatively, 5 mg PO if client is of low weight. Limit use to 7 to 10 days; re-evaluate if drug is needed for more than 2 to 3 weeks. *Elderly clients*: Initially, 5 mg PO daily at bedtime; doses greater than 10 mg not recommended.

Half-life

1 hour

Common Adverse Reactions

CNS: Headache, amnesia, anxiety, dizziness
GI: Abdominal pain, anorexia, constipation, dry mouth
Skin: Photosensitivity reactions

Key Interactions

Decreased drug bioavailability with: Carbamazepine, phenobarbital, phenytoin, rifampin, other CYP3A4 inducers
Increased drug bioavailability with: Cimetidine
Increased risk for CNS depression with: CNS depressants, imipramine, thioridazine, alcohol
Delayed drug absorption with: High-fat foods, heavy meals

Nursing Considerations

- Give immediately before bedtime or after client has gone to bed and had difficulty falling asleep. Zaleplon works rapidly.
- Monitor clients using this drug who have compromised respiratory function from illness or who are elderly or debilitated. These clients are more sensitive to respiratory depression.

- Start treatment only after carefully evaluating clients, because sleep disturbances may signify an underlying physical or psychiatric disorder.
- Be aware that adverse reactions are usually dose-related. Consult prescriber about dose reduction if adverse reactions occur.
- Inform client that drug works rapidly and he or she should take it only immediately before bedtime or after he or she has gone to bed and had trouble falling asleep.
- Advise client to take drug only if he or she will be able to sleep for at least 4 undisturbed hours.
- Caution client that drowsiness, dizziness, light-headedness, and coordination problems occur most often within 1 hour after taking drug.
- Advise client to avoid activities that require mental alertness until CNS adverse reactions are known.
- Urge client to avoid alcohol use while using the drug and to notify prescriber before taking other prescription or over-the-counter drugs.
- Instruct client not to take drug after a high-fat or heavy meal.
- Advise client to report sleep problems that continue despite use of drug.
- Notify client that dependence can occur and that this drug is recommended for short-term use only.
- Notify client that insomnia may recur for a few nights after stopping the drug, but it should resolve on its own.
- Warn client that drug may cause changes in behavior and thinking, including outgoing, strange, or aggressive behavior; loss of personal identity; confusion; agitation; hallucinations; worsened depression; or suicidal thoughts. Tell client to notify prescriber immediately if these symptoms occur.

zolpidem tartrate (Ambien, Ambien CR)

Drug Class
Sedative-hypnotic

Indications and Dosage

Insomnia (short-term therapy; *see p. 437*)	*Adults*: 10 mg (immediate-release form) or 12.5 mg (extended-release form) PO immediately before bedtime. *Elderly clients*: 5 mg (immediate-release form) or 6.25 mg (extended-release form) PO immediately before bedtime. Maximum daily dose of 10 mg (immediate-release form) or 6.25 mg (extended-release form).

Half-life

2.5 hours

Common Adverse Reactions

CNS: Headache, amnesia, change in dreams, daytime drowsiness, dizziness, hangover
CV: Palpitations
GI: Constipation, diarrhea, dry mouth
Other: Flu-like syndrome

Key Interactions

Increased CNS depression with: CNS depressants, alcohol
Decreased drug effect with: Rifampin

Nursing Considerations

- Use zolpidem only for short-term management of insomnia, usually 7 to 10 days.
- Use the smallest effective dose for each client.
- Take precautions to prevent hoarding by clients who are depressed, suicidal, or drug dependent, or who have a history of drug abuse.
- Alert: Do not crush or divide extended-release tablets; instruct client similarly.

- Instruct client to take drug immediately before going to bed; onset of action is rapid. Caution client not to take drug with or immediately after meals.
- Tell client to avoid alcohol while using the drug.
- Caution client to avoid activities that require mental alertness or physical coordination during therapy.

Antidepressants

Overview

Primary Indications

Major depression (*see p. 383*), depressive phases of bipolar disorder (*see p. 388*), and depressive symptoms not associated with major depression.

Other Indications

Anxiety disorders, such as panic disorder (*see p. 312*), obsessive-compulsive disorder (*see p. 305*), social phobia, generalized anxiety disorder (*see p. 300*), and posttraumatic stress disorder (*see p. 324*).

Signs and Symptoms

Symptoms indicating a possible need for antidepressants include dysphoria, change in appetite and energy, anhedonia (lack of interest in routine activities), difficulty concentrating, hopelessness, and suicidality.

Major Categories

- Tricyclic antidepressants (TCAs): Inhibit neuronal uptake of serotonin and norepinephrine, act as anticholinergics at central nervous system (CNS) and peripheral receptors, and act as sedatives

- amitriptyline (*see p. 187*)
- amoxapine
- clomipramine (*see p. 192*)
- desipramine (*see p. 194*)
- doxepin (*see p. 196*)
- imipramine (*see p. 204*)
- maprotiline (*see p. 206*)
- nortriptyline (*see p. 210*)
- protriptyline
- trimipramine
- Monoamine-oxidase inhibitors (MAOIs): Inhibit monoamine oxidase-A
  - isocarboxazide
  - phenelzine (*see p. 214*)
  - tranylcypromine (*see p. 219*)
- Designer drugs: Selective serotonin reuptake inhibitors (SSRIs) block neuronal transport of serotonin and inhibit reuptake of serotonin only; selective reuptake inhibitors (SRIs) inhibit reuptake of dopamine, norepinephrine, or both; selective norepinephrine reuptake inhibitors (SNRIs) inhibit reuptake of norepinephrine
  - citalopram (*see p. 191*)
  - duloxetine (*see p. 198*)
  - escitalopram (*see p. 200*)
  - fluóxetine (*see p. 201*)
  - fluvoxamine (*see p. 203*)
  - nefazodone (*see p. 209*)
  - paroxetine (*see p. 212*)
  - sertraline (*see p. 217*)
- Atypical antidepressants: Affect noradrenergic and serotonergic neurotransmission
  - bupropion (*see p. 188*)
  - mirtazapine (*see p. 208*)
  - trazodone (*see p. 220*)
  - venlafaxine (*see p. 222*)
- Other drugs used for refractory depression
  - pramipexole
  - selegiline (*see p. 216*)

Key Drug Monographs
amitriptyline hydrochloride
Drug Class
TCA

Indications and Dosage

Depression (*see p. 383*)	*Adults*: 50 to 100 mg PO at bedtime (hs), increasing to 150 mg daily to a maximum dose of 300 mg if needed. *Elderly adults and adolescents*: 20 mg PO three times daily (tid) and 20 mg at bedtime.

Half-life
Not established; highly variable

Common Adverse Reactions
Central nervous system (CNS): Stroke, seizures, ataxia, tremor, insomnia, restlessness, drowsiness, weakness, fatigue
Cardiovascular (CV): Orthostatic hypotension, tachycardia
Gastrointestinal (GI): Dry mouth
Genitourinary (GU): Urine retention, altered libido
Metabolic: Hypoglycemia, hyperglycemia

Key Interactions
Enhanced CNS depression with: Barbiturates, CNS depressants, alcohol use
Increased tricyclic antidepressants (TCA) levels with: Cimetidine, fluoxetines, fluvoxamine, hormonal contraceptives, paroxetine, sertraline
Possible life-threatening hypertension with: Clonidine
Severe excitation, hyperpyrexia, or seizures with: High doses of MAOIs
Possible life-threatening arrhythmias with: Quinolones
Increased risk of seizures with: Evening primrose
Possible serotonin syndrome with: St. John's wort, SAM-e, yohimbe
Increased risk of photosensitivity with: Sun exposure

Nursing Considerations

- Alert: Do not use in children younger than 12 years; drug may increase risk of suicidal thinking and behavior in children and adolescents with major depressive disorder.
- Monitor for sedation and anticholinergic effects.
- Monitor glucose levels periodically.
- Assess for mood changes and suicidal tendencies; provide client with only a minimum supply of the drug.
- Alert: Do not withdraw the drug abruptly; warn client not to stop drug abruptly.
- Advise client to take the full dose at bedtime; warn of possible orthostatic hypotension on arising.
- Instruct client to avoid alcohol while using the drug.
- Warn client to avoid activities requiring alertness and physical coordination until CNS effects are known.
- Suggest use of sugarless hard candy, gum, or saliva substitutes for dry mouth.
- Advise clients to wear sunblock and protective clothing, and to avoid prolonged exposure to strong sunlight to prevent photosensitivity.
- Inform clients that it may take as long as 30 days to achieve full therapeutic effect.

buproprion (Wellbutrin, Wellbutrin SR, Wellbutrin XL, Zyban)

Drug Class

Atypical antidepressant

Indications and Dosage

Depression (see p. 383)	*Adults*: *Immediate-release form*: 100 mg PO two times daily (bid), increasing after 3 days to 100 mg PO tid if needed; increase to 150 mg tid if no improvement after several weeks of therapy; no single dose should exceed 150 mg; allow at least 6 hours between doses; maximum dose of 450 mg daily.

	Adults: *Sustained-release form*: 150 mg PO every morning, increasing to target dose of 150 mg PO bid, as tolerated as early as day 4 of dosing, with at least 8 hours between doses to a maximum dose of 400 mg daily. *Adults*: *Extended-release form*: 150 mg PO every morning, increasing to target dose of 300 mg PO daily as tolerated as early as day 4 of dosing, allowing at least 24 hours between doses to a maximum dose of 450 mg daily. *Adults with severe hepatic cirrhosis*: No more than 75 mg immediate-release form PO daily, 100 mg sustained-release form PO daily, 150 mg sustained-release PO every other day, or 150 mg extended-release PO every other day.
Smoking cessation aid	*Adults*: 150 mg (Zyban) PO daily for 3 days, increasing to a maximum dose of 300 mg daily in two divided doses at least 8 hours apart.

Half-life

8 to 24 hours

Common Adverse Reactions

CNS: Abnormal dreams, insomnia, headache, sedation, tremor, agitation, dizziness
CV: Tachycardia, arrhythmias, hypertension, hypotension
EENT: Blurred vision, rhinitis
GI: Constipation, nausea, vomiting, anorexia, dry mouth
Metabolic: Weight loss, weight gain
Integumentary: Excessive sweating

Key Interactions

Increased risk of adverse reactions with: Amantadine, levelodopa
Possible lowering of seizure threshold with: Antidepressants, antipsychotics, systemic corticosteroids, theophylline, alcohol
Decreased drug effectiveness with: Carbamazepine, phenobarbital, phenytoins
Increased risk of drug toxicity with: MAOIs
Increased risk of photosensitivity with: Sun exposure

Nursing Considerations

- Many clients experience a period of increased restlessness, including agitation, insomnia, and anxiety, especially at start of therapy.
- Alert: To minimize risk of seizures, do not exceed maximum recommended dose.
- Alert: Carefully monitor client for worsening depression or suicidal thoughts, especially at the beginning of therapy and during dosage changes. Clients with major depression may experience worsened depression and suicidal thoughts.
- In switching client from regular- or sustained-release to extended-release tablets, give the same total daily dose (when possible) as the once-daily dosage provided.
- Closely monitor clients with history of bipolar disorder. Antidepressants can cause manic episodes during the depressed phase of bipolar disorder. This may be less likely with bupropion than with other antidepressants.
- Begin smoking cessation treatment while client is still smoking; approximately 1 week is needed to achieve steady drug levels; stop the smoking cessation treatment if client has not progressed toward abstinence by week 7. Treatment usually lasts up to 12 weeks. Client can stop taking the drug without tapering off.
- Alert: Explain that excessive use of alcohol, abrupt withdrawal from alcohol or other sedatives, and addiction to cocaine, opiates, or stimulants during therapy increase risk of seizures. Seizure risks also are higher in clients using over-the-counter (OTC) stimulants, with anorexia, and with diabetes who use oral antidiabetic drugs or insulin.
- Advise client to consult prescriber before taking other prescription or OTC drugs.
- Advise client to avoid hazardous activities that require alertness and physical coordination until effects of drug are known.
- Alert: Advise client that Zyban and Wellbutrin contain the same active ingredient and shouldn't be used together.
- Tell client that it may take 4 weeks to reach full antidepressant effect.

- Alert: Advise client to report mood swings or suicidal thoughts immediately. Tell client not to chew, crush, or divide tablets.
- Inform client that tablets may have an odor.

citalopram hydrobromide (Celexa)

Drug Class
SSRI

Indications and Dosage

Depression (*see p. 383*)	*Adults*: Initially, 20 mg PO once daily, increasing to 40 mg daily after no less than 1 week to a maximum recommended dose of 40 mg daily. *Elderly*: 20 mg daily PO with adjustment to 40 mg daily only for unresponsive clients.

Half-life
35 hours

Common Adverse Reactions
CNS: Somnolence, insomnia, suicide attempt, anxiety, agitation, dizziness, paresthesia, migraine, impaired concentration
CV: Tachycardia, orthostatic hypotension, hypotension
GI: Dry mouth, nausea, diarrhea, anorexia, dyspepsia, vomiting, abdominal pain
GU: Ejaculation disorder, impotence
Skin: Rash, pruritus
Other: Increased sweating, yawning, decreased libido

Key Interactions
Increased risk of serotonin syndrome with: Amphetamines, buspirone, dextromethorphan, dihydroergotamine, MAOIs, meperidine, other SSRIs or SNRIs (duloxetine, venlajaxine), St. John's wort, tramadol, trazodone, TCAs, tryptophan
Increased risk of additive effects with: CNS drugs and alcohol
Decreased drug clearance (increasing risk of toxicity) with: Drugs that inhibit cytochrome P-450 isoenzymes 3A4 and 2CI9 for increased adverse effects

Nursing Considerations

- Tell client that he or she may take the drug in the morning or evening without regard to meals. If drowsiness occurs, he or she should take drug in the evening.
- Teach client to allow an orally disintegrating tablet to dissolve on the tongue, then swallow, with or without water. Tell client not to cut, crush, or chew the tablet.
- Alert: Drug may increase risk of suicidal thinking and behavior in children and adolescents with major depression or other psychiatric disorders. Closely supervise high-risk clients at start of drug therapy, because the possibility of a suicide attempt inherently accompanies depression and may persist until remission is significant. Reduce risk of overdose by limiting amount of drug available per refill.
- Alert: Do not confuse Celexa with Celebrex or Cerebyx.
- Ensure that at least 14 days has elapsed between MAOI therapy and citalopram therapy.
- Inform client that improvement may take 1 to 4 weeks. Advise client to continue therapy as prescribed and not to stop the drug abruptly.
- Instruct client to exercise caution when driving or operating hazardous machinery; drug may impair judgment, thinking, and motor skills.
- Advise client to avoid alcohol ingestion and to consult prescriber before taking other prescription or OTC drugs.

clomipramine hydrochloride (Anafranil)

Drug Class
TCA

Indications and Dosage

Obsessive-compulsive disorder (see p. 305)	Adults: Initially, 25 mg PO daily with meals, gradually increased to 100 mg daily in divided doses during first 2 weeks; increased to maximum dose of 250 mg daily in divided doses with meals, as needed (p.r.n.). After adjustment, give total daily dose at bedtime.

	Children and adolescents: Initially, 25 mg PO daily with meals, gradually increased over first 2 weeks to a daily maximum of 3 mg/kg or 100 mg PO in divided doses, whichever is smaller.
Panic disorders with or without agoraphobia (*see p. 311*)	*Adults*: 12.5 to 150 mg PO daily; maximum dose of 200 mg.
Depression (*see p. 383*), chronic pain	100 to 250 mg PO daily.
Cataplexy and related narcolepsy	25 to 200 mg PO daily.

Half-life

Parent compound: 32 hours
Active metabolite: 69 hours

Common Adverse Reactions

CNS: Somnolence, tremor, dizziness, headache, insomnia, nervousness, myoclonus, fatigue, seizures
EENT: Pharyngitis, rhinitis, visual changes
GI: Dry mouth, constipation, nausea, dyspepsia, increased appetite, anorexia, abdominal pain
GU: Urinary hesitancy, dysmenorrhea, ejaculation failure, impotence
Metabolic: Weight gain
Musculoskeletal: Myalgia

Key Interactions

Decreased antidepressant effect with: Barbiturates
Increased antidepressant effect and possible toxicity with: Cimetidine, fluoxetine, fluvoxamine, paroxetine, sertraline
Severe life-threatening hypertension with: Clonidine
Increased hypertensive effect with: Epinephrine, norepinephrine
Increased CNS depression with: CNS depressants, alcohol ingestion
Risk for hyperpyretic crisis, seizures, coma, or death with: MAOIs
Risk of life-threatening arrhythmias with: Quinolones
Reduced seizure threshold with: Evening primrose oil

Risk of serotonin syndrome with: St. John's wort, SAM-e, yohimbe

Increased risk of photosensitivity with: Sun exposure

Nursing Considerations

- Monitor mood and watch for suicidal tendencies. Allow client to have only the minimal amount of drug. Alert: Drug may increase risk of suicidal thinking and behavior in children and adolescents with major depression or other psychiatric disorder.
- Do not withdraw drug abruptly. Stop drug gradually several days before surgery because clients may suffer hypertensive episodes during surgery.
- Relieve dry mouth with sugarless candy or gum. Client may need saliva substitutes.
- Alert: Do not confuse clomipramine with chlorpromazine or clomiphene, or Anafranil with enalapril, nafarelin, or alfentanil.
- Warn client to avoid hazardous activities requiring alertness and physical coordination, especially during adjustment. Daytime sedation and dizziness may occur.
- Tell client to avoid alcohol while using the drug.
- Advise client to wear sunblock and protective clothing, and to avoid prolonged exposure to strong sunlight to prevent oversensitivity to the sun.

desipramine hydrochloride (Norpramin)

Drug Class
TCA

Indications and Dosage

Depression (*see p. 383*)	*Adults*: 100 to 200 mg PO daily in divided doses, increasing to a maximum daily dose of 300 mg. Alternatively, give entire dose at bedtime. *Adolescents and elderly clients*: 25 to 100 mg PO daily in divided doses, increasing gradually to maximum of 150 mg daily, if needed.

Half-life
Unknown

Common Adverse Reactions
CNS: Drowsiness, dizziness, seizures
CV: Tachycardia, orthostatic hypotension
EENT: Blurred vision
GI: Dry mouth, constipation, nausea, vomiting, anorexia
Metabolic: Hypoglycemia
Skin: Photosensitivity reactions
Other: Sudden death in children

Key Interactions
Increased CNS depression with: Barbiturates, CNS depressants, alcohol ingestion
Increased risk for drug toxicity with: Cimetidine, fluoxetine, fluvoxamine, paroxetine, sertraline
Risk for life-threatening hypertension with: Clonidine
Increased hypertensive effect with: Epinephrine, norepinephrine
Risk for hyperpyrexia or seizures with: MAOIs
Risk for life-threatening arrhythmias with: Quinolones
Decreased seizure threshold with: Evening primrose oil
Risk for serotonin syndrome with: St. John's wort, SAM-e, yohimbe
Increased risk for photosensitivity reactions with: Sun exposure

Nursing Considerations
• Monitor for mood changes and suicidal tendencies; if signs and symptoms of psychosis appear, notify prescriber. Alert: Drug may increase risk of suicidal thinking and behavior in children and adolescents with major depression or other psychiatric disorders.
• Monitor client for nausea, headache, and malaise after abrupt withdrawal of long-term therapy; do not withdraw abruptly.
• Because client may suffer hypertensive episodes during surgery, stop drug gradually several days before surgery.
• Recommend sugarless hard candy or gum to relieve dry mouth. Client may need saliva substitutes.
• Alert: Norpramin may contain tartrazine.
• Alert: Do not confuse desipramine with disopyramide or imipramine.

- Advise client to take full dose at bedtime to avoid daytime sedation; if insomnia occurs, tell the client to take the drug in the morning.
- Warn client to avoid hazardous activities that require alertness and physical coordination until effects of drug are known.
- Advise client to call prescriber if they have fever and sore throat. Blood counts may be necessary.
- Tell client to avoid alcohol and to consult prescriber before taking other prescription or OTC drugs.
- Advise client to wear sunblock and protective clothing, and to avoid prolonged exposure to strong sunlight.

doxepin hydrochloride (Sinequan)

Drug Class

TCA

Indications and Dosage

Depression (*see p. 383*)	*Adults*: Initially, 75 mg PO daily, with a usual dosage ranging from 75 to 150 mg daily to maximum dose of 300 mg daily in divided doses. Alternatively, give entire maintenance dose once daily, at maximum of 150 mg.
Anxiety (*see p. 300*)	*Adults*: Initially, 75 mg PO daily, with a usual dosage ranging from 75 to 150 mg daily to maximum dose of 300 mg daily in divided doses. Alternatively, give entire maintenance dose once daily, at maximum of 150 mg.

Half-life

6 to 8 hours

Common Adverse Reactions

CNS: Drowsiness, dizziness, seizures
CV: Orthostatic hypotension, tachycardia
EENT: Blurred vision, tinnitus
GI: Dry mouth, constipation, nausea, vomiting, anorexia
Metabolic: Hypoglycemia
Skin: Diaphoresis, rash, photosensitivity reactions

Key Interactions

Increased CNS depression with: Barbiturates, CNS depressants, alcohol ingestion
Increased risk for drug toxicity with: Cimetidine, fluoxetine, fluvoxamine, paroxetine, sertraline
Risk for life-threatening hypertension with: Clonidine
Increased hypertensive effect with: Epinephrine, norepinephrine
Risk for hyperpyrexia or seizures with: MAOIs
Risk for life-threatening arrhythmias with: Quinolones
Decreased seizure threshold with: Evening primrose oil
Risk for serotonin syndrome with: St. John's wort, SAM-e, yohimbe
Increased risk for photosensitivity reactions with: Sun exposure

Nursing Considerations

- Monitor for mood changes and suicidal tendencies; if signs and symptoms of psychosis appear, notify prescriber. Alert: Drug may increase risk of suicidal thinking and behavior in children and adolescents with major depression or other psychiatric disorders.
- Monitor for nausea, headache, and malaise after abrupt withdrawal of long-term therapy; do not withdraw abruptly.
- Because client may suffer hypertensive episodes during surgery, stop drug gradually several days before surgery.
- Recommend sugarless hard candy or gum to relieve dry mouth. Client may need saliva substitutes.
- Alert: Be aware that drug has strong anticholinergic effects and is one of the strongest sedating TCAs. Adverse anticholinergic effects can occur rapidly.
- Alert: Do not confuse doxepin with doxazosin, digoxin, doxapram, or Doxidan; do not confuse Sinequan with saquinavir.
- Advise client to take full dose at bedtime to avoid daytime sedation; if insomnia occurs, tell the client to take drug in the morning.
- Inform client that maximum effect may not be evident for 2 to 3 weeks.
- Tell client to dilute oral concentrate with 4 ounces (120 ml) of water, milk, or juice (orange, grapefruit, tomato, prune, or pineapple, but not grape); the client should not mix the preparation with carbonated beverages.

- Tell client to take full dose at bedtime, but warn of possible morning dizziness upon standing up quickly.
- Warn client to avoid hazardous activities that require alertness and physical coordination until effects of drug are known.
- Tell client to avoid alcohol and to consult prescriber before taking other prescription or OTC drugs.
- Advise client to wear sunblock and protective clothing, and to avoid prolonged exposure to strong sunlight.

duloxetine hydrochloride (Cymbalta)

Drug Class
SNRI

Indications and Dosage

Major depression (*see p. 383*)	*Adults*: Initially, 20 mg PO bid increased to a maximum of 60 mg PO once daily or divided in two equal doses.
Neuropathic pain related to diabetic peripheral neuropathy	*Adults*: 60 mg PO once daily.

Half-life
12 hours

Common Adverse Reactions
CNS: Dizziness, fatigue, headache, insomnia, somnolence, suicidal thoughts
GI: Constipation, diarrhea, dry mouth, nausea, decreased appetite
Metabolic: Hypoglycemia

Key Interactions
Increased levels of both drugs with: Type 1C antiarrhythmics (flecainide, propafenone), phenothiazines
Increased risk for adverse effects with: CNS drugs
Increased drug levels with: CYP 1A2 inhibitors (cimetidine, fluvoxamine, certain quinolones), CYP2D6 inhibitors (fluoxetine, paroxetine, quinidine)
Increased risk for hyperthermia with: MAOIs

Increased risk for serious ventricular arrhythmias and sudden death with: Thioridazine

Increased levels of TCAs with: TCAs (amitriptyline, nortriptyline, imipramine)

Increased risk of serotonin syndrome with: Triptans

Increased risk of liver damage with: Alcohol

Nursing Considerations

- Instruct client to swallow capsules whole, not to chew, crush, or open them because they have an enteric coating.
- Monitor for worsening of depression or suicidal behavior, especially when therapy starts or dosage changes. Alert: Drug may increase risk of suicidal thinking and behavior in children and adolescents with major depression or other psychiatric disorder.
- Be aware that treatment of overdose is symptomatic. Do not induce emesis; perform gastric lavage or administer activated charcoal soon after ingestion or if client remains symptomatic, because the drug undergoes extensive distribution. Forced diuresis, dialysis, hemoperfusion, and exchange transfusion are not useful. Contact a poison control center for information.
- Provide extended monitoring when giving the drug with TCAs because duloxetine metabolism will be prolonged.
- Periodically reassess client to determine the need for continued therapy.
- If client takes the drug for depression, explain that it may take 1 to 4 weeks to notice an effect.
- Decrease dosage gradually; watch for symptoms that may arise when drug is stopped, such as dizziness, nausea, headache, paresthesia, vomiting, irritability, and nightmares.
- If intolerable symptoms arise when decreasing or stopping drug, restart at previous dose and decrease more gradually.
- Monitor blood pressure periodically during treatment.
- Alert: Warn families or caregivers to report signs of worsening depression (eg, agitation, irritability, insomnia, hostility, impulsivity) and suicidal behavior to prescriber immediately.
- Tell client to consult prescriber or pharmacist if the client plans to take other prescription or OTC drugs or an herbal or other dietary supplement.

• Urge client to avoid activities that are hazardous or require mental alertness until the drug's effects are known.

escitalopram oxalate (Lexapro)

Drug Class
SSRI

Indications and Dosage

| Major depression (*see p. 383*) | *Adults*: Initially, 10 mg PO once daily, increasing to 20 mg if needed after at least 1 week. |
| Generalized anxiety disorder (*see p. 300*) | *Adults*: Initially, 10 mg PO once daily, increasing to 20 mg if needed after at least 1 week. |

Half-life
27 to 32 hours

Common Adverse Reactions
CNS: Suicidal behavior
GI: Nausea, diarrhea, constipation, indigestion, abdominal pain

Key Interactions
Increased risk of bleeding with: Aspirin, NSAIDs, other drugs known to affect coagulation
Increased drug clearance with: Carbamazepine
Increased drug level with: Cimetidine
Risk for additive effects with: Citalopram, alcohol, CNS drugs
Increased risk for serotonin syndrome with: MAOIs, triptans, tramadol
Increased levels of co-administered drug with: Desipramine, other drugs metabolized by CYP2D6
Enhanced serotonergic drug effect with: Lithium

Nursing Considerations
• Evaluate client for history of drug abuse; observe for signs of misuse or abuse.

- Tell client that he or she may take the drug in the morning or evening without regard to meals.
- Closely monitor client at high risk for suicide. Alert: Drug may increase risk of suicidal thinking and behavior in children and adolescents with major depression or other psychiatric disorder.
- Alert: Do not confuse escitalopram with estazolam.
- Periodically reassess client to determine need for maintenance treatment and appropriate dosing.
- Inform client that symptoms should improve gradually over several weeks, rather than immediately. Explain that although symptoms may improve within 1 to 4 weeks, client should continue drug as prescribed.
- Advise client to avoid alcohol and to use caution while driving or operating hazardous machinery because of drug's potential to impair judgment, thinking, and motor skills.
- Instruct client to consult healthcare provider before taking other prescription or OTC drugs.

fluoxetine (Prozac, Sarafem)

Drug Class

SSRI

Indications and Dosage

Depression (*see p. 383*), obsessive-compulsive disorder (*see p. 305*)	*Adults*: 20 mg PO daily in the morning; increase dosage on the basis of response to a maximum daily dose of 80 mg. *Children 7 to 17 years (OCD)*: 10 mg PO daily; increase to 20 mg daily after 2 weeks; dosage range 20 to 60 mg daily. *Children 8 to 18 years (depression)*: 10 mg PO daily for 1 week; increased to 20 mg daily.
Depression (older adult)	*Adults 65 years and older*: Initially, 20 mg PO daily in the morning; increase dosage on the basis of response; doses may be given morning and noon up to maximum daily dose of 80 mg.
Maintenance therapy for depression (client stabilized)	*Adults*: 90 mg (Prozac) once weekly, starting dose 7 days after last daily dose of 20 mg.

Bulimia nervosa (short- and long-term treatment; *see p. 366*)	*Adults*: 60 mg daily in the morning
Panic disorder (with or without agoraphobia [*see p. 311*]; short-term treatment)	*Adults*: 10 mg PO daily for 1 week; increase dose as needed to 20 mg daily up to maximum daily dose of 60 mg.
Anorexia nervosa (weight-restored clients; *see p. 357*)	*Adults*: 40 mg PO daily.
Depressive phases of bipolar disorder (*see p. 388*)	*Adults*: 20 to 60 mg PO daily.
Cataplexy	*Adults*: 20 mg PO once or twice daily along with CNS stimulant therapy.
Alcohol dependence	*Adults*: 60 mg PO daily.
Premenstrual dysphoric disorder	*Adults*: 20 mg (Sarafem) PO daily (every day of menstrual cycle or starting 14 days before anticipated onset of menses through first full day of menses; repeating with each new cycle).

Half-life

2 to 3 days

Common Adverse Reactions

CNS: Nervousness, somnolence, anxiety, insomnia, headache, drowsiness, tremor, dizziness, asthenia, suicidal behavior
GI: Nausea, diarrhea, dry mouth, anorexia, increased appetite
GU: Sexual dysfunction

Key Interactions

Increased risk of serotonin syndrome with: Amphetamines, buspirone, dextromethorphan, dihydroergotamine, lithium salts, MAOIs, meperidine, other SSRIs or SNRIs (duloxetine, venlafaxine), St. John's wort, tramadol, trazodone, TCAs, tryptophan
Increased CNS effects with: Benzodiazepines, lithium, TCAs, alcohol
Increased sedative and hypnotic effects with: St. John's wort

Nursing Considerations

- Use antihistamines or topical corticosteroids to treat rashes or pruritus.

- Watch for weight change during therapy, particularly in underweight clients or those with bulimia.
- Record mood changes. Watch for suicidal tendencies.
- *Alert:* Drug may increase risk of suicidal thinking and behavior in children and adolescents with major depression or other psychiatric disorder.
- Drug has a long half-life; monitor client for adverse effects for up to 2 weeks after client stops taking the drug.
- Tell client to avoid taking the drug in the afternoon, because doing so commonly causes nervousness and insomnia.
- Drug may cause dizziness or drowsiness. Warn client to avoid driving and other hazardous activities that require alertness and good psychomotor coordination until effects of drug are known.
- Tell client to consult prescriber before taking other prescription or OTC drugs.
- Advise client that a full therapeutic effect may take 4 weeks or longer.

fluvoxamine maleate (Luvox)

Drug Class
SSRI

Indications and Dosage

Obsessive-compulsive disorder (*see p. 305*)	*Adults*: Initially, 50 mg PO daily at bedtime, increasing by 50 mg qid 4 to 7 days to a maximum daily dose of 300 mg. Give total daily amounts above 100 mg in two divided doses. *Children 8 to 17 years*: Initially, 25 mg PO daily at bedtime, increasing by 25 mg qid 4 to 7 days to a maximum daily dose of 200 mg for clients 8 to 11 years old and 300 mg daily for those 11 to 17 years old. Give total daily dose amounts of more than 50 mg in two divided doses.

Half-life
17 hours

Common Adverse Reactions

CNS: Agitation, headache, asthenia, somnolence, insomnia, nervousness, dizziness

GI: Nausea, diarrhea, constipation, dyspepsia, vomiting, dry mouth, anorexia

Key Interactions

Decreased clearance of co-administered drug with: Benzodiazepines, theophylline, warfarin
Increased level of co-administered drug with: Carbamazepine, clozapine, methadone, metoprolol, propranolol, theophylline, TCAs
Risk for bradycardia with: Diltiazem
Increased drug effects with: Lithium, tryptophan
Risk for serotonin syndrome with: Tramadol, MAOIs
Prolonged QTc interval with: Pimozide, thioridazine
Increased CNS effects with: Alcohol
Decreased drug effectiveness with: Smoking

Nursing Considerations

- Give drug with or without food.
- Assess mood changes. Monitor client for suicidal tendencies.
- Alert: Do not use for treatment of major depression in children younger than 18 years, because of an increased risk of suicidal behavior.
- Inform client that he or she may need several weeks of therapy to obtain full therapeutic effect. Once improvement occurs, advise client not to stop drug until directed by prescriber.
- Suggest that client keep a diary of changes in mood or behavior. Tell client to report suicidal thoughts immediately.
- Alert: Do not confuse fluvoxamine with fluoxetine.
- Warn client to avoid hazardous activities until CNS effects of drug are known.
- Advise client to check with prescriber before taking OTC drugs; drug interactions can occur.

imipramine hydrochloride (Tofranil), imipramine pamoate (Tofranil-PM)

Drug Class

TCA

Indications and Dosage

| Depression (*see p. 383*) | *Adults*: 75 to 100 mg PO daily in divided doses, increasing by 25 to 50 mg to a maximum daily dose of 200 mg for outpatients and 300 mg for hospitalized clients. Give entire dose at bedtime.
Adolescents and elderly clients: Initially, 30 to 40 mg daily to a maximum dose not to exceed 100 mg daily. |
| Childhood enuresis | *Children 5 years and older*: 25 mg PO 1 hour before bedtime; if no improvement in 1 week, increase dose to 50 mg if child is younger than 12 years old or to 75 mg for children 12 years and older. In either case, maximum daily dose is 2.5 mg/kg. |

Half-life

11 to 25 hours

Common Adverse Reactions

CNS: Drowsiness, dizziness, seizures, stroke
CV: Orthostatic hypotension, tachycardia, ECG changes, myocardial infarction, arrhythmias, heart block
EENT: Blurred vision
GI: Dry mouth, constipation
GU: Urine retention
Metabolic: Hypoglycemia
Skin: Photosensitivity reactions

Key Interactions

Increased CNS effects with: Barbiturates, CNS depressants, alcohol
Increased drug level with: Cimetidine, fluoxetine, fluvoxamine, paroxetine, sertraline
Risk for life-threatening hypertension with: Clonidine
Increased hypertensive effects with: Epinephrine, norepinephrine
Possible hyperpyretic crisis with: MAOIs
Increased risk for life-threatening arrhythmias with: Quinolones

Decreased seizure threshold with: Evening primrose oil
Increased risk of serotonin syndrome with: St. John's wort, SAM-e, yohimbe
Decreased drug effectiveness with: Smoking
Increased risk of photosensitivity with: Sun exposure

Nursing Considerations

- Tell client to take full dose at bedtime, but warn of possible morning dizziness upon standing up quickly.
- Do not withdraw drug abruptly; monitor client for nausea, headache, and malaise after abrupt withdrawal of long-term therapy; these symptoms do not indicate addiction.
- Alert: Because of hypertensive episodes during surgery in clients receiving TCAs, stop drug gradually several days before surgery.
- Record mood changes. Monitor client for suicidal tendencies, and allow only a minimum supply of drug. Alert: Drug may increase risk of suicidal thinking and behavior in children and adolescents with major depression or other psychiatric disorder. If signs or symptoms of psychosis occur or increase, expect prescriber to reduce dosage.
- Recommend sugarless hard candy or gum to relieve dry mouth. Saliva substitutes may be useful.
- Alert: Tofranil and Tofranil-PM may contain tartrazine; do not confuse imipramine with desipramine.
- Tell client to avoid alcohol and to consult prescriber before taking other prescription or OTC drugs.
- Warn client to avoid hazardous activities that require alertness and physical coordination until effects of the drug are known.
- To prevent oversensitivity to the sun, advise client to wear sunblock and protective clothing, and to avoid prolonged exposure to strong sunlight.

maprotiline hydrochloride (Ludiomil)

Drug Class

Tetracyclic antidepressant

Indications and Dosage

Depression, mild to moderate (*see p. 383*)	*Adults*: Initially, 75 mg daily PO in outpatients, mainlining initial dose for 2 weeks, then gradually increasing dose in 24-mg intervals up to 150 mg to 225 mg daily.
Depression, severe	*Adults*: Initially 100 mg to 150 mg daily PO in hospitalized clients, possibly gradually increasing dose to 225 mg daily if needed.

Half-life

27 to 58 hours

Common Adverse Reactions

CNS: Sedation, anticholinergic effects, confusion, disturbed concentration
CV: Orthostatic hypotension
GI: Dry mouth, constipation, nausea

Key Interactions

Increased risk of seizures with: Benzodiazepines
Additive anticholinergic effects with: Anticholinergics, sympathomimetics
Increased risk of cardiotoxicity with: Thyroid medications

Nursing Considerations

- Monitor for mood changes and suicidal tendencies; allow only a minimum supply of drug.
- Alert: Do not confuse Ludiomil with Lomotil.
- Be aware that effectiveness typically requires approximately 3 weeks, although client may see some improvement in 3 to 7 days.
- Administer most of the dose at bedtime if drowsiness or anticholinergic effects are severe.
- Anticipate the need for complete blood count if client develops sore throat, fever, or signs of infection.
- Tell client to avoid alcohol and to consult prescriber before taking other prescription or OTC drugs.

- Warn client to avoid hazardous activities that require alertness and physical coordination until effects of the drug are known.
- To prevent oversensitivity to the sun, advise client to wear sunblock and protective clothing, and to avoid prolonged exposure to strong sunlight.

mirtazapine (Remeron, Remeron Soltab)

Drug Class

Tetracyclic antidepressant

Indications and Dosage

Depression (*see p. 383*)	*Adults*: Initially, 15 mg PO at bedtime to a maintenance dose of 15 to 45 mg daily

Half-life

Approximately 20 to 40 hours

Common Adverse Reactions

CNS: Somnolence, suicidal behavior
GI: Increased appetite, dry mouth, constipation
Metabolic: Weight gain

Key Interactions

Increased CNS effects with: Diazepam, other CNS depressants, alcohol
Possible fatal reactions with: MAOIs

Nursing Considerations

- Monitor mood changes. Watch for suicidal tendencies. Alert: Drug may increase risk of suicidal thinking and behavior in children and adolescents with major depression or other psychiatric disorder.
- Do not use within 14 days of MAOI therapy.
- Instruct client to remove oral disintegrating tablets from blister pack and place immediately on tongue. Advise client not to break or split tablet.
- Caution client not to perform hazardous activities if the drug causes drowsiness.

- Tell client to report signs and symptoms of infection, such as fever, chills, sore throat, irritation of the mucous membranes, or flu-like syndrome.
- Instruct client not to use alcohol or other CNS depressants and not to take other drugs without prescriber's approval.

nefazodone hydrochloride

Drug Class
Phenylpiperazine

Indication and Dosage

Depression (*see p. 383*)	*Adults*: Initially, 200 mg daily PO in two divided doses, increasing dosage by 100 to 200 mg daily at intervals of at least 1 week, p.r.n.; usual dosage range is 300 to 600 mg daily. *Elderly clients*: Initially, 100 mg daily PO in two divided doses.

Half-life
2 to 4 hours

Common Adverse Reactions
CNS: Headache, somnolence, dizziness, asthenia, insomnia, light-headedness, confusion, suicidal behavior
GI: Dry mouth, nausea, constipation, liver failure
GU: Prolonged erections

Key Interactions
Potentiation of co-administered drug with: Alprazolam, triazolam
Altered CNS activity with: CNS drugs, alcohol
Increased risk of co-administered drug toxicity with: Cyclosporine, digoxin, haloperidol, HMG CoA-reductase inhibitors
Increased risk of serotonin syndrome with: MAOIs, tramadol, St. John's wort

Nursing Considerations
- Monitor mood changes; watch for evidence of suicidal thoughts or tendencies.

- Alert: Drug may cause hepatic failure. Do not start in clients with active liver disease or elevated baseline transaminase level. Although pre-existing hepatic disease doesn't increase the likelihood of hepatic failure, baseline abnormalities can complicate monitoring. Stop drug if clinical signs and symptoms of hepatic dysfunction appear, such as AST or ALT level exceeding three times the upper limit of normal. Do not restart therapy.
- Perform a thorough risk-versus-benefit assessment before using the drug to treat depression, considering the risk for hepatic failure and emergence of suicidal thoughts and attempts.
- Inform client that he or she may need several weeks of therapy to obtain full antidepressant effect. Once improvement occurs, advise client not to stop drug until directed by prescriber.
- Warn client not to engage in hazardous activity until effects of drug are known.
- Alert: Teach client the signs and symptoms of liver problems, including yellowed skin or eyes, appetite loss, GI complaints, and malaise. Tell client to report these adverse events to prescriber immediately.
- Instruct client to avoid alcohol and to notify prescriber before taking OTC drugs.

nortriptyline hydrochloride (Aventyl, Pamelor)

Drug Class
TCA

Indications and Dosage

| Depression (see p. 383) | *Adults*: 25 mg PO tid or qid, gradually increasing dosage to a maximum of 150 mg daily. Give entire dose at bedtime. Monitor level when doses above 100 mg daily are given. *Adolescents and elderly clients*: 30 to 50 mg daily given once or in divided doses. |

Half-life

18 to 24 hours

Common Adverse Reactions

CNS: Drowsiness, dizziness, seizures, stroke
CV: Tachycardia, heart block, myocardial infarction
EENT: Blurred vision
GI: Constipation
GU: Urine retention
Hematologic: Agranulocytosis, thrombocytopenia
Metabolic: Hypoglycemia
Skin: Photosensitivity reactions

Key Interactions

Increased CNS depression with: Barbiturates, CNS depressants, alcohol
Increased drug level with: Cimetidine, fluoxetine, fluvoxamine, paroxetine, sertraline
Risk of life-threatening hypertension with: Clonidine
Increased hypertensive effect with: Epinephrine, norepinephrine
Increased risk of hyperpyrexia or seizures with: MAOIs
Increased risk of life-threatening arrhythmias with: Quinolones
Decreased seizure threshold with: Evening primrose oil
Risk for serotonin syndrome with: St. John's wort, SAM-e, yohimbe
Decreased drug level with: Smoking
Increased risk for photosensitivity with: Sun exposure

Nursing Considerations

- Because clients using TCAs may suffer hypertensive episodes during surgery, stop drug gradually several days before surgery.
- Monitor for mood changes and evidence of suicidal tendencies. Allow only a minimum supply of the drug. If signs or symptoms of psychosis occur or increase, expect to reduce dosage.
- Advise client to take full dose at bedtime to reduce risk of dizziness upon standing quickly. Urge client not to stop the drug suddenly.
- Warn client to avoid activities that require alertness and physical coordination until effects of drug are known.

- Recommend use of sugarless hard candy or gum to relieve dry mouth. Client may need saliva substitutes.
- Tell client to consult prescriber before taking other prescription or OTC drugs.
- To prevent oversensitivity to the sun, advise client to wear sunblock and protective clothing, and to avoid prolonged exposure to strong sunlight.

paroxetine hydrochloride (Paxil, Paxil CR)

Drug Class
SSRI

Indications and Dosage

Depression (*see p. 383*)	*Adults*: Initially, 20 mg PO daily, preferably in morning, as indicated; if no improvement, increasing dose by 10 mg daily at intervals of at least 1 week to a maximum of 50 mg daily. If using controlled-release form, initially, 25 mg PO daily, increasing dose by 12.5 mg daily at weekly intervals to a maximum of 62.5 mg daily. *Elderly clients*: Initially, 10 mg PO daily, preferably in morning, as indicated; if no improvement, increase dose by 10 mg daily at weekly intervals, to a maximum of 40 mg daily. If using controlled-release form, start therapy at 12.5 mg PO daily. Do not exceed 50 mg daily.
Obsessive-compulsive disorder (*see p. 305*)	*Adults*: Initially, 20 mg PO daily, preferably in morning, increasing dose by 10 mg daily at weekly intervals to a recommended daily dose of 40 mg; maximum daily dose is 60 mg.
Panic disorder (*see p. 311*)	*Adults*: Initially, 10 mg PO daily, increasing dose by 10 mg at no less than 1-week intervals to maximum of 60 mg daily. Or, 12.5 mg Paxil CR PO as a single daily dose, usually in the morning, with or without food, increasing dose at intervals of at least 1 week by 12.5 mg daily, up to a maximum of 75 mg daily.

Social anxiety disorder	*Adults*: Initially, 20 mg PO daily, preferably in morning, with a range of 20 to 60 mg daily, adjusting dosage to maintain client on lowest effective dose. Or, 12.5 mg Paxil CR PO as a single daily dose, usually in the morning, with or without food, increasing dosage at weekly intervals in increments of 12.5 mg daily, up to a maximum of 37.5 mg daily.
Generalized anxiety disorder (*see p. 300*)	*Adults*: 20 mg PO daily initially, increasing dose by 10 mg per day weekly up to 50 mg daily.
Post-traumatic stress disorder (*see p. 324*)	*Adults*: 20 mg PO daily initially, increasing dose by 10 mg daily at intervals of at least 1 week; maximum daily dose is 50 mg PO.
Premenstrual dysphoric disorder	*Adults*: Initially, 12.5 mg Paxil CR PO as a single daily dose, usually in the morning, with or without food, daily or during the luteal phase of the menstrual cycle, with dose changes occurring at intervals of at least 1 week; maximum dose is 25 mg PO daily.

Half-life

Approximately 24 hours

Common Adverse Reactions

CNS: Asthenia, dizziness, headache, insomnia, somnolence, tremor, nervousness, suicidal behavior

GI: Dry mouth, nausea, constipation, diarrhea

GU: Ejaculatory disturbances, sexual dysfunction, decreased libido

Skin: Diaphoresis

Key Interactions

Increased risk of serotonin syndrome with: Amphetamines, buspirone, dextromethorphan, dihydroergotamine, lithium salts, MAOIs, meperidine, other SSRIs or selective serotonin-norepinephrine reuptake inhibitors (duloxetine, venlafaxine), tramadol, trazodone, TCAs, tryptophan, triptans

Increased risk for adverse effects with: Cimetidine
Increased level of co-administered drug with: Digoxin
Increased risk for anticholinergic effects with: Procyclidine
Increased risk for serious ventricular arrhythmias with: Thioridazine
Increased risk for bleeding with: Warfarin
Increased sedative-hypnotic effects with: St. John's wort

Nursing Considerations

- Monitor for mood changes and suicidal tendencies, and allow only a minimum supply of drug. Alert: Drug may increase risk of suicidal thinking and behavior in children and adolescents with major depression or other psychiatric disorder. Suicidal behavior in clients taking the drug hasn't been definitively attributed to its use. If signs or symptoms of psychosis occur or increase, expect prescriber to reduce dosage.
- Periodically reassess client taking Paxil CR for premenstrual dysphoric disorder to determine the need for continued treatment.
- Advise client that the drug may be taken with or without food, usually in the morning; tell client not to break, crush, or chew controlled-release tablets.
- Monitor client for complaints of sexual dysfunction.
- Alert: Do not stop drug abruptly. Withdrawal or discontinuation syndrome may occur if client stops the drug abruptly. Symptoms include headache, myalgia, lethargy, and general flu-like symptoms. Taper drug slowly over 1 to 2 weeks.
- Alert: Do not confuse paroxetine with paclitaxel, or Paxil with Doxil, paclitaxel, Plavix, or Taxol.
- Warn client to avoid activities that require alertness and good coordination until effects of drug are known.
- Tell client to avoid alcohol and to consult prescriber before taking other prescription or OTC drugs or herbal medicines.

phenelzine (Nardil)

Drug Class
MAOI

Indications and Dosage

Depression (see p. 383)	*Adults*: 15 mg PO tid, increasing dosage to at least 60 mg daily rapidly on the basis of client tolerance; after achieving maximum benefit, slowly reduce dosage over several weeks; maintenance dose of 15 mg daily or every other day.

Half-life
Unknown

Common Adverse Reactions
CNS: Dizziness, vertigo, headache, overactivity, hyperreflexia, tremors, muscle twitching, mania, hypomania, jitteriness, confusion, memory impairment, weakness, fatigue, drowsiness, restlessness, increased anxiety, agitation
CV: Hypertensive crisis, orthostatic hypotension, disturbed cardiac rate and rhythm
EENT: Blurred vision
GI: Constipation, diarrhea, nausea, abdominal pain, dry mouth, anorexia, weight changes

Key Interactions
Risk of hypertensive crisis with: TCAs, sympathomimetics, amphetamines, other anorexiants, tyramine-containing foods
Increased hypoglycemic effect with: Insulin and oral sulfonylureas
Increased risk of serotonin syndrome with: SSRIs or other serotonergic agents

Nursing Considerations
* Monitor vital signs, including blood pressure, closely for changes.
* Alert: Have phentolamine or another alpha-adrenergic blocker readily available to treat hypertensive crisis.
* Advise client to avoid foods with tyramine.
* Instruct client to take the drug exactly as prescribed and not to discontinue the drug abruptly or without consulting the prescriber.

- Warn client to avoid activities that require alertness and physical coordination until effects of drug are known.
- Tell client to avoid alcohol and to consult prescriber before taking other prescription or OTC drugs or herbal medicines.

selegiline (Emsam, Eldepryl, Zelapar)

Drug Class
MAOI (type B)

Indications and Dosage

Major depression (*see p. 383*)	*Adults*: One patch daily; initially 6 mg daily, increasing in increments of 3 mg daily at intervals of 2 or more weeks to a maximum daily dose of 12 mg. *Elderly*: 6 mg daily.

Half-life
2 to 10 hours

Common Adverse Reactions
CNS: Headache, insomnia, dizziness
CV: Arrhythmias
GI: Nausea
Skin: Application site reaction

Key Interactions
Increased risk of serotonin syndrome with: Citalopram, duloxetine, fluoxetine, fluvoxamine, nefazodone, paroxetine, sertraline, venlafaxine
Increased serotonergic effects with: St. John's wort
Risk for hypertensive crisis with: Bupropion, cyclobenzaprine, dextromethorphan, meperidine, methadone, mirtazapine, MAOIs, propoxyphene, sympathomimetic amines, tramadol, TCAs, tyramine-containing foods
Increased drug levels with: Carbamazepine, oxcarbazepine

Nursing Considerations
- Alert: Do not confuse selegiline with Stelazine or Eldepryl with enalapril.

- Monitor for mood changes. Drug may increase the risk of suicidal thinking in children and adolescents.
- Monitor client with major depression for worsening symptoms and suicidal behavior, especially during first few weeks of therapy.
- Monitor vital signs, including blood pressure, closely for changes.
- Advise client to avoid foods with tyramine.
- Instruct client to take the drug exactly as prescribed and not to discontinue the drug abruptly or without consulting the prescriber.
- Encourage client to avoid exposing transdermal system to direct external heat sources and not to cut the transdermal system into smaller pieces.
- Warn client to avoid activities that require alertness and physical coordination until effects of drug are known.
- Tell client to avoid alcohol and to consult prescriber before taking other prescription or OTC drugs or herbal medicines.

sertraline hydrochloride (Zoloft)

Drug Class
SSRI

Indications and Dosage

Depression (*see p. 383*)	*Adults*: 50 mg PO daily, adjusting dosage as needed and tolerated to a range of 50 to 200 mg daily.
Obsessive-compulsive disorder (*see p. 305*)	*Adults*: 50 mg PO once daily; if no improvement, increasing dosage, up to 200 mg daily. *Children 6 to 17 years old*: Initially, 25 mg PO daily in clients 6 to 12 years old, or 50 mg PO daily in those 13 to 17 years old. Increase dosage p.r.n., up to 200 mg daily at intervals of no less than 1 week.

Panic disorder (*see p. 311*)	*Adults*: Initially, 25 mg PO daily, increasing dosage to 50 mg PO daily after 1 week; if no improvement, increasing dosage to a maximum of 200 mg daily.
Premenstrual dysphoric disorder	*Adults*: Initially, 50 mg daily PO, either continuously or only during the luteal phase of the menstrual cycle; if no response, increasing dosage to 50 mg per menstrual cycle, up to 150 mg daily for use throughout the menstrual cycle or 100 mg daily for luteal phase doses. If a 100-mg daily dose has been established with luteal phase dose, use a 50-mg daily adjustment for 3 days at the beginning of each luteal phase.
Social anxiety disorder	*Adults*: Initially, 25 mg PO once daily, increasing dosage to 50 mg PO once daily after 1 week of therapy to a dose range between 50 and 200 mg daily.

Half-life
26 hours

Common Adverse Reactions
CNS: Fatigue, headache, tremor, dizziness, insomnia, somnolence, suicidal behavior
GI: Dry mouth, nausea, diarrhea, loose stools, dyspepsia
GU: Male sexual dysfunction

Key Interactions
Increased risk of serotonin syndrome with: Amphetamines, buspirone, dextromethorphan, dihydroergotamine, lithium salts, MAOIs, meperidine, other SSRIs or SNRIs (duloxetine, venlafaxine), sumatriptan, tramadol, trazodone, TCAs, triptans, tryptophan, St. John's wort
Increased drug clearance with: Cimetidine
Decreased clearance of co-administered drug with: Benzodiazepines, tolbutamide
Increased risk for bleeding with: Warfarin

Nursing Considerations

- Give drug once daily, either in morning or evening, with or without food.
- Advise client to mix the oral concentrate with 4 oz of water, ginger ale, lemon or lime soda, lemonade, or orange juice only, and to take the dose right away.
- Record mood changes. Monitor client for suicidal tendencies, and allow only a minimum supply of drug. Alert: Drug may increase risk of suicidal thinking and behavior in children and adolescents with major depression or other psychiatric disorder.
- Advise client to use caution when performing hazardous tasks that require alertness.
- Tell client to avoid alcohol and to consult prescriber before taking OTC drugs.
- Instruct client to avoid stopping drug abruptly.

tranylcypromine (Parnate)

Drug Class

MAOI

Indications and Dosage

Major depression (*see p. 383*) without melancholia	*Adults*: 30 mg daily PO in divided doses, increasing dosages daily in increments of 10 mg if no improvement within 2 to 3 weeks; increased to a maximum of 60 mg daily.

Half-life

Unknown

Common Adverse Reactions

CNS: Dizziness, vertigo, headache, overactivity, hyperreflexia, tremors, muscle twitching, mania, hypomania, jitteriness, confusion, memory impairment, weakness, fatigue, drowsiness, restlessness, increased anxiety, agitation

CV: Hypertensive crisis, orthostatic hypotension, disturbed cardiac rate and rhythm
EENT: Blurred vision
GI: Constipation, diarrhea, nausea, abdominal pain, dry mouth, anorexia, weight changes

Key Interactions

Risk of hypertensive crisis with: TCAs, sympathomimetics, amphetamines, other anorexiants, tyramine-containing foods
Increased hypoglycemic effect with: Insulin and oral sulfonylureas
Increased risk of serotonin syndrome with: SSRIs or other serotonergic agents

Nursing Considerations

- Monitor vital signs, including blood pressure, closely for changes.
- Alert: Have phentolamine or another alpha-adrenergic blocker readily available to treat hypertensive crisis.
- Monitor liver function tests periodically during therapy.
- Advise client to avoid foods containing tyramine.
- Instruct client to take the drug exactly as prescribed and not to discontinue it abruptly or without consulting the prescriber.
- Warn client to avoid activities that require alertness and physical coordination until effects of drug are known.

trazodone hydrochloride (Desyrel)

Drug Class

Triazolopyridine derivative (other)

Indications and Dosage

Depression (*see p. 383*)-	*Adults*: Initially, 150 mg PO daily in divided doses, increasing by 50 mg daily every 3 to 4 days, p.r.n., with doses ranging from 150 to 400 mg daily; maximum dosage of 600 mg daily for inpatients and 400 mg daily for outpatients.

Half-life

First phase: 3 to 6 hours
Second phase: 5 to 9 hours

Common Adverse Reactions

CNS: Drowsiness, dizziness
CV: Orthostatic hypotension
GI: Dry mouth
GU: Priapism

Key Interactions

Increased risk of serotonin syndrome with: Amphetamines, buspirone, dextromethorphan, dihydroergotamine, lithium salts, meperidine, SSRIs or SNRIs (duloxetine, venlafaxine), sumatriptan, tramadol, TCAs, tryptophan, St. John's wort
Increased hypotensive effect with: Antihypertensives
Increased CNS depression with: Clonidine, CNS depressants, alcohol
Increased sedation with: Ginkgo biloba
Decreased drug level with: CYP3A4 inducers (carbamazepine)
Increased drug level with: CYP3A4 inhibitors (ketoconazole), protease inhibitors (amprenavir, atazanavir, fosamprenavir, indinavir, lopinavir, nelfinavir, ritonavir, saquinavir)
Increased level of co-administered drug with: Digoxin, phenytoin

Nursing Considerations

- Give after meals or a light snack for optimal absorption and to decrease risk of dizziness.
- Monitor mood changes. Assess client for suicidal tendencies; allow only minimum supply of drug. Alert: Drug may increase the risk of suicidal thinking and behavior in children and adolescents with major depression or other psychiatric disorder.
- Alert: Do not confuse trazodone hydrochloride with tramadol hydrochloride.
- Alert: Tell client to report priapism (a persistent, painful erection) right away, because client may need immediate intervention.
- Warn client to avoid activities that require alertness and physical coordination until effects of the drug are known.

venlafaxine hydrochloride (Effexor, Effexor XR)

Drug Class
SNRI

Indications and Dosage

Depression (*see p. 383*)	*Adults*: Initially, 75 mg PO daily in two or three divided doses with food, increasing as tolerated and needed by 75 mg daily every 4 days. For outpatients with moderate depression, usual maximum is 225 mg daily; in certain clients with severe depression, dose may be as high as 375 mg daily. For extended-release capsules, 75 mg PO daily in a single dose. For some clients, it may be desirable to start at 37.5 mg PO daily for 4 to 7 days before increasing to 75 mg daily. Dosage may be increased by 75 mg daily every 4 days to maximum of 225 mg daily.
Generalized anxiety disorder (*see p. 300*)	*Adults*: Initially, 75-mg extended-release capsule PO daily in a single dose. For some clients, it may be desirable to start at 37.5 mg PO daily for 4 to 7 days before increasing to 75 mg daily. Dosage may be increased by 75 mg daily every 4 days to maximum of 225 mg daily.
Panic disorder (*see p. 311*)	*Adults*: Initially, 37.5 mg extended-release capsule PO daily for 1 week, increasing dosage to 75 mg daily. If client isn't responding, may increase dosage by up to 75 mg daily in no less than weekly intervals p.r.n., to a maximum dosage of 225 mg daily.
Social anxiety disorder	*Adults*: Initially, 75-mg extended-release capsule daily; some clients may start at 37.5 mg PO daily for 4 to 7 days before increasing dosage p.r.n. by 75 mg daily every 4 days to a maximum dose of 225 mg daily.
Prevention of relapse of major depression	*Adults*: 100 to 200 mg PO regular-release form or 75 to 225 mg PO daily of extended-release form.

Half-life

5 hours

Common Adverse Reactions

CNS: Asthenia, headache, somnolence, dizziness, nervousness, insomnia, suicidal behavior
GI: Nausea, constipation, dry mouth, anorexia
GU: Abnormal ejaculation
Skin: Diaphoresis

Key Interactions

Increased risk of serotonin syndrome with: MAOIs, tramadol, triptans
Increased risk of stimulation with: Yohimbe

Nursing Considerations

- Alert: Closely monitor client with depression for signs and symptoms of clinical worsening and suicidal ideation, especially at the beginning of therapy and with dosage adjustments. Drug may increase risk of suicidal thinking and behavior in children and adolescents with major depression or other psychiatric disorder.
- Carefully monitor blood pressure. Drug therapy may cause sustained, dose-dependent increases in blood pressure.
- Monitor weight, particularly for underweight clients with depression.
- If medication is to be stopped, inform client who has taken the drug for 6 weeks or longer that the drug will be stopped gradually by tapering dosage over a 2-week period as instructed by prescriber. Alert: Do not abruptly stop the drug.
- Tell client to avoid alcohol and to consult prescriber before taking other prescription or OTC drugs.

Mood Stabilizers

Overview

Primary Indications

Bipolar disorder (*see p. 388*), impulse-control disorders (*see p. 375*)

Signs and Symptoms

Symptoms indicating a possible need for mood stabilizers include episodes of mania characterized by extreme mood swings, with irritability or sudden outbursts of misplaced rage; episodes of major depression; and episodes of hypomania.

Major Categories

- Lithium salt (*see p. 231*)
- Anticonvulsants
  - carbamazepine (*see p. 225*)
  - divalproex sodium (*see p. 227*)
  - gabapentin (*see p. 228*)
  - lamotrigine (*see p. 229*)
  - oxcarbazepine (*see p. 233*)
- Agents for refractory mania
  - topiramate (*see p. 235*)

- Other drugs used for acute mania (atypical antipsychotics)
  - aripiprazole (*see p. 238*)
  - olanzapine (*see p. 251*)
  - quetiapine (*see p. 256*)
  - risperidone (*see p. 258*)
  - ziprasidone (*see p. 266*)

Key Drug Monographs

carbamazepine (Carbatrol, Epilol, Equetro, Tegretol, Tegretol-XR)

Drug Class

Anticonvulsant

Indications and Dosage

Acute mania; mixed episodes associated with bipolar I disorder (*see p. 388*)	*Adults*: Initially, 200 mg Equetro PO twice a day (bid), increasing by 200 mg daily to achieve therapeutic response.

Half-life

Single dose: 25 to 65 hours
Long-term use: 8 to 29 hours

Common Adverse Reactions

Central nervous system (CNS): Ataxia, dizziness, drowsiness, vertigo, worsening of seizures
Cardiovascular (CV): Arrhythmias, arteriovenous block, heart failure
Gastrointestinal (GI): Nausea, vomiting
Hematologic: Agranulocytosis, aplastic anemia, thrombocytopenia
Hepatic: Hepatitis
Skin: Erythema multiforme, Stevens-Johnson syndrome

Key Interactions

Increased drug level with: Cimetidine, danazol, diltiazem, fluoxetine, fluvoxamine, isoniazid, macrolides, propoxyphene, valproic acid, verapamil

Increased drug level and possible toxicity with: Clarithromycin, erythromycin, troleandomycin, lamotrigine, nefazodone

Decreased level of co-administered drug with: Doxycycline, felbamate, haloperidol, hormonal contraceptives, phenytoin, theophylline, tiagabine, topiramate, valproate, warfarin

Increased risk for CNS toxicity with: Lithium

Increased risk for depressant and anticholinergic effects with: Monoamine oxidase inhibitors

Decreased drug level with: Phenobarbital, phenytoin, primidone

Nursing Considerations

- Administer the drug with food to minimize gastric upset; if using suspension form, tell client to shake container before measuring dose; tell client not to crush or chew extended-release form.
- Inform client that Tegretol XR tablet coating may appear in stool because it is not absorbed.
- Obtain baseline determinations of urinalysis, blood urea nitrogen and iron levels, liver function studies, complete blood count, and platelet and reticulocyte counts; monitor periodically.
- Shake oral suspension well before measuring dose.
- If necessary, sprinkle contents of extended-release capsules over applesauce if client has difficulty swallowing them. Capsules and tablets should not be crushed or chewed, unless labeled as chewable.
- Expect to gradually increase dose to minimize adverse reactions.
- Monitor blood levels of drug; therapeutic level is 4 to 12 μg/mL.
- Alert: Watch for signs of anorexia or subtle appetite changes, which may indicate excessive drug level.
- Alert: Do not confuse Tegretol or Tegretol-XR with Topamax, Toprol XL, or Toradol; do not confuse Carbatrol with carvedilol.
- Advise client to keep tablets in the original container tightly closed and away from moisture. Some formulations may harden when exposed to excessive moisture so that less is available in the body, decreasing seizure control.
- Advise client to notify prescriber immediately if fever, sore throat, mouth ulcers, or easy bruising or bleeding occurs.
- Tell client that drug may cause mild to moderate dizziness and drowsiness when first taken. Advise client to avoid

hazardous activities until effects disappear, usually within 3 to 4 days.

divalproex sodium (Depakote, Depakote EF, Depakote sprinkle)

Drug Class
Anticonvulsant

Indications and Dosage

Mania	*Adults*: Initially, 750 mg Depakote daily PO in divided doses, or 25 mg/kg Depakote ER once daily to a maximum daily dose of 60 mg/kg.

Half-life
6 to 16 hours

Common Adverse Reactions

CNS: Asthenia, dizziness, headache, insomnia, nervousness, somnolence, tremor

Ear, eye, nose, and throat (EENT): Blurred vision, diplopia

GI: Abdominal pain, anorexia, diarrhea, dyspepsia, nausea, vomiting, pancreatitis

Hematologic: Bone marrow suppression, hemorrhage, thrombocytopenia

Hepatic: Hepatotoxicity

Skin: Alopecia, flu-like syndrome, infection, erythema multiforme, hypersensitivity reactions, Stevens-Johnson syndrome

Key Interactions

Increased risk for toxicity with: Aspirin, chlorpromazine, cimetidine, erythromycin, felbamate

Increased CNS depression with: Benzodiazepines, other CNS depressants, alcohol

Increased risk for toxicity of co-administered drug with: Carbamazepine

Increased level of co-administered drug with: Lamotrigine, phenobarbital, phenytoin
Decreased drug level with: Lamotrigine, phenytoin, rifampin

Nursing Considerations

- Obtain liver function test results, platelet count, and prothrombin time (PT) and international normalized ratio (INR) before starting therapy; monitor these values periodically.
- Keep in mind that divalproex sodium has a lower risk of adverse GI reactions.
- Alert: Fatal hepatotoxicity may follow nonspecific symptoms such as malaise, fever, and lethargy. If these symptoms occur during therapy, notify prescriber at once because clients who might be developing hepatic dysfunction must stop taking drug.
- Notify prescriber if client develops tremors; client may need a dosage reduction.
- Monitor drug level. Therapeutic level is 50 to 100 µg/mL.
- Tell client to take drug with food or milk to reduce adverse effects. Advise client not to chew capsules to avoid irritation of mouth and throat.
- Tell client to either swallow capsules whole or open them carefully, sprinkling the contents on a teaspoonful of soft food. Tell client to swallow immediately without chewing.
- Warn client not to stop drug therapy abruptly.
- Advise client to avoid driving and other potentially hazardous activities that require mental alertness until drug's CNS effects are known.
- Urge client to call prescriber if malaise, weakness, lethargy, facial swelling, loss of appetite, or vomiting occurs.

gabapentin (Neurontin, Gabarone)

Drug Class

Anticonvulsant

Indications and Dosage

Bipolar disorder (*see p. 388*), adjunct for refractory mania (off-label use)	*Adults:* Initially, 300 mg PO three time daily, titrating upward as needed, ranging from 1800 to 3600 mg/day.

Half-life

5 to 7 hours

Common Adverse Reactions

CNS: Ataxia, dizziness, fatigue, somnolence, insomnia
EENT: Diplopia
Hematologic: Leukopenia

Key Interactions

Decreased drug absorption with: Antacids
Increased drug level and decreased level of co-administered drug with: Hydrocodone

Nursing Considerations

- Give first dose at bedtime to minimize drowsiness, dizziness, fatigue, and ataxia.
- If drug is to be stopped or another drug substituted, do so gradually over at least 1 week.
- Inform client that the drug may be taken without regard to meals.
- Warn client to avoid driving and operating heavy machinery until drug's CNS effects are known.

lamotrigine (Lamictal)

Drug Class

Anticonvulsant

Indications and Dosage

Bipolar disorder (*see p. 388*)	*Adults*: Initially, 25 mg PO once daily for 2 weeks; then 50 mg PO once daily for 2 weeks. Dosage may then be doubled at weekly intervals to maintenance dosage of 200 mg daily. *Adults taking carbamazepine or other hepatic enzyme-inducing drugs without valproic acid*: Initially, 50 mg PO once daily for 2 weeks; then 100 mg daily in two divided doses for 2 weeks. Dosage is then increased by 100 mg weekly to maintenance dosage of 400 mg daily, given in two divided doses. *Adults taking valproic acid*: Initially, 25 mg PO every other day for 2 weeks; then 25 mg PO once daily for 2 weeks. Dosage may then be doubled at weekly intervals to maintenance dosage of 100 mg daily.

Half-life

14.5 to 70.25 hours (dependent on dosage schedule and use of other anticonvulsants)

Common Adverse Reactions

CNS: Ataxia, dizziness, headache, somnolence, seizures
EENT: Blurred vision, diplopia, rhinitis
GI: Nausea, vomiting
Skin: Rash, Stevens-Johnson syndrome, toxic epidermal necrolysis

Key Interactions

Decreased drug effect with: Acetaminophen, carbamazepine, ethosuximide, oxcarbazepine, phenobarbital, phenytoin, primidone
Decreased drug level with: Oral contraceptives containing estrogen, rifampin
Possible additive effects with: Folate inhibitors, such as co-trimoxazole and methotrexate
Decreased drug clearance with: Valproic acid

Nursing Considerations

- Do not stop drug abruptly; taper drug over at least 2 weeks.
- Alert: Stop drug at first sign of rash, unless rash is clearly not related to the use of this drug.
- Reduce lamotrigine dose if drug is added to a multidrug regimen that includes valproic acid.
- Advise client taking chewable dispersible tablets to swallow them whole, chew them, or disperse them in water or diluted fruit juice. If client is chewing tablets, give a small amount of water or diluted fruit juice to aid in swallowing.
- Alert: Do not confuse lamotrigine with lamivudine or Lamictal with Lamisil, Ludiomil, labetalol, or Lomotil.
- Inform client that drug may cause rash. Combination of valproic acid and lamotrigine may cause a serious rash. Tell client to report rash or signs or symptoms of hypersensitivity promptly because the symptoms may warrant stopping drug.
- Warn client not to engage in hazardous activity until drug's CNS effects are known.

lithium carbonate (Eskalith, Eskalith CR, Lithane, Lithobid, Lithonate, Lithotabs, Quilonum)

Drug Class
Mood stabilizer

Indications and Dosage

Mania	*Adults*: 300 to 600 mg PO up to four times daily. Alternatively, 900-mg controlled-release tablets PO every 12 hours; increasing dosage on the basis of blood levels to achieve optimal dosage. Recommended therapeutic lithium levels are 1 to 1.5 mEq/L for acute mania and 0.6 to 1.2 mEq/L for maintenance therapy.

Half-life
17 to 36 hours

Common Adverse Reactions

CNS: Fatigue, lethargy, coma, epileptiform seizures, muscle weakness, fine hand tremors

CV: Arrhythmias, bradycardia

GI: Vomiting, anorexia, diarrhea, thirst

Genitourinary: Polyuria, renal toxicity with long-term use

Hematologic: Leukocytosis with leukocyte count of 14,000 to 18,000/mm^3

Key Interactions

Increased drug level with: Angiotensin-converting enzyme inhibitors

Increased risk for toxicity with: Thiazide diuretics

Increased drug excretion with: Aminophylline, sodium bicarbonate, urine alkalinizers

Decreased drug levels with: Calcium channel blockers (verapamil), caffeine

Increased drug effect with: Carbamazepine, fluoxetine, methyldopa, nonsteroidal anti-inflammatory drugs, probenecid

Increased risk for prolonged paralysis or weakness with: Neuromuscular blockers

Increased risk for CNS toxicity with: Carbamazepine

Increased risk for hypothyroidism with: Iodide salts

Nursing Considerations

• Alert: Drug has a narrow therapeutic margin of safety. Determining drug level is crucial to safe use. Monitor drug level 8 to 12 hours after first dose, the morning before second dose is given, two or three times weekly for the first month, and then weekly to monthly during maintenance therapy.

• Alert: Be aware that when drug level is less than 1.5 mEq/L, adverse reactions are usually mild. Mild to moderate toxic reactions occur with levels from 1.5 to 2 mEq/L; moderate to severe toxic reactions occur with levels from 2 to 2.5 mEq/L; life-threatening toxicity occurs when levels are greater than 2.5 mEq/L.

• Monitor baseline ECG, thyroid and renal studies, and electrolyte levels.

- Check fluid intake and output, especially when surgery is scheduled.
- Alert: Weigh client daily; check for edema or sudden weight gain; adjust fluid and salt ingestion to compensate if excessive loss occurs from protracted diaphoresis or diarrhea. Under normal conditions, client's fluid intake should be 2.5 to 3 L daily, and client should follow a balanced diet with adequate salt intake.
- Check urine-specific gravity and report levels below 1.005, which may indicate diabetes insipidus.
- Monitor glucose levels closely in clients with diabetes because lithium alters glucose tolerance.
- Perform outpatient follow-up monitoring of thyroid and renal functions every 6 to 12 months. Palpate thyroid to check for enlargement.
- Tell client to take drug with plenty of water and after meals to minimize GI upset.
- Emphasize importance of having regular blood tests to determine drug levels; even slightly high values can be dangerous.
- Warn client and caregivers to expect transient nausea, large amounts of urine, thirst, and discomfort during first few days of therapy and to watch for evidence of toxicity (diarrhea, vomiting, tremor, drowsiness, muscle weakness, incoordination); instruct client to withhold one dose and call prescriber if signs and symptoms of toxicity appear, but warn the client not to stop drug abruptly.
- Warn client to avoid hazardous activities that require alertness and good psychomotor coordination until the drug's CNS effects are known.
- Tell client not to switch brands or take other prescription or OTC drugs without prescriber's guidance.
- Tell client to wear or carry medical identification at all times.

oxcarbazepine (Trileptal)

Drug Class
Anticonvulsant

Indications and Dosage

Bipolar disorder (*see p. 388*)	*Adults:* Initially, 300 mg PO bid, increasing dose to 1200 mg bid.

Half-life

Drug: 2 hours
Active metabolite: 9 hours

Common Adverse Reactions

CNS: Abnormal gait, ataxia, dizziness, fatigue, headache, somnolence, tremor, vertigo
EENT: Abnormal vision, diplopia, nystagmus
GI: Abdominal pain, nausea, vomiting, rectal hemorrhage
Respiratory: Upper respiratory tract infection

Key Interactions

Decreased drug effectiveness with: Phenytoin, carbamazepine, phenobarbital, valproic acid, verapamil
Decreased level of co-administered drug with: Felodipine, hormonal contraceptives
Increased CNS effects with: Alcohol

Nursing Considerations

- Administer the drug without regard to food or meals.
- Shake oral suspension well. Mix suspension with water or help client swallow suspension directly from syringe.
- Alert: Between 25 and 30% of clients with history of hypersensitivity reaction to carbamazepine develop hypersensitivities to oxcarbazepine. Ask client about carbamazepine hypersensitivity and stop drug immediately if signs or symptoms of hypersensitivity occur.
- Watch for signs and symptoms of hyponatremia, including nausea, malaise, headache, lethargy, confusion, and decreased sensation.

- Monitor sodium level in clients receiving oxcarbazepine for maintenance treatment, especially those receiving other therapies that may decrease sodium levels.
- Alert: Multiorgan hypersensitivity reactions may occur. Tell client to report fever and swollen lymph nodes to prescriber. Serious skin reactions, including Stevens-Johnson syndrome and toxic epidermal necrosis, can occur. Advise client to immediately report skin rashes to prescriber.
- Caution client to avoid driving and other potentially hazardous activities that require mental alertness until effects of drug are known.

topiramate (Topamax)

Drug Class
Anticonvulsant

Indications and Dosage

Bipolar disorder (off-label use; *see p. 388*)	*Adults:* Initially, 25 to 50 mg/day, increasing to a target range of 100 to 200 mg/day.

Half-life
21 hours

Common Adverse Reactions
CNS: Ataxia, confusion, difficulty with memory, dizziness, fatigue, nervousness, paresthesia, psychomotor slowing, somnolence, speech disorders, tremor, generalized tonic-clonic seizures, suicide attempts
EENT: Abnormal vision, diplopia, nystagmus
GI: Anorexia, nausea
Hematologic: Leukopenia
Metabolic: Weight loss
Respiratory: Upper respiratory tract infection

Key Interactions

Decreased drug level with: Carbamazepine, valproic acid, phenytoin

Risk for renal calculi formation with: Carbonic anhydrase inhibitors (acetazolamide, dichlorphenamide)

Increased CNS depression with: CNS depressants, alcohol

Decreased effect of co-administered drug with: Hormonal contraceptives

Nursing Considerations

• Administer drug without regard to food or meals. Avoid crushing or breaking tablets because this drug has a bitter taste.

• Have client swallow capsules whole or carefully open and sprinkle contents on a teaspoonful of soft food. Tell client to swallow immediately without chewing.

• Drug may infrequently cause oligohydrosis and hyperthermia. Monitor client closely, especially in hot weather.

• Measure baseline and periodic bicarbonate levels. If metabolic acidosis develops and persists, consider reducing the dose, gradually stopping the drug, or alkali treatment.

• Alert: Stop drug if client experiences acute myopia and secondary angle-closure glaucoma.

• Alert: Do not confuse Topamax with Toprol-XL, Tegretol, or Tegretol-XR.

• Tell client to drink plenty of fluids during therapy to minimize risk of forming renal calculi (kidney stones).

• Advise client not to drive or operate hazardous machinery until CNS effects of drug are known. Drug can cause sleepiness, dizziness, confusion, and concentration problems. Tell women of childbearing age that drug may decrease effectiveness of hormonal contraceptives. Advise women using hormonal contraceptives to report change in menstrual patterns.

• Urge client to notify prescriber immediately if they experience changes in vision.

Antipsychotics

Overview

Primary Indications

Treatment of severe thought disorders such as schizophrenia (*see p. 488*)

Other Indications

Acute and chronic confusion that commonly accompanies psychoses, extreme aggression, and dementia (*see p. 338*)

Signs and Symptoms

Symptoms indicating a need for antipsychotic agents include disorganized speech and behavior, flat or inappropriate affect, delusions, hallucinations, and catatonia.

Major Categories

- Typical (traditional) antipsychotics: Block dopamine receptors in the brain, thus altering the release and turnover of dopamine.
  - chlorpromazine (*see p. 240*)
  - fluphenazine (*see p. 246*)
  - haloperidol (*see p. 248*)

- loxapine (*see p. 250*)
- perphenazine (*see p. 254*)
- thioridazine (*see p. 260*)
- thiothixene (*see p. 262*)
- trifluoperazine (*see p. 264*)
- Atypical antipsychotics: Simultaneous blocking of dopamine and serotonin receptors; may account for their increased efficacy in improving negative symptoms
  - aripiprazole (*see p. 238*)
  - clozapine (*see p. 242*)
  - olanzapine (*see p. 251*)
  - quetiapine (*see p. 256*)
  - risperidone (*see p. 258*)
  - symbyax
  - ziprasidone (*see p. 266*)

Key Drug Monographs

aripiprazole (Abilify)

Drug Class

Atypical antipsychotic

Indications and Dosage

Schizophrenia (*see p. 488*)	*Adults*: Initially, 10 to 15 mg PO daily, increasing to a maximum daily dose of 30 mg if needed, after at least 2 weeks.
Bipolar mania including manic and mixed episodes	*Adults*: Initially, 30 mg PO once daily, possibly reducing dose to 15 mg daily based on client tolerance.
Agitation associated with phrenia or bipolar I disorder, mixed or manic	*Adults*: 5.25 to 15 mg by deep schizo-intramuscular (IM) injection; recommended dose is 9.75 mg; possible second dose after 2 hours, if needed. Safety of giving more frequently than every 2 hours or a total daily dose more than 30 mg is unknown. Switch to oral form as soon as possible.

Half-life

Approximately 75 hours in clients with normal metabolism; 6 days in client who cannot metabolize the drug through CYP2D6

Common Adverse Reactions

Central nervous system (CNS): Headache, anxiety, insomnia, light-headedness, somnolence, akathisia, increased suicide risk, neuroleptic malignant syndrome (NMS), seizures, suicidal thoughts, tardive dyskinesia

Cardiovascular (CV): Bradycardia

Gastrointestinal (GI): Nausea, vomiting, constipation, anorexia, dry mouth

Key Interactions

Increased antihypertensive effect with: Antihypertensives

Decreased drug level with: Carbamazepine and other CYP3A4 inducers

Increased risk of serious toxic effects with: Ketoconazole and other CYP3A4 inhibitors

Increased risk of drug toxicity with: Potential CYP2D6 inhibitors (fluoxetine, paroxetine, quinidine)

Increased drug level with: Grapefruit juice

Increased CNS effects with: Alcohol

Nursing Considerations

- Administer the smallest dose for the shortest time; periodically reevaluate for need for continuing. Do not administer intravenous (IV) or subcutaneously.
- Give drug without regard to meals.
- Warn client not to take the drug with grapefruit juice.
- Advise client that improvement will be gradual over several weeks.
- Alert: NMS may occur. Monitor client for hyperpyrexia, muscle rigidity, altered mental status, irregular pulse or blood pressure, tachycardia, diaphoresis, and cardiac dysrhythmias; if signs and symptoms of NMS occur, immediately stop drug and notify prescriber.
- Monitor client for signs and symptoms of tardive dyskinesia. The elderly, especially women, are at highest risk of developing this adverse effect.

- Alert: Monitor clients with diabetes regularly for signs and symptoms of hyperglycemia. Obtain baseline and periodic fasting blood glucose levels.
- Alert: Monitor for symptoms of metabolic syndrome (significant weight gain and increased body mass index, hypertension, hyperglycemia, hypercholesterolemia, and hypertriglyceridemia).
- Give prescriptions only for small quantities of drug to reduce risk of overdose.
- Substitute the oral solution on a milligram-by-milligram basis for the 5-, 10-, 15-, or 20-mg tablets, up to 25 mg. Give 25 mg of solution to clients taking 30-mg tablets. Tell clients to store solution in refrigerator.
- Advise client to use caution while driving or operating hazardous machinery, because the drug may impair judgment, thinking, or motor skills.

chlorpromazine

Drug Class
Typical antipsychotic

Indications and Dosage

Psychosis, mania	*Adults:* For hospitalized clients with acute disease, 25 mg IM, with an additional 24 to 50 mg IM in 1 hour if needed, increasing over several days to 400 mg every 4 to 6 hours and switching to oral therapy as soon as possible. Alternatively, 25 mg PO three times daily (tid) initially, gradually increasing to 400 mg daily in divided doses. For outpatients, 30 to 75 mg daily in two to four divided doses, increasing dosage by 20 to 50 mg twice weekly until symptoms are controlled. *Children 6 months and older:* 0.55 mg/kg PO every 4 to 6 hours or IM every 6 to 8 hours; or 1.1 mg/kg. Maximum IM dose in children younger than 5 years old or who weigh less than 22.7 kg (50 lb) is 40 mg. Maximum IM dose in children 5 to 12 years old or who weigh 22.7 to 45.4 kg (50 to 100 lb) is 75 mg.

Half-life

20 to 24 hours

Common Adverse Effects

CNS: Extrapyramidal reactions, sedation, tardive dyskinesia, pseudoparkinsonism, NMS, seizures

CV: Orthostatic hypotension, tachycardia

GI: Dry mouth, constipation, nausea

Genitourinary (GU): Urine retention

Hematologic: Leukopenia, agranulocytosis, aplastic anemia, thrombocytopenia

Skin: Mild photosensitivity reactions, pain at IM injection site

Key Interactions

Decreased drug absorption with: Antacids

Increased anticholinergic activity with: Anticholinergics such as tricyclic antidepressants, antiparkinsonian drugs

Decreased seizure threshold with: Anticonvulsants

Decreased antihypertensive effect with: Centrally acting antihypertensives

Increased CNS depression with: CNS depressants, alcohol

Increased CNS sedation with: Meperidine

Increased risk for severe reactions with: Electroconvulsive therapy, insulin

Increased levels of both drugs with: Propranolol

Decreased anticoagulant effects with: Warfarin

Risk for photosensitivity reactions with: St. John's wort

Nursing Considerations

- Obtain baseline blood pressure measurements before therapy and monitor blood pressure regularly. Watch for orthostatic hypotension, especially with parenteral administration. Monitor blood pressure before and after IM administration; keep client supine for 1 hour afterward and have client rise slowly.
- Alert: Wear gloves when preparing solutions and avoid contact with skin and clothing. Oral liquid and parenteral forms can cause contact dermatitis.

- Slight yellowing of injection or concentrate is common and doesn't affect potency. Discard markedly discolored solutions.
- Protect liquid concentrate from light. Dilute with fruit juice, milk, or semisolid food just before giving.
- Give deep IM only in upper outer quadrant of buttocks. Consider giving injection by Z-track method. Massage slowly afterward to prevent sterile abscess. Injection stings. Rotate injection sites.
- Monitor clients for tardive dyskinesia, which may occur after prolonged use. It may not appear until months or years later and may disappear spontaneously or persist for life, despite stopping drug.
- After abrupt withdrawal of long-term therapy, monitor for gastritis, nausea, vomiting, dizziness, or tremor.
- Alert: Watch for evidence of NMS (extrapyramidal effects, hyperthermia, autonomic disturbance), which is rare but usually fatal.
- If jaundice, symptoms of blood dyscrasia (fever, sore throat, infection, cellulitis, weakness), or persistent (longer than a few hours) extrapyramidal reactions develop, or if such reactions occur in children or pregnant women, withhold dose and notify prescriber.
- Alert: Don't withdraw drug abruptly unless required by severe adverse reactions.
- Alert: Don't confuse chlorpromazine with clomipramine or with chlorpropamide, a hypoglycemic.
- Advise clients receiving drug by any method other than by mouth to remain lying down for 1 hour afterward and to rise slowly.
- Caution clients to avoid alcohol while taking drug.
- Tell client to wear sunblock and protective clothing to avoid oversensitivity to the sun. This drug is more likely to cause sun sensitivity than other drugs in its class.
- Suggest the use of sugarless gum or hard candy to relieve dry mouth.

clozapine (Clozaril, FazaClo)

Drug Class

Atypical antipsychotic

Indications and Dosage

Schizophrenia (severely ill clients unresponsive to other therapies *see p. 488*); risk reduction of recurrent suicidal behavior in schizophrenia or schizoaffective disorders	*Adults*: Initially, 12.5 mg PO once daily or bid (if using orally disintegrating tablet, cut in half and discard the unused half), adjusting dose upward by 25 to 50 mg daily (if tolerated) to 300 to 450 mg daily by end of 2 weeks. Individual dosage is based on response, client tolerance, and adverse reactions. Subsequent dosage shouldn't be increased more than once or twice weekly and shouldn't exceed 50- to 100-mg increments. Maximum daily dose is 900 mg.

Half-life

Appears proportional to dose and may range from 8 to 12 hours

Common Adverse Reactions

CNS: Drowsiness, sedation, dizziness, vertigo, headache, seizures
CV: Tachycardia, cardiomyopathy, myocarditis, pulmonary embolism, cardiac arrest
GI: Constipation, excessive salivation
Hematologic: Leukopenia, agranulocytosis, granulocytopenia, eosinophilia
Metabolic: Hyperglycemia
Respiratory: Respiratory arrest

Key Interactions

Increased anticholinergic effects with: Anticholinergics
Increased hypotensive effects with: Antihypertensives
Increased risk of sedation, cardiac and respiratory arrest with: Benzodiazepines
Bone marrow toxicity with: Bone marrow suppressants
Increased drug level and risk for toxicity with: Citalopram, fluoroquinolones, fluoxetine, fluvoxamine, paroxetine, sertraline, ritonavir
Increased risk for additive effects with: Psychoactive drugs
Increased levels of co-administered drug with: Digoxin, other highly protein-bound drugs, warfarin
Risk for decreased drug level with: Phenytoin, St. John's wort, smoking
Increased CNS depression with: Alcohol

Nursing Considerations

- Alert: Drug carries significant risk of agranulocytosis. If possible, give client at least two trials of standard antipsychotic before starting clozapine.
- Obtain baseline white blood cell count (WBC) and differential counts before clozapine therapy. Baseline WBC count must be at least $3500/mm^3$, and baseline absolute neutrophil count (ANC) must be at least $2000/mm^3$. Monitor WBC and ANC values weekly for at least 4 weeks after stopping the drug, regardless of the frequency of monitoring when therapy stopped.
- During the first 6 months of therapy, monitor client weekly and dispense no more than a 1-week supply of the drug. If client maintains acceptable WBC ($3500/mm^3$ or higher) and ANC ($2000/mm^3$ or higher) values during the first 6 months of continuous therapy, reduce monitoring to every other week. After 6 months of every-other-week monitoring without interruption by leukopenia, reduce frequency of monitoring WBC and ANC to monthly.
- If WBC count drops below $3500/mm^3$ after therapy begins or drops substantially from baseline, monitor client closely for signs and symptoms of infection. If WBC count is 3000 to $3500/mm^3$ and granulocyte count is above $1500 mm^3$, perform WBC and differential count twice weekly. If WBC count drops to $2000/mm^3$ to $3000/mm^3$ or granulocyte count drops to $1000/mm^3$ to $1500/mm^3$, interrupt therapy and notify prescriber. Monitor WBC and differential daily until WBC exceeds $3000/mm^3$ and ANC exceeds $1500/mm^3$, and monitor client for signs and symptoms of infection.
- Continue monitoring WBC and differential counts twice weekly until WBC count exceeds $3500/mm^3$ and ANC exceeds $2000/mm^3$. Then, restart therapy with weekly monitoring for 1 year before returning to the usual monitoring schedule of every 2 weeks for 6 months and then every 4 weeks.
- If WBC count drops below $2000/mm^3$ and granulocyte count drops below $1000/mm^3$, anticipate need for protective isolation. Client may need bone marrow aspiration to assess bone marrow function. Future clozapine therapy is contraindicated.

- Tell client about the need for weekly blood tests to check for blood-cell deficiency. Advise client to report flu-like symptoms, fever, sore throat, lethargy, malaise, or other signs of infection.
- Alert: Drug increases risk of fatal myocarditis, especially during, but not limited to, the first month of therapy. In clients with suspected myocarditis (unexplained fatigue, dyspnea, tachypnea, chest pain, tachycardia, fever, palpitations, and other signs or symptoms of heart failure or ECG abnormalities, such as ST-T wave abnormalities or arrhythmias), stop therapy immediately and do not restart.
- Monitor fasting blood glucose levels as a baseline and periodically because drug may cause hyperglycemia. Monitor clients with diabetes regularly.
- Alert: Monitor client for metabolic syndrome, which includes symptoms of significant weight gain and increased body mass index, hypertension, hyperglycemia, hypercholesterolemia, and hypertriglyceridemia.
- Monitor for signs and symptoms of cardiomyopathy.
- Be aware that some clients experience transient fever higher than 100.4°F (38.0°C), especially in the first 3 weeks of therapy. Monitor these clients closely.
- After abrupt withdrawal of long-term therapy, abrupt recurrence of psychosis is possible.
- If therapy must be stopped, withdraw drug gradually over 1 or 2 weeks. If changes in medical condition (including development of leukopenia) require that drug be stopped immediately, monitor client closely for recurrence of psychosis.
- If reinstating therapy in a client who has withdrawn from the drug, follow usual guidelines for dosage increase. Re-exposure to drug may increase severity and risk of adverse reactions. If therapy was stopped because WBC counts were below $2000/mm^3$ or granulocyte counts were below $1000/mm^3$, do not restart.
- Alert: Do not confuse clozapine with clonidine, clofazimine, or Klonopin.
- Warn client to avoid hazardous activities that require alertness and good coordination while taking drug. Urge client to rise slowly to avoid dizziness.

- Tell client to check with prescriber before taking alcohol or non-prescription drugs; advise that smoking may decrease the effectiveness of the drug.

fluphenazine decanoate (Modecate, Prolixin Decanoate); fluphenazine hydrochloride (Prolixin, Prolixin Concentrate)

Drug Class
Typical antipsychotic

Indications and Dosage

Psychosis	*Adults*: Initially, 0.5 to 10 mg fluphenazine hydrochloride PO daily in divided doses every 6 to 8 hours, possibly increasing cautiously to 20 mg to a maintenance dose of 1 to 5 mg PO daily. IM doses are one third to one half of PO doses. Usual IM dose is 1.25 mg. Give more than 10 mg daily with caution. Alternatively, 12.5 to 25 mg of fluphenazine decanoate IM or subcutaneously every 1 to 6 weeks for a maintenance dose of 25 to 100 mg, as needed (p.r.n.). *Elderly clients*: 1 to 2.5 mg fluphenazine hydrochloride PO daily.

Half-life
Hydrochloride: 15 hours
Decanoate: 7 to 10 days

Common Adverse Reactions
CNS: Extrapyramidal reactions, tardive dyskinesia, pseudoparkinsonism, seizures, NMS
EENT: Blurred vision
GI: Dry mouth, constipation
GU: Urine retention
Hematologic: Leukopenia, agranulocytosis, aplastic anemia, thrombocytopenia
Skin: Mild photosensitivity reactions

Key Interactions

Decreased absorption with: Antacids
Increased anticholinergic effects with: Anticholinergics
Increased neurologic adverse reactions with: Barbiturates, lithium
Possible decreased antihypertensive effect with: Centrally acting antihypertensives
Increased CNS depression with: CNS depressants, alcohol
Increased risk for photosensitivity with: St. John's wort, sun exposure

Nursing Considerations

- Alert: Be aware that Prolixin Concentrate and Permitil Concentrate are 10 times more concentrated than Prolixin elixir (5 mg/mL versus 0.5 mg/mL). Check dosage order carefully.
- Alert: Wear gloves when preparing solutions with oral liquid and parenteral forms; avoid contact with skin and clothing to reduce risk of contact dermatitis.
- Protect drug from light. Slight yellowing of injection solution or concentrate is common and doesn't affect potency. Discard markedly discolored solutions.
- Dilute liquid concentrate with water, fruit juice, milk, or semisolid food just before administration.
- For long-acting form (decanoate), which is an oil preparation, use a dry needle of at least 21 G. Allow 24 to 96 hours for onset of action. Note and report to prescriber adverse reactions in clients taking this form.
- Monitor client for tardive dyskinesia, which may occur after prolonged use. It may not appear until months or years later and may disappear spontaneously or persist for life, despite ending use of the drug.
- Alert: Watch for signs and symptoms of NMS (extrapyramidal effects, hyperthermia, autonomic disturbance), which is rare but usually fatal. NMS may not be related to length of drug use or type of neuroleptic; more than 60% of affected clients are men.
- Withhold dose and notify prescriber if client (especially children or pregnant women) develops signs or symptoms of blood dyscrasia (fever, sore throat, infection, cellulitis, weakness) or extrapyramidal reactions persisting longer than a few hours.

- Don't withdraw drug abruptly unless serious adverse reactions occur.
- Alert: Prolixin may contain tartrazine.
- Warn client to avoid activities that require alertness and physical coordination until effects of drug are known; warn client to avoid alcohol while using the drug.
- Tell client to relieve dry mouth with sugarless gum or hard candy.
- Advise client to wear sunblock and protective clothing to avoid sensitivity to the sun.
- Tell client that drug may discolor urine.

haloperidol (Haldol), haloperidol decanoate (Haldol Decanoate), haloperidol lactate (Haldol, Haldol Concentrate, Haloperidol Intensol)

Drug Class
Typical antipsychotic

Indications and Dosage

Psychotic disorders	*Adults and children older than 12 years:* Dosage varies; initially, 0.5 to 5 mg PO bid or tid; alternatively, 2 to 5 mg IM lactate every 4 to 8 hours, although hourly administration may be needed until control is obtained. Maximum, 100 mg PO daily. *Children 3 to 12 years old who weigh 15 to 40 kg (33 to 88 lb):* Initially, 0.5 mg PO daily divided bid or tid, possibly increasing dose by 0.5 mg at 5- to 7-day intervals, depending on therapeutic response and client tolerance. Maintenance dose, 0.05 to 0.15 mg/kg PO daily given in two to three divided doses. Severely disturbed children may need higher doses.
Chronic psychosis requiring prolonged therapy	*Adults:* 50 to 100 mg IM decanoate every 4 weeks.
Nonpsychotic behavior disorders	*Children 3 to 12 years old:* 0.05 to 0.075 mg/kg PO daily, in two or three divided doses to a maximum dose of 6 mg daily.

| Tourette syndrome | *Adults*: 0.5 to 5 mg PO bid, tid, or p.r.n.
Children 3 to 12 years old: 0.05 to 0.075 mg/kg PO daily, in two or three divided doses.
Elderly clients: 0.5 to 2 mg PO bid or tid; increase gradually, p.r.n. |
| Delirium | *Adults*: 1 to 2 mg IV lactate every 2 to 4 hours. Severely agitated clients may require higher doses.
Elderly clients: 0.25 to 0.5 mg IV every 4 hours. |

Half-life

Oral form: 24 hours
IM form: 21 hours

Common Adverse Reactions

CNS: Severe extrapyramidal reactions, tardive dyskinesia, NMS, seizures
CV: Torsades de pointes with IV use
GI: Dry mouth, anorexia, constipation, diarrhea
GU: Urine retention, menstrual irregularities, priapism
Hematologic: Leukopenia

Key Interactions

Increased anticholinergic effects with: Anticholinergics
Increased drug level with: Azole antifungals, buspirone, macrolides
Decreased drug level with: Carbamazepine, rifampin
Increased CNS depression with: CNS depressants, alcohol
Increased risk for lethargy and confusion with: Lithium
Increased risk for dementia with: Methyldopa

Nursing Considerations

- Protect drug from light. Slight yellowing of injection solution or concentrate is common and does not affect potency. Discard very discolored solutions.
- When switching from tablets to decanoate injection, give 10 to 15 times the oral dose once a month (maximum 100 mg).
- Dilute oral dose with water or beverage (eg, orange juice, apple juice, tomato juice, cola) immediately before administration.

- Alert: Do not give decanoate form intravenously. Only the lactate form can be given intravenously.
- Monitor for tardive dyskinesia, which may occur after prolonged use. It may not appear until months or years later and may disappear spontaneously or persist for life, despite ending use of drug.
- Alert: Watch for signs and symptoms of NMS (extrapyramidal effects, hyperthermia, autonomic disturbance), which is rare but usually fatal.
- Do not withdraw drug abruptly unless severe adverse reactions occur.
- Alert: Do not confuse Haldol with Halcion or Halog; be aware that Haldol may contain tartrazine.
- Although this drug is the least sedating of the antipsychotics, warn client to avoid activities that require alertness and physical coordination until effects of drug are known. Also warn client to avoid alcohol during therapy.
- Tell client to relieve dry mouth with sugarless gum or hard candy.

loxapine succinate (Loxitane)

Drug Class
Typical antipsychotic

Indications and Dosage

Psychotic disorders	*Adults*: 10 mg PO bid to qid, rapidly increasing to 60 to 100 mg PO daily for most clients; dosage varies. *Elderly clients*: Initially, 5 mg PO bid.

Half-life
8 hours

Common Adverse Reactions
CNS: Extrapyramidal reactions, sedation, tardive dyskinesia, NMS, seizures

CV: Orthostatic hypotension
EENT: Blurred vision
GI: Dry mouth, constipation, nausea
GU: Urine retention
Hematologic: Leukopenia, agranulocytosis, thrombocytopenia

Key Interactions

Increased risk for CNS depression with: CNS depressants, alcohol
Increased anticholinergic effects with: Anticholinergics
Inhibition of vasopressor effect of co-administered drug with: Epinephrine

Nursing Considerations

- Obtain baseline blood pressure measurements before starting therapy and monitor pressure regularly.
- Monitor client for tardive dyskinesia, which may occur after prolonged use. It may not appear until months or years later and may disappear spontaneously or persist for life, despite ending use of drug.
- Alert: Watch for evidence of NMS (extrapyramidal effects, hyperthermia, autonomic disturbance), a rare but deadly disorder.
- Warn client to avoid activities that require alertness and physical coordination until effects of drug are known. Also urge client to avoid alcohol.
- Advise client to report bruising, fever, or sore throat immediately.
- Warn client to get up slowly to avoid dizziness upon standing quickly.
- Tell client to relieve dry mouth with sugarless gum or hard candy.
- Recommend periodic eye examinations.

olanzapine (Zyprexa, Zyprexa Zydis)

Drug Class

Atypical antipsychotic

Indications and Dosage

Schizophrenia (*see p. 488*)	*Adults*: Initially, 5 to 10 mg PO once daily with the goal of 10 mg daily within several days of starting therapy. Safety of dosages greater than 20 mg daily has not been established.
Acute mania linked to bipolar I disorder (short-term; *see p. 388*)	*Adults*: Initially, 10 to 15 mg PO daily, increasing dosage p.r.n. in 5-mg daily increments at intervals of 24 hours or more to a maximum dose of 20 mg PO daily for a duration of 3 to 4 weeks.
Acute mania linked to bipolar I disorder (short-term with lithium or valproate)	*Adults*: 10 mg PO once daily (dosage range is 5 to 20 mg daily) for a duration of 6 weeks.
Bipolar I disorder (long-term)	*Adults:* 5 to 20 mg PO daily.
Bipolar mania (adjunct to lithium or valproate)	*Adults*: 10 mg PO daily.
Agitation from schizophrenia and bipolar I mania	*Adults*: 10 mg IM (range 2.5 to 10 mg) with subsequent doses of up to 10 mg given 2 hours after the first dose or 4 hours after the second dose, up to 30 mg IM daily. If maintenance therapy is required, convert client to 5 to 20 mg PO daily.

Half-life

21 to 54 hours

Common Adverse Reactions

CNS: Somnolence, insomnia, parkinsonism, dizziness, NMS, suicide attempt
CV: Orthostatic hypotension
GI: Constipation, dry mouth, dyspepsia, weight gain
Hematologic: Leukopenia
Metabolic: Hyperglycemia, fever

Key Interactions

Increased risk for hypotension with: Antihypertensives, alcohol, benzodiazepines

Increased drug clearance with: Carbamazepine, omeprazole, rifampin, smoking

Increased drug level with: Ciproflaxin, fluoxetine

Increased risk for toxicity with: Fluvoxamine

Increased risk for CNS depression with: CNS depressants, alcohol, diazepam

Increased risk for drug antagonism with: Levodopa, dopamine agonists

Decreased drug level with: St. John's wort

Nursing Considerations

- Administer oral form without regard to food.
- To reconstitute for IM injection, dissolve contents of one vial with 2.1 mL sterile water for injection to yield a clear yellow solution (5 mg/mL). Store at room temperature and administer within 1 hour of reconstitution. Discard any unused solution.
- Discard IM solution if particulate matter and discoloration occur.
- Monitor client for abnormal body temperature regulation, especially if they exercise, are exposed to extreme heat, take anticholinergics, or are dehydrated.
- Obtain baseline and periodic liver function test results.
- Monitor for weight gain.
- Alert: Watch for evidence of NMS (hyperpyrexia, muscle rigidity, altered mental status, autonomic instability), which is rare but usually fatal. Stop drug immediately; monitor and treat client as needed.
- Monitor for tardive dyskinesia, which may occur after prolonged use. It may not appear until months or years later and may disappear spontaneously or persist for life, despite ending use of drug.
- Periodically reevaluate the long-term usefulness of olanzapine.
- Monitor client after IM injection. Clients who feel dizzy or drowsy after IM injection should remain recumbent until they can be assessed for orthostatic hypotension and bradycardia; clients should rest until the feeling passes.

- Alert: Do not confuse olanzapine with olsalazine or Zyprexa with Zyrtec.
- Caution client to avoid hazardous tasks until full effects of drug are known and to avoid alcohol.
- Tell client to rise slowly to avoid dizziness upon standing up quickly.
- Warn client against exposure to extreme heat; drug may impair body's ability to reduce temperature.
- Inform client that they may gain weight.

perphenazine (Trilafon)

Drug Class
Typical antipsychotic

Indications and Dosage

Psychosis (nonhospitalized clients)	*Adults and children older than 12 years*: Initially, 4 to 8 mg PO tid, reducing dosage as soon as possible to minimum effective dose.
Psychosis (hospitalized clients)	*Adults and children older than 12 years*: Initially, 8 to 16 mg PO bid, tid, or qid, increasing to 64 mg daily, p.r.n.; alternatively, 5 to 10 mg IM every 6 hours, p.r.n. Maximum dose, 30 mg.

Half-life
9 to 12 hours

Common Adverse Reactions
CNS: Extrapyramidal reactions, tardive dyskinesia, seizures, NMS
CV: Orthostatic hypotension
EENT: Blurred vision
GI: Dry mouth, constipation
GU: Urine retention
Hematologic: Leukopenia, agranulocytosis, thrombocytopenia
Skin: Mild photosensitivity reactions

Key Interactions

Decreased drug absorption with: Antacids

Decreased drug effect with: Barbiturates

Increased drug level with: Fluoxetine, paroxetine, sertraline, tricyclic antidepressants

Increased CNS depression with: CNS depressants, alcohol

Increased neurologic adverse effects with: Lithium

Increased risk for photosensitivity with: St. John's wort, sun exposure

Nursing Considerations

- Obtain baseline blood pressure measurements before starting therapy; monitor pressure regularly. Watch for orthostatic hypotension, especially with parenteral administration. Keep client supine for 1 hour after giving drug; tell client to change positions slowly.
- Protect drug from light. Slight yellowing of injection or concentrate is common and does not affect potency. Discard markedly discolored solutions.
- Wear gloves when preparing liquid forms to prevent contact dermatitis; keep drug away from skin and clothes.
- Dilute liquid concentrate with fruit juice, milk, carbonated beverage, or semisolid food just before giving. Do not use colas, black coffee, grape juice, apple juice, or tea, because turbidity or precipitation may result.
- Administer by deep IM injection only in upper outer quadrant of buttocks. Massage slowly afterward to prevent sterile abscess. Injection may sting.
- Monitor for tardive dyskinesia, which may occur after prolonged use. It may not appear until months or years later, and it may disappear spontaneously or persist for life, despite ending use of drug.
- Alert: Watch for evidence of NMS (extrapyramidal effects, hyperthermia, autonomic disturbance), which is rare but deadly.
- Monitor therapy with weekly bilirubin levels during first month, periodic blood tests (CBC tests and liver function tests), and ophthalmic tests (long-term use).

- Withhold dose and notify prescriber if jaundice, symptoms of blood dyscrasia (fever, sore throat, infection, cellulitis, weakness), or persistent extrapyramidal reactions (longer than a few hours) develop.
- Do not withdraw drug abruptly unless severe adverse reactions occur.
- Tell client which beverages may be used with oral concentrate.
- Warn client to avoid activities that require alertness or phyical coordination until effects of drug are known. Also advise client to avoid alcohol.
- Tell client to wear sunblock and protective clothing to avoid oversensitivity to the sun.
- Advise client to relieve dry mouth with sugarless gum or hard candy.

quetiapine fumarate (Seroquel)

Drug Class
Atypical antipsychotic

Indications and Dosage

Depression secondary to bipolar disorder	*Adults*: Give drug PO once daily at bedtime to reach 300 mg/day by day 4. Day 1, give 50 mg; day 2, give 100 mg; day 3, give 200 mg; day 4, give 300 mg.
Psychotic symptom management	*Adults*: Initially, 25 mg PO bid, increasing in increments of 25 to 50 mg bid or tid on days 2 and 3, as tolerated to a target range of 300 to 400 mg daily divided into two or three doses by day 4. *Elderly clients*: Give lower dosages, adjust more slowly, and monitor client carefully in first dosing period.
Acute manic episodes (short-term with bipolar I disorder *see p. 388*; monotherapy or adjunct therapy with lithium or divalproex)	*Adults*: Initially, 50 mg PO bid, increasing dosages in increments of 100 mg daily in two divided doses up to 200 mg PO bid on day 4; usual dose of 400 to 800 mg daily. *Elderly clients:* Give lower dosages, adjust more slowly, and monitor client carefully in first dosing period.

Half-life
6 hours

Common Adverse Reactions
CNS: Dizziness, headache, somnolence, NMS, seizures
CV: Orthostatic hypotension
Hematologic: Leukopenia
Metabolic: Weight gain, hyperglycemia

Key Interactions
Increased antihypertensive effect with: Antihypertensives
Increased drug clearance with: Carbamazepine, glucocorticoids, phenobarbital, phenytoin, rifampin, thioridazine
Increased CNS effects with: CNS depressants, alcohol, lorazepam
Risk for antagonism of co-administered drug with: Dopamine agonists, levodopa
Decreased drug clearance with: Erythromycin, fluconazole, itraconazole, ketoconazole

Nursing Considerations
- Administer drug without regard to food or meals.
- Give client the lowest appropriate quantity of drug to reduce risk of overdose.
- Alert: Watch for evidence of NMS (extrapyramidal effects, hyperthermia, autonomic disturbance), which is rare but deadly.
- Monitor client for tardive dyskinesia, which may occur after prolonged use. It may not appear until months or years later and may disappear spontaneously or persist for life, despite ending use of drug.
- Assess clients with diabetes regularly; hyperglycemia may occur.
- Monitor client for weight gain.
- Advise client about risk of dizziness upon standing up quickly. The risk is greatest during the 3- to 5-day period of first dosage adjustment, when resuming treatment, and when increasing dosages.
- Tell client to avoid becoming overheated or dehydrated.
- Warn client to avoid activities that require mental alertness until effects of drug are known, especially during first dosage adjustment or dosage increases.

- Tell client to notify prescriber about other prescription or over-the-counter drugs they are taking or plan to take.
- Urge client to avoid alcohol while taking drug.

risperidone (Risperdal, Risperdal Consta, Risperdal M-Tab)

Drug Class
Atypical antipsychotic

Indications and Dosage

Schizophrenia (short-term treatment; *see p. 488*)	*Adults*: Initially, 1 mg PO bid, increasing by 1 mg bid on days 2 and 3 of treatment to a target dose of 3 mg bid. Alternatively, 1 mg PO on day 1, increase to 2 mg once daily on day 2, and 4 mg once daily on day 3, waiting at least 1 week before adjusting dosage further, with adjustments of 1 to 2 mg. Maximum, 8 mg daily.
Schizophrenia (12-week therapy)	*Adults*: Establishment of tolerance to oral risperidone, then 25 mg deep IM gluteal injection every 2 weeks; alternating injections between the two buttocks. Adjust dose no more frequently than every 4 weeks. Maximum, 50 mg IM every 2 weeks. Continue oral antipsychotic for 3 weeks after first IM injection. Then stop oral therapy.
Schizophrenia relapse delay	*Adults*: Initially, 1 mg PO on day 1, increasing to 2 mg once daily on day 2, and 4 mg once daily on day 3; dosage range of 2 to 8 mg daily.
Acute mania or mixed episodes from bipolar I disorder (monotherapy or combination therapy with lithium or valproate; *see p. 388* 3-week treatment)	*Adults*: 2 to 3 mg PO once daily, adjusting dose by 1 mg daily to a range of 1 to 6 mg daily.

Autistic disorder (for irritability, including aggression, self-injury, and temper tantrums)	*Adolescents and children 5 years and older who weigh at least 20 kg (44 lb)*: Initially, 0.5 mg PO once daily or divided bid, increasing dose to 1 mg after 4 days with further dosage increases in 0.5 mg increments at intervals of at least 2 weeks. *Children 5 years and older who weigh less than 20 kg*: Initially, 0.25 mg PO once daily or divided bid, with dose increases to 0.5 mg after 4 days, with further increases in 0.25-mg increments at intervals of at least 2 weeks. Increase cautiously in children who weigh less than 15 kg (33 lbs).

Half-life

3 to 20 hours

Common Adverse Reactions

CNS: Akathisia, somnolence, dystonia, headache, insomnia, agitation, anxiety, pain, parkinsonism, NMS, suicide attempt
EENT: Rhinitis
GI: Constipation, nausea, vomiting, dyspepsia, abdominal pain
Metabolic: Weight gain, hyperglycemia

Key Interactions

Increased antihypotensive effect with: Antihypertensives
Increased drug clearance with: Carbamazepine
Decreased drug clearance and risk for toxicity with: Clozapine
Increased risk for adverse reactions with: Fluoxetine, paroxetine
Increased CNS depression with: CNS depressants, alcohol

Nursing Considerations

- Administer the drug without regard to food or meals.
- Alert: Obtain baseline blood pressure measurements before starting therapy; monitor regularly. Watch for orthostatic hypotension, especially during first dosage adjustment.
- Monitor clients for tardive dyskinesia, which may occur after prolonged use. It may not appear until months or years later and

may disappear spontaneously or persist for life, despite ending use of drug.

- Alert: Watch for evidence of the rare but potentially fatal NMS (extrapyramidal effects, hyperthermia, autonomic disturbance).
- Asses blood glucose levels regularly in clients with diabetes. Life-threatening hyperglycemia may occur.
- Periodically reevaluate drug's risks and benefits, especially during prolonged use.
- To reconstitute IM injection, inject premeasured diluent into vial and shake vigorously for at least 10 seconds. Suspension appears uniform, thick, and milky; particles are visible, but no dry particles remain. Drug should be used immediately, but may be refrigerated up to 6 hours of reconstitution. If more than 2 minutes pass before injection, shake vigorously again. See manufacturer's package insert for more detailed instructions.
- Refrigerate IM injection kit and protect it from light. Drug can be stored at temperatures less than 77°F (25°C) for no more than 7 days before administration.
- Continue oral therapy for the first 3 weeks of IM injection therapy until injections take effect; then stop oral therapy.
- Monitor client for weight gain.
- Alert: Do not confuse risperidone with reserpine.
- Warn client to avoid activities that require alertness until effects of drug are known. Also urge client to avoid alcohol.
- Instruct client to rise slowly, avoid hot showers, and use other precautions to avoid fainting when starting therapy.
- Advise client to use caution in hot weather to prevent heatstroke.

thioridazine hydrochloride

Drug Class

Typical antipsychotic

Indications and Dosage

Schizophrenia (clients nonresponsive to at least two other antipsychotic agents; *see p. 488*)	*Adults*: Initially, 50 to 100 mg PO tid, increasing gradually to 800 mg daily in divided doses, p.r.n. *Children 2 to 12 years old*: Initially, 0.5 mg/kg daily in divided doses, increasing gradually to optimal therapeutic effect and maximum dose of 3 mg/kg daily.

Half-life

20 to 40 hours

Common Adverse Reactions

CNS: Tardive dyskinesia, sedation, NMS
CV: Orthostatic hypotension, prolonged QTc interval, torsades de pointes
EENT: Ocular changes, blurred vision
GI: Dry mouth, constipation
GU: Urine retention
Hematologic: Transient leukopenia, agranulocytosis
Skin: Mild photosensitivity reactions

Key Interactions

Decreased drug absorption with: Antacids
Increased risk for arrhythmias with: Anti-arrhythmics (amiodarone, bretylium, disopyramide, dofetilide, procainamide, quinidine, sotalol), duloxetine, fluoxetine, fluvoxamine, paroxetine, pimozide, pindolol, propranolol, other drugs that inhibit CYP2D6 enzyme, quinolones
Decreased drug effect with: Barbiturates, lithium
Decreased antihypertensive effect with: Centrally acting antihypertensives
Increased CNS depression with: CNS depressants, alcohol
Increased risk for photosensitivity with: St. John's wort, sun exposure

Nursing Considerations

- Alert: Before therapy, obtain baseline ECG and potassium level. Clients with a QTc interval greater than 450 ms shouldn't receive drug; clients with a QTc interval greater than 500 ms should stop the drug.
- Alert: The drug is not used as first-line treatment of schizophrenia because of the risk of life-threatening adverse reactions. Different liquid formulations have different concentrations. Check dosage carefully.
- Wear gloves when preparing solutions with oral liquid and parenteral forms; avoid contact with skin and clothing to reduce risk of contact dermatitis.
- Dilute liquid concentrate with water or fruit juice just before giving.
- Shake suspension well before using.
- Monitor client for tardive dyskinesia, which may occur after prolonged use. It may not appear until months or years later and may disappear spontaneously or persist for life, despite ending use of drug.
- Alert: Watch for evidence of the rare but deadly NMS (extrapyramidal effects, hyperthermia, autonomic disturbance).
- Monitor periodic blood tests (CBC and liver function) and ophthalmic tests (long-term use).
- Withhold dose and notify prescriber if jaundice, blood dyscrasia (fever, sore throat, infection, cellulitis, weakness), or persistent extrapyramidal reactions develop.
- Alert: Do not confuse thioridazine with Thorazine.
- Warn client to avoid activities that require alertness and to watch for dizziness when standing quickly; encourage client to change positions slowly and avoid alcohol.
- Instruct client to report symptoms of dizziness, palpitations, or fainting to prescriber.
- Tell client that drug may discolor urine.
- Advise client to relieve dry mouth with sugarless gum or hard candy.
- Instruct client to wear sunblock and protective clothing outdoors.

thiothixene (Navane)

Drug Class
Typical antipsychotic

Indications and Dosage

Psychosis (mild to moderate)	*Adults*: Initially, 2 mg PO tid, gradually increased to 15 mg daily, p.r.n.
Psychosis (severe)	*Adults*: Initially, 5 mg PO bid, increasing gradually to 20 to 30 mg daily, p.r.n., to a maximum dose of 60 mg daily.

Half-life

20 to 40 hours

Common Adverse Reactions

CNS: Extrapyramidal reactions, drowsiness, tardive dyskinesia, NMS
CV: Hypotension
EENT: Blurred vision
GI: Dry mouth, constipation
GU: Urine retention
Hematologic: Agranulocytosis, transient leukopenia
Skin: Mild photosensitivity reactions

Key Interactions

Increased CNS depression with: CNS depressants, alcohol
Increased risk of photosensitivity with: Sun exposure

Nursing Considerations

- Wear gloves when preparing solutions with oral liquid and parenteral forms; avoid contact with skin and clothing to reduce risk of contact dermatitis.
- Dilute liquid concentrate with fruit juice, milk, or semisolid food just before giving.
- Monitor client for tardive dyskinesia, which may occur after prolonged use; it may not appear until months or years later, and may disappear spontaneously or persist for life, despite stopping drug.
- Alert: Watch for evidence of NMS (extrapyramidal effects, hyperthermia, autonomic disturbance), which is rare but deadly.
- Monitor periodic CBC tests, liver and renal function tests, and ophthalmic tests for long-term use.

- Watch for orthostatic hypotension. Keep client supine for 1 hour after drug administration; tell client to change positions slowly.
- Withhold dose and notify prescriber if jaundice, blood dyscrasia (fever, sore throat, infection, cellulitis, weakness), or persistent extrapyramidal reactions develop, especially in pregnant women.
- Do not withdraw drug abruptly unless severe adverse reactions occur.
- Alert: Do not confuse Navane with Nubain or Norvasc.
- Warn client to avoid activities that require alertness until effects of drug are known.
- Tell client to watch for dizziness upon standing quickly. Advise to change positions slowly.
- Tell client to avoid alcohol use during therapy.
- Instruct client to wear sunblock and protective clothing outdoors.

trifluoperazine hydrochloride

Drug Class
Typical antipsychotic

Indications and Dosage

| Anxiety | *Adults*: 1 to 2 mg PO bid, to a maximum of 6 mg daily; do not give drug for longer than 12 weeks for anxiety. |
| Schizophrenia (*see p. 488*), other psychotic disorders | *Adults*: In outpatients, 1 to 2 mg PO bid; in hospitalized clients, 2 to 5 mg PO bid, gradually increased until therapeutic response occurs. *Children 6 to 12 years*: For hospitalized or closely supervised clients, 1 mg PO daily or bid, possibly gradually increased to 15 mg daily, if needed. |

Half-life
20 to 40 hours

Common Adverse Reactions
CNS: Extrapyramidal reactions, tardive dyskinesia, NMS
CV: Orthostatic hypotension

EENT: Blurred vision
GI: Dry mouth, constipation
GU: Urine retention
Hematologic: Transient leukopenia, agranulocytosis
Skin: Photosensitivity reactions

Key Interactions

Decreased absorption with: Antacids
Decreased drug effect with: Barbiturates, lithium
Decreased antihypertensive effect with: Centrally acting antihypertensives
Increased CNS depression with: CNS depressants, alcohol
Increased levels of both drugs with: Propranolol
Increased risk for photosensitivity with: St. John's wort, sun exposure

Nursing Considerations

- Wear gloves when preparing liquid forms.
- Watch for orthostatic hypotension. Keep client supine for 1 hour after giving drug; tell client to change positions slowly.
- Monitor client for tardive dyskinesia, which may occur after prolonged use. It may not appear until months or years later and may disappear spontaneously or persist for life, despite ending use of drug.
- Alert: Watch for evidence of NMS (extrapyramidal effects, hyperthermia, autonomic disturbance), which is rare but deadly.
- Monitor periodic CBC and liver function tests, and ophthalmic tests (long-term use).
- Withhold dose and notify prescriber if jaundice, signs and symptoms of blood dyscrasia (fever, sore throat, infection, cellulitis, weakness), or persistent (longer than a few hours) extrapyramidal reactions develop.
- Do not withdraw drug abruptly unless severe adverse reactions occur.
- Alert: Do not confuse trifluoperazine with triflupromazine.
- Warn client to avoid activities that require alertness until effects of drug are known and to avoid alcohol while taking drug.

- Instruct client to properly dilute liquid.
- Tell client to wear sunblock and protective clothing outdoors.
- Advise client to relieve dry mouth with sugarless gum or hard candy.

ziprasidone (Geodon)

Drug Class

Atypical antipsychotic

Indications and Dosage

Schizophrenia (symptomatic treatment; *see p. 488*)	*Adults*: Initially, 20 mg bid with food, adjusting dosage as necessary but no more frequently than every 2 days; to allow for lowest possible doses, the interval should be several weeks to assess symptom response. Effective dosage range is usually 20 to 80 mg bid. Maximum dosage is 100 mg bid.
Acute agitation with schizophrenia (for rapid control)	*Adults*: 10 to 20 mg IM p.r.n., up to a maximum dose of 40 mg daily. Doses of 10 mg may be given every 2 hours; doses of 20 mg may be given every 4 hours.
Acute bipolar mania (manic and mixed episodes with or without psychotic features; *see p. 388*)	*Adults*: 40 mg PO bid, with food, on day 1, increasing to 60 to 80 mg PO bid, with food, on day 2; then adjusting dosage on the basis of client response from 40 to 80 mg bid, with food.

Half-life

2.25 to 7 hours

Common Adverse Reactions

CNS: Dizziness, headache, somnolence, suicide attempt
CV: Bradycardia, QT interval prolongation, orthostatic hypotension
GI: Nausea, constipation

Key Interactions

Increased risk for life-threatening arrhythmias with: Anti-arrhythmics (amiodarone, bretylium, disopyramide, dofetilide,

procainamide, quinidine, sotalol), arsenic trioxide, cisapride, dolasetron, droperidol, levomethadyl, mefloquine, pentamidine, phenothiazines, pimozide, quinolones, tacrolimus, drugs that decrease potassium or magnesium (diuretics)
Increased hypotensive effect with: Antihypertensives
Decreased drug level with: Carbamazepine
Increased drug level with: Itraconazole, ketoconazole

Nursing Considerations

- Give the drug with food to achieve optimal effects.
- Monitor for signs and symptoms of hyperglycemia, especially in clients with diabetes. Clients at risk for diabetes should undergo fasting blood glucose testing at baseline and periodically during treatment. Monitor all clients for symptoms of hyperglycemia, including excessive hunger or thirst, frequent urination, and weakness. Hyperglycemia may be reversible when drug is stopped.
- Alert: Assess for dizziness, palpitations, or syncope, which may be symptoms of a life-threatening arrhythmia, such as torsades de pointes. Provide cardiac evaluation and monitoring in clients who experience these symptoms. Stop drug in clients with a QT interval of more than 500 ms.
- Alert: Do not give to clients with electrolyte disturbances (eg, hypokalemia, hypomagnesemia) because these conditions increase the risk of arrhythmia.
- Monitor for life-threatening NMS (hyperpyrexia, muscle rigidity, altered mental status, and autonomic instability) or tardive dyskinesia. Assess abnormal involuntary movement before starting therapy, at dosage changes, and periodically thereafter, to monitor client for tardive dyskinesia.
- Monitor for abnormal body temperature regulation, especially if client is exercising strenuously, exposed to extreme heat, also receiving anticholinergics, or subject to dehydration.
- Tell client that symptoms may not improve for 4 to 6 weeks.
- To prepare IM ziprasidone, add 1.2 mL sterile water for injection to the vial and shake vigorously until drug is completely dissolved. Do not mix injection with other medicinal products or with solvents other than sterile water for injection.

- Tell client to immediately report signs or symptoms of dizziness, fainting, irregular heartbeat, or relevant heart problems to prescriber.
- Advise client to report any recent episodes of diarrhea, abnormal movements, sudden fever, muscle rigidity, or change in mental status.

11

Cognitive Enhancers

Overview

Primary Indication

Dementia to (1) stabilize memory, language, and orientation and (2) promote the client's ability to cope with daily life, slowing down the loss of skills resulting in a decrease in apathy or indifference

Signs and Symptoms

- Symptoms that indicate a possible need for cognitive enhancers include changes in memory, language, and orientation, as well as difficulties with coping with daily life.
- Temporary benefits (disappear if client stops treatment for a few weeks) peak in improvement 3 months after initiating therapy, with slow return to starting point over 9 to 12 months.

Major Category

- Cholinesterase inhibitors
  - donepezil (*see p. 270*)
  - galantamine (*see p. 271*)
  - rivastigmine (*see p. 272*)
  - tacrine (no longer actively marketed by manufacturer)

Key Drug Monographs
donepezil hydrochloride (Aricept)
Drug Class

Cholinesterase inhibitor

Indications and Dosage

Alzheimer dementia (mild to severe; *see p. 338*)	*Adults*: Initially, 5 mg PO daily at bedtime, increasing to 10 mg daily if needed after 4 to 6 weeks.

Half-life

70 hours

Common Adverse Reactions

Central nervous system (CNS): Headache, insomnia, seizures, dizziness, chest pain, hypertension, vasodilation, atrial fibrillation, hot flashes, hypotension

Gastrointestinal (GI): Nausea, diarrhea, vomiting, anorexia, abdominal pain, dyspepsia

Musculoskeletal: Muscle cramps

Skin: Rash

Key Interactions

Decreased drug effects with: Anticholinergics

Possible synergistic effect with: Anticholinesterases, cholinomimetics

Possible increased rate of drug elimination with: Carbamazepine, dexamethasone, phenobarbital, phenytoin, rifampin

Possible additive effects with: Bethanechol, succinylcholine

Nursing Considerations

- Administer drug each day at bedtime.
- Alert: Do not confuse Aricept with Ascriptin.
- Stress that drug does not alter underlying degenerative disease but can temporarily stabilize or relieve symptoms. Effectiveness depends on taking drug at regular intervals.
- Provide small, frequent meals if GI upset is distressing.

- Advise clients and caregivers to report immediately significant adverse effects or changes in overall health status and to inform healthcare team that clients are taking drug before they receive anesthesia.
- Tell client to avoid over-the-counter cold or sleep remedies because of risk of increased anticholinergic effects.

galantamine hydrobromide (Razadyne)

Drug Class
Cholinesterase inhibitor

Indications and Dosage

Alzheimer dementia (mild to moderate; *see p. 338*)	*Adults*: Initially, 4 mg bid, preferably with morning and evening meals. If dose is well tolerated after minimum of 4 weeks of therapy, increase dosage to 8 mg bid; further increase to 12 mg bid may be attempted, but only after at least 4 weeks of therapy at the previous dosage. Dosage range is 16 to 24 mg daily in two divided doses. Alternatively, 8 mg extended-release capsule PO once daily in the morning with food, increasing to 16 mg PO once daily after a minimum of 4 weeks with further increases up to 24 mg once daily after a minimum of 4 weeks, on the basis of client response and tolerability.

Half-life
Approximately 7 hours

Common Adverse Reactions
CNS: Insomnia, dizziness, fatigue
Cardiovascular (CV): Bradycardia, syncope
GI: Diarrhea, nausea, vomiting, anorexia, abdominal pain, dyspepsia, anorexia

Key Interactions
Decreased drug clearance with: Amitriptyline, fluoxetine, fluvoxamine, quinidine

Antagonism of anticholinergic activity with: Anticholinergics
Possible synergistic effect with: Cholinergics (such as bethanechol, succinylcholine)
Increased drug bioavailability with: Cimetidine, clarithromycin, erythromycin, ketoconazole, paroxetine

Nursing Considerations

- Give Razadyne tablets twice daily; give extended-release form capsule once daily. Always verify any prescription that suggests a different dosing schedule.
- Drug may cause bradycardia and heart block. Consider all clients at risk for adverse effects on cardiac conduction.
- Give drug with food and antiemetics; ensure adequate fluid intake to decrease the risk of nausea and vomiting.
- Use proper technique when dispensing the oral solution with the dosing syringe. Dispense measured amount into a beverage and give right away.
- If drug is stopped for several days or longer, restart at the lowest dose and gradually increase, at 4-week or longer intervals, to the previous dosage level.
- Advise caregiver to give drug with morning and evening meals (for the conventional form), or only in the morning (for the extended-release form).
- Inform client that nausea and vomiting are common adverse effects.
- Urge clients or caregivers to report slow heartbeat immediately.
- Advise clients and caregivers that, although drug may improve cognitive function, it doesn't alter the underlying disease process.

rivastigmine tartrate (Exelon)

Drug Class

Cholinesterase inhibitor

Indications and Dosage

Alzheimer dementia (mild to moderate; *see p. 338*)	*Adults*: Initially, 1.5 mg PO bid with food, increasing to 3 mg bid after 2 weeks, if tolerated, then increasing to 4.5 mg bid and 6 mg bid, as tolerated. Effective dosage range of 6 to 12 mg daily to a maximum dose of 12 mg daily.
Dementia (mild to moderate) associated with Parkinson disease	*Adults*: Initially, 1.5 mg PO bid, possibly increasing, as tolerated, to 3 mg bid, then 4.5 mg bid, and finally 6 mg bid after a minimum of 4 weeks at each dose.

Half-life

Approximately 1.5 hours (clients with normal renal function)

Common Adverse Reactions

CNS: Dizziness, insomnia, headache, syncope, fatigue, asthenia, malaise, somnolence, tremor, insomnia, confusion, abnormal thinking
CV: Bradycardia
GI: Nausea, vomiting, diarrhea, anorexia, abdominal pain, dyspepsia, constipation, flatulence

Key Interactions

Possible synergistic effect with: Bethanechol, succinylcholine, other neuromuscular-blocking drugs or cholinergic antagonists
Increased drug clearance with: Smoking
Increased risk of GI bleeding with: Nonsteroidal anti-inflammatory drugs

Nursing Considerations

- Administer rivastigmine with food in the morning and evening.
- Expect significant GI adverse effects (such as nausea, vomiting, anorexia, and weight loss). These effects are less common during maintenance doses.

- Monitor client for evidence of active or occult GI bleeding.
- Dramatic memory improvement is unlikely. As disease progresses, the benefits of drug may decline.
- Monitor client for severe nausea, vomiting, and diarrhea, which may lead to dehydration and weight loss.
- Advise client that memory improvement may be subtle and that drug more likely slows future memory loss.
- Caution client to consult prescriber before using any over-the-counter drugs.

12

Stimulants/Nonstimulants

Overview

Primary Indications

Attention deficit/hyperactivity disorder (ADHD) in children and adults, narcolepsy

Other Indications

Augmentation of treatment for depression

Signs and Symptoms

Symptoms that indicate possible need for stimulants include inattention, hyperactivity, and impulsivity; excessive daytime sleepiness; and cataplexy.

Major Categories

- Amphetamines
  - dextroamphetamine (*see p. 280*)
  - lisdexamfetamine dimesylate (*see p. 281*)
  - mixed amphetamine salts (dextroamphetamine and amphetamine; *see p. 286*)

- Other stimulants
  - dexmethylphenidate (*see p. 277*)
  - methylphenidate (*see p. 283*)
  - modafinil (*see p. 288*)
  - pemoline (*see p. 289*)
- Selective norepinephrine reuptake inhibitors (SNRIs)
  - atomoxetine (*see p. 276*)

Key Drug Monographs

atomoxetine hydrochloride (Strattera)

Drug Class
SNRI

Indications and Dosage

ADHD (*see p. 548*)	*Adults, children, and adolescents who weigh more than 70 kg (154 lb)*: Initially, 40 mg PO daily; increase after at least 3 days to a total of 80 mg/day PO, as a single dose in the morning or two evenly divided doses in the morning and late afternoon or early evening; then increasing total dose to a maximum of 100 mg if needed after 2 to 4 weeks. *Children who weigh 70 kg or less*: Initially, 0.5 mg/kg PO daily, increasing to a total daily dose of 1.2 mg/kg PO as a singe dose in the morning or two evenly divided doses in the morning and late afternoon or early evening after a minimum of 3 days. Not to exceed 1.4 mg/kg or 100 mg daily, whichever is less.

Half-life
21.5 hours

Common Adverse Reactions
Central nervous system (CNS): Headache, insomnia, dizziness
Gastrointestinal (GI): Abdominal pain, constipation, nausea, vomiting, decreased appetite, dry mouth, flatulence
Respiratory: Cough

Key Interactions

Increased risk for cardiovascular effects with: Albuterol

Increased risk for neuroleptic malignant syndrome with: Monoamine oxidase inhibitors (MAOIs)

Risk for hypertension with: Pressor agents

Increased drug level with: Strong CYP2D6 inhibitors (paroxetine, fluoxetine, quinidine)

Nursing Considerations

- Periodically re-evaluate clients taking drug long term to determine drug's usefulness.
- Alert: Assess children and adolescents closely for worsening of condition, agitation, irritability, suicidal thinking or behaviors, and unusual changes in behavior, especially the first few months of therapy or when dosage is increased or decreased.
- Monitor growth during treatment. If growth or weight gain is unsatisfactory, consider interrupting therapy.
- Alert: Severe liver injury may progress to liver failure. Notify prescriber of any sign of liver injury: yellowing of the skin or the sclera of the eyes, pruritus, dark urine, upper right-sided tenderness or unexplained flu-like syndrome.
- Monitor blood pressure and pulse at baseline, after each dose increase, and during treatment periodically.
- Be aware that drug can be stopped without tapering.
- Tell client to use caution when operating a vehicle or machinery or engaging in activities that require alertness until the effects of drug are known.

dexmethylphenidate hydrochloride
(Focalin, Focalin XR)

Drug Class
CNS stimulant

Indications and Dosage

ADHD (see p. 548)	**Immediate-release form:**
	Adults and children 6 years and older:
	• For clients who are not now taking methylphenidate, initially administer 2.5 mg PO twice daily (bid), given at least 4 hours apart, increasing weekly by 2.5 to 5 mg daily, up to a maximum of 20 mg daily in divided doses.
	• For clients who are now taking methylphenidate, initially give half the current methylphenidate dosage, up to a maximum of 20 mg PO daily in divided doses.
	Extended-release form:
	Adults:
	• For clients who are not now taking dexmethylphenidate or methylphenidate, or who are on stimulants other than methylphenidate, give 10 mg PO once daily in the morning, adjusting in weekly increments of 10 mg to a maximum dose of 20 mg daily.
	• For clients who are now taking methylphenidate, initially give half the total daily dose of methylphenidate.
	• Clients who are now taking the immediate-release form of dexmethylphenidate may be switched to the same daily dose of extended-release form. Maximum daily dose is 20 mg.
	Children 6 years and older:
	• For clients who are not now taking dexmethylphenidate or methylphenidate, or who are on stimulants other than methylphenidate, give 5 mg PO once daily in the morning, adjusting in weekly increments of 5 mg to a maximum daily dose of 20 mg.
	• For clients who are now taking methylphenidate, initially give half the total daily dose of methylphenidate.
	• Clients who are now taking the immediate-release form of dexmethylphenidate may be switched to the same daily dose of extended-release form. Maximum daily dose is 20 mg.

Half-life

2.2 hours

Common Adverse Reactions

CNS: Headache, anxiety, feeling jittery

Cardiovascular (CV): Tachycardia

Ears, eyes, nose, and throat (EENT): Blurred vision
GI: Anorexia, abdominal pain, nausea

Key Interactions

Increased level and possible inhibition of co-administered drug with: Anticoagulants, phenobarbital, phenytoin, primidone, tricyclic antidepressants (TCAs)
Decreased effectiveness of co-administered drug with: Antihypertensives
Increased risk of serious adverse reactions with: Clonidine, other centrally acting alpha agonists
Increased risk for hypertensive crisis with: MAOIs

Nursing Considerations

- Obtain a detailed client history, including a family history for mental disorders, family suicide, ventricular arrhythmias, or sudden death.
- Refer client for psychological, educational, and social support.
- Administer drug before 6 pm if insomnia is a problem.
- If client experiences difficulty swallowing capsule, empty the contents of the capsule onto a spoonful of applesauce and give immediately.
- Alert: Tell client not to cut, crush, or chew the contents of the extended-release beaded capsule.
- Stress the importance of taking the correct dose of drug at the same time every day. Periodically reevaluate the long-term usefulness of the drug. Expect to interrupt drug dosage periodically in children to evaluate condition and determine the need for continued therapy.
- Monitor complete blood count and differential and platelet counts during prolonged therapy.
- Stop treatment or reduce dosage if symptoms worsen or adverse reactions occur.
- Monitor children for growth and weight gain. If growth slows or weight gain is lower than expected, stop drug.
- Routinely monitor blood pressure and pulse.
- If seizures occur, stop drug.
- Report accidental overdose immediately.

- Alert: Warn client that misuse of amphetamines can have serious effects, including sudden death.
- Advise parents to monitor child for medication abuse or sharing. Also inform parents to watch for increased aggression or hostility and to report worsening behavior.
- Caution client to expect blurred vision or difficulty with accommodation and to exercise caution while performing activities that require a clear visual field.

dextroamphetamine sulfate (Dexedrine, Dexedrine Spansule, DextroStat)

Drug Class
Amphetamine

Indications and Dosage

Narcolepsy	*Adults*: 5 to 60 mg PO daily in divided doses. *Children 6 to 12 years old*: 5 mg PO daily, increasing by 5 mg at weekly intervals as needed (p.r.n.). *Children 12 years and older*: 10 mg PO daily, increasing by 10 mg at weekly intervals, p.r.n., with first dose on awakening and additional doses (one or two) given at intervals of 4 to 6 hours.
ADHD (*see p. 548*)	*Children 6 years and older*: 5 mg PO once daily or bid, increasing by 5 mg weekly p.r.n. (rarely necessary to exceed 40 mg/day). *Children 3 to 5 years old*: 2.5 mg PO daily, increasing by 2.5 mg at weekly intervals, p.r.n.

Half-life
10 to 12 hours

Common Adverse Reactions
CNS: Insomnia, nervousness, restlessness, dizziness, overstimulation
CV: Tachycardia, palpitations, arrhythmias, hypertension
GI: Dry mouth, taste perversion, diarrhea, weight loss
Genitourinary (GU): Impotence

Key Interactions

Increased drug effect with: Acetazolamide, alkalizing drugs, antacids, sodium bicarbonate, caffeine

Decreased drug level with: Acidifying drugs, ammonium chloride, ascorbic acid

Increased risk for hypertensive crisis and CNS effects with: MAOIs

Possible decreased glucose level with: Insulin, oral hypoglycemics

Decreased absorption of co-administered drug with: Phenobarbital, phenytoin

Nursing Considerations

- Obtain a detailed client history, including a family history for mental disorders, family suicide, ventricular arrhythmias, or sudden death.
- Give drug at least 6 hours before bedtime to avoid sleep interference.
- Alert: Drug has a high abuse potential and may cause dependence.
- Expect to interrupt therapy periodically in children to assess response and continued need.
- Give only the lowest amount of drug to client to reduce risk of overdose.
- Alert: Do not confuse Dexedrine with dextran or Excedrin.
- Alert: Warn client that the misuse of amphetamines can cause serious cardiovascular adverse events, including sudden death.
- Warn client to avoid activities that require alertness, clear visual field, or physical coordination until CNS effects of drug are known.
- Tell client that they may get tired as drug effects wear off.
- Ask client to report signs and symptoms of excessive stimulation.
- Inform parents that children may show increased aggression or hostility and to report any worsening of behavior.
- Advise client to avoid intake of caffeine-containing products.

lisdexamfetamine dimesylate (Vyvanse)

Drug Class

Amphetamine

Indications and Dosage

ADHD (*see p. 548*)	*Children 6 to 12 years old*: Initiation of treatment or switch from another medication: 30 mg PO in the morning, increasing daily dose by 10 to 20 mg at weekly intervals. Alternatively, initial dose may be lowered, starting at 20 mg PO daily in the morning. Maximum daily dose should not exceed 70 mg/day.

Half-life

1 hour

Common Adverse Reactions

CNS: Dizziness, irritability, insomnia

CV: Palpitations, tachycardia, hypertension

GI: Upper abdominal pain, decreased appetite, dry mouth, nausea, vomiting, weight loss

Key Interactions

Increased drug effect with: Acetazolamide, alkalizing drugs, antacids, sodium bicarbonate, caffeine

Decreased drug level with: Acidifying drugs, ammonium chloride, ascorbic acid

Increased risk for hypertensive crisis and CNS effects with: MAOIs

Possible decreased glucose level with: Insulin, oral antidiabetics

Decreased absorption of co-administered drug with: Phenobarbital, phenytoin, ethosuximide

Decreased stimulant effect with: Chlorpromazine, lithium

Nursing Considerations

- Administer once daily in the morning without regard to food or meals.
- Stress the importance of taking the correct dose of drug at the same time every day.
- Periodically re-evaluate therapy. Expect to interrupt drug dosage periodically in children to evaluate condition and determine the need for continued therapy.

- Monitor children for growth and weight gain. If growth slows or weight gain is lower than expected, stop drug.
- Give only the lowest amount of drug to client to reduce risk of overdose.
- Alert: Warn client that the misuse of amphetamines can cause serious cardiovascular adverse events, including sudden death.
- Warn client to avoid activities that require alertness, clear visual field, or physical coordination until CNS effects of drug are known.
- Ask client and parents to report signs and symptoms of excessive stimulation.

methylphenidate hydrochloride (Concerta, Metadate CD, Metadate ER, Methylin, Methylin ER, Ritalin, Ritalin LA, Ritalin-SR); methylphenidate transdermal system (Daytrana)

Drug Class

CNS stimulant

Indications and Dosage

ADHD (*see p. 548*)	*Children 6 years and older*: Initially, 5 mg PO bid immediate-release form before breakfast and lunch, increasing by 5 to 10 mg weekly, p.r.n., until an optimum daily dose of 2 mg/kg is reached, not to exceed 60 mg/day. To use Ritalin-SR, Metadate ER, and Methylin ER tablets in place of immediate-release methylphenidate tablets, calculate methylphenidate dosage in 8-hour intervals.
	Concerta
	Adolescents 13 to 17 years old not currently taking methylphenidate, or clients taking other stimulants: 18 mg PO extended-release once daily in the morning, adjusting dosage by 18 mg weekly to a maximum of 72 mg PO and not to exceed 2 mg/kg once daily in the morning.
	Children 6 to 12 years old not currently taking methylphenidate or clients taking stimulants other than methylphenidate: 18 mg extended-release PO once daily in the morning, adjusting dosage by 18 mg weekly to a maximum of 54 mg daily in the morning.

Adolescents and children 6 years and older currently taking methylphenidate: If previous methylphenidate dosage was 5 mg bid or three times daily (tid) or 20 mg sustained-release, give 18 mg PO every morning. If previous dosage was 10 mg bid or tid or 40 mg sustained-release, give 36 mg PO every morning. If previous dosage was 15 mg bid or tid or 60 mg sustained-release, give 54 mg PO every morning. Maximum conversion daily dose is 54 mg. When conversion complete, adjust adolescents 13 to 17 years old to maximum dose of 72 mg once daily (not to exceed 2 mg/kg).

Metadate CD

Children 6 years and older: Initially, 20 mg PO daily before breakfast, increasing by 10 to 20 mg weekly to a maximum of 60 mg daily.

Ritalin LA

Children 6 years and older: 20 mg PO once daily, increasing by 10 mg weekly to a maximum of 60 mg daily. If previous methylphenidate dosage was 10 mg bid or 20 mg sustained-release, give 20 mg PO once daily. If previous methylphenidate dosage was 15 mg bid, give 30 mg PO once daily. If previous methylphenidate dosage was 20 mg bid or 40 mg sustained-release, give 40 mg PO once daily. If previous methylphenidate dosage was 30 mg bid or 60 mg sustained-release, give 60 mg PO once daily.

Daytrana

Children 6 to 12 years: Initially, apply one 10-mg patch to clean, dry, nonirritated skin on the hip, alternating sites daily. Avoid the waistline or where tight clothing may rub it off. Apply 2 hours before desired effect and remove 9 hours later. Increase dose weekly as needed to a maximum of 30 mg daily. Base final dose and wear time on client response.

Narcolepsy

Adults: 10 mg PO bid or tid immediate-release, 30 to 45 minutes before meals. Dosage varies; average is 40 to 60 mg/day. To use Ritalin-SR, Metadate ER, or Methylin ER tablets in place of immediate-release methylphenidate tablets, calculate the dose of methylphenidate in 8-hour intervals.

Half-life

Immediate-release formulation: 1 to 3 hours
Extended-release formulation: 3 to 8 or 8 to 12 hours
Transdermal: 3 to 4 hours

Common Adverse Reactions

CNS: Nervousness, headache, insomnia, seizures
CV: Tachycardia, bradycardia, hypertension, hypotension
GI: Nausea, abdominal pain, anorexia, decreased appetite, vomiting
Hematologic: Thrombocytopenia, thrombocytopenic purpura, leukopenia
Skin: Exfoliative dermatitis, erythema multiforme

Key Interactions

Increased level of co-administered drug with: Anticonvulsants (such as phenobarbital, phenytoin, primidone), selective serotonin reuptake inhibitors, TCAs (imipramine, clomipramine, desipramine), warfarin
Increased risk for serious adverse effects with: Centrally acting alpha-2 agonists, clonidine
Decreased antihypertensive effect with: Centrally acting antihypertensives
Increased risk for hypertensive crisis with: MAOIs
Increased drug effect with: Caffeine

Nursing Considerations

- Give last daily dose at least 6 hours before bedtime to prevent insomnia and after meals to reduce appetite-suppressant effects. Drug may trigger Tourette syndrome in children.
- Administer Metadate CD or Ritalin LA to be swallowed whole; if necessary, sprinkle contents of the capsule onto a small amount of cool applesauce and give immediately.
- Alert: Warn client to take chewable tablet with at least 8 ounces of water. Not using enough water to swallow tablet may cause tablet to swell and block throat, causing choking.
- Monitor client, especially at start of therapy. Observe for signs of excessive stimulation. Monitor blood pressure.

- Check complete blood count as well as differential and platelet counts with long-term use, particularly if client shows signs or symptoms of hematologic toxicity (fever, sore throat, easy bruising).
- Monitor height and weight in children on long-term therapy. Drug may delay growth spurt, but children will attain normal height when drug is stopped.
- Monitor client for tolerance or psychological dependence.
- Warn client against chewing sustained-release tablets.
- Caution client to avoid activities that require alertness or good psychomotor coordination until CNS effects of drug are known.
- Advise client to avoid beverages containing caffeine while taking drug.
- Tell parents to apply patch immediately after opening and not to use if pouch seal is broken; they should press firmly in place for about 30 seconds using the palm of the hand, being sure there is good contact with the skin, especially around the edges. When patch is applied correctly, children may shower, bathe, or swim as usual.
- Encourage parents to use the application chart provided with patch carton to keep track of application and removal.
- Tell parents to remove patch sooner than 9 hours if children have decreased evening appetite or difficulty sleeping. Tell parents that the effects of the patch last for several hours after removal.
- Inform parents that, if patch comes off, they may apply a new one on a different site, but the total wear time for that day should be 9 hours. Upon removal, parents should fold patch in half so the sticky sides adhere to each other, and then flush the patch down the toilet or dispose of in a lidded container.
- Tell parents, if the applied patch is missing, to ask children when or how the patch came off.
- Tell parents to notify prescriber if children develop bumps, swelling, or blistering at the application site or experience blurred vision or other serious side effects.

mixed amphetamine salts (dextroamphetamine and amphetamine; Adderall, Adderall XL)

Drug Class
Amphetamine

Indications and Dosage

ADHD (*see p. 548*)	*Children 3 to 5 years old*: Initially, 2.5 mg PO daily, increasing by 2.5 mg at weekly intervals until optimal response. *Children 6 years and older*: Initially, 5 mg once or twice daily, increasing daily dosage by 5 mg at weekly intervals until optimal response. Give first dose on awakening; additional doses (1 or 2) at intervals of 4 to 6 hours.
Narcolepsy	*Children 12 years and older*: 5 to 60 mg per day in divided doses, based on individual response.

Half-life

9 to 14 hours

Common Adverse Reactions

CNS: Overstimulation, restlessness, dizziness, insomnia

CV: Palpitations, tachycardia, hypertension

GI: Dry mouth, unpleasant taste, diarrhea, constipation, anorexia, weight loss

GU: Impotence

Key Interactions

Decreased drug absorption with: Guanethidine, reserpine, glutamic acid, ascorbic acid, fruit juices

Increased drug effect with: Acetazolamide, alkalizing drugs, antacids, sodium bicarbonate, caffeine

Decreased drug level with: Acidifying drugs, ammonium chloride, ascorbic acid

Increased risk for hypertensive crisis and CNS effects with: MAOIs

Possible decreased glucose level with: Insulin, oral antidiabetics

Decreased absorption of co-administered drug with: Phenobarbital, phenytoin, ethosuximide

Decreased stimulant effect with: Lithium, haloperidol

Nursing Considerations

- Give drug exactly as prescribed. Instruct client and parents that client should take the first dose early in the morning upon awakening.
- Obtain a detailed client history, including a family history for mental disorders, family suicide, ventricular arrhythmias, or sudden death.
- Alert: Drug has a high potential for abuse and may cause dependence. Give only the lowest amount to client to reduce risk of overdose.
- Expect to interrupt therapy periodically in children to assess response and continued need.
- Alert: Warn client that misuse of amphetamines can cause serious cardiovascular adverse events, including sudden death.
- Warn client to avoid activities that require alertness, clear visual field, or good coordination until CNS effects of drug are known.
- Ask client to report signs and symptoms of excessive stimulation.
- Inform parents that children may show increased aggression or hostility and to report any worsening of behavior.

modanifil (Provigil)

Drug Class
CNS stimulant

Indications and Dosage

Narcolepsy, obstructive sleep apnea	200 mg PO daily as a single dose in the morning.

Half-life
15 hours

Common Adverse Reactions
CNS: Headache, nervousness, dizziness, insomnia
CV: Arrhythmias, hypotension
EENT: Rhinitis
GI: Nausea, diarrhea, dry mouth, anorexia

Key Interactions

Altered drug level with: Carbamazepine, phenobarbital, rifampin, itraconazole, ketoconazole, and other inducers of CYP3A4

Decreased level of co-administered drug with: Cyclosporine, theophylline

Increased level of co-administered drug with: Diazepam, phenytoin, propranolol, warfarin, other drugs metabolized by CYP2C19

Decreased effect of co-administered drug with: Hormonal contraceptives

Increased antidepressant effect with: TCAs (clomipramine, desipramine)

Nursing Considerations

- Monitor blood pressure closely, especially in clients with hypertension.
- Be aware that food has no effect on overall bioavailability but may delay absorption of drug by 1 hour.
- Caution client that use of hormonal contraceptives (including depot or implantable contraceptives) with modafinil tablets may reduce contraceptive effectiveness. Recommend an alternative method of contraception during modafinil therapy and for 1 month after drug is stopped.
- Instruct client to confer with prescriber before taking prescription or over-the-counter drugs.
- Tell client to avoid alcohol while taking drug.
- Warn client to avoid activities that require alertness or physical coordination until CNS effects of drug are known.

pemoline (Cyclert)

Drug Class

CNS stimulant

Indications and Dosage

ADHD (*see p. 548*)	*Adults and children older than 6 years*: Initially, 37.5 mg/day PO as a single morning dose, increasing gradually by 18.75 mg at weekly intervals until response; not to exceed 112.5 mg/day.

Half-life

12 hours

Common Adverse Reactions

CNS: Insomnia, headache, dizziness, somnolence

GI: Anorexia, weight loss, nausea, abdominal discomfort, elevations of liver enzymes

Key Interactions

Increased CNS stimulation with: CNS stimulants

Nursing Considerations

- Administer drug as a single oral dose each morning.
- Periodically re-evaluate client if taking drug for extended periods to determine usefulness.
- Monitor growth during long-term treatment.
- Alert: Monitor liver function tests every 2 weeks during long-term therapy. Severe liver injury may progress to liver failure. Notify prescriber of any sign of liver injury: yellowing of the skin or sclera of the eyes, pruritus, dark urine, upper right-sided tenderness, or unexplained flu-like syndrome.
- Give the smallest amount of drug to minimize risk of overdose.
- Tell client to use caution when operating a vehicle or machinery or engaging in activities that require alertness until the effects of drug are known.

13

Miscellaneous Drugs

Overview

Various drugs primarily indicated for use with other disorders have been found effective in treating psychiatric disorders or associated problems, such as extrapyramidal reactions, neuroleptic malignant syndrome, and management of alcohol abstinence. Major categories include the following:

- Antiparkinsonian agents
  - amantadine (*see p. 291*)
  - benztropine (*see p. 293*)
  - biperiden (*see p. 294*)
  - bromocriptine mesylate (*see p. 295*)
- Enzyme (aldehyde dehydrogenase) inhibitor
  - disulfiram (*see p. 296*)

Key Drug Monographs
amantadine hydrochloride (Symmetrel)
Drug Class
Antiparkinsonian agent

Indications and Dosage

Drug-induced extrapyramidal reactions	*Adults*: 100 mg PO twice daily (bid), possibly increasing up to 300 mg/day in divided doses.

Half-life

Approximately 15 to 24 hours

Common Adverse Reactions

Central nervous system (CNS): Dizziness, insomnia, irritability, light-headedness
Cardiovascular (CV): Heart failure
Gastrointestinal (GI): Nausea, anorexia

Key Interactions

Increased anticholinergic effects with: Anticholinergics
Increased drug level and risk of toxicity with: Co-trimoxazole, quinidine, thiazide diuretics, triamterene
Increased CNS effects with: Alcohol

Nursing Considerations

- Alert: Monitor mental status closely for changes, especially in older adults, who are more susceptible to adverse neurologic effects.
- Monitor for possible suicidal ideation and worsening of psychiatric problems.
- Alert: Do not confuse amantadine with rimantadine.
- Alert: Tell client to take drug exactly as prescribed; failure to do so may result in serious adverse reactions or death.
- If insomnia occurs, tell client to take drug several hours before bedtime.
- If client becomes dizzy upon standing, instruct client not to stand or change positions too quickly.
- Instruct client to notify prescriber of adverse reactions, especially dizziness, depression, anxiety, nausea, and urine retention.

- Caution client to avoid activities that require mental alertness until effects of drug are known.
- Advise client to avoid alcohol while taking drug.

benztropine mesylate (Cogentin)

Drug Class

Antiparkinsonian agent, anticholinergic

Indications and Dosage

Drug-induced extrapyramidal disorders (except tardive dyskinesia)	*Adults*: 1 to 4 mg PO or intramuscular (IM) injection once or twice daily.
Acute dystonic reaction	*Adults*: 1 to 2 mg intravenous (IV) or IM injection; then 1 to 2 mg PO bid to prevent recurrence.

Half-life

Unknown

Common Adverse Reactions

CNS: Confusion, memory impairment, nervousness, disorientation
CV: Tachycardia
Ears, eyes, nose, and throat (EENT): Dilated pupils, blurred vision
GI: Dry mouth, constipation
Genitourinary (GU): Urine retention, hesitancy

Key Interactions

Increased anticholinergic effects with: Amantadine, phenothiazines, tricyclic antidepressants (TCAs)
Decreased effectiveness of co-administered drug with: Cholinergics (donepezil, galantamine, rivastigmine, tacrine), antipsychotic agents

Nursing Considerations

- Monitor vital signs carefully. Watch closely for adverse reactions, especially in elderly or debilitated clients. Call prescriber promptly if adverse reactions occur.

- Alert: At certain doses, drug produces atropine-like toxicity, which may aggravate tardive dyskinesia.
- Watch for intermittent constipation and abdominal distension and pain, which may indicate onset of paralytic ileus.
- Monitor elderly clients closely, because they are more prone to severe adverse effects.
- Alert: Never stop drug abruptly. Reduce dosage gradually.
- Warn client to avoid activities that require alertness until CNS effects of drug are known.
- If client takes a single daily dose, tell client to do so at bedtime.
- Advise client to report signs and symptoms of urinary hesitancy or urine retention.
- Suggest the use of cool drinks, ice chips, sugarless gum, or hard candy to relieve dry mouth.
- Advise client to limit activities in hot weather, because drug-induced lack of sweating may cause overheating.

biperiden

Drug Class
Antiparkinsonian agent, anticholinergic

Indications and Dosage

Extrapyramidal symptoms associated with phenothiazine therapy	*Adults*: 2 mg PO one to three times daily. Alternatively, 2 mg IM or IV, repeating every 30 minutes until symptoms resolve, not to exceed four consecutive doses in 24 hours.

Half-life
18 to 24 hours

Common Adverse Reactions
CNS: Disorientation, confusion, light-headedness, dizziness
EENT: Blurred vision, mydriasis
GI: Dry mouth, constipation

GU: Urinary retention, hesitancy
Skin: Flushing, decreased sweating

Key Interactions

Increased anticholinergic effects with: Other anticholinergics, phenothiazines, TCAs
Decreased effectiveness of co-administered drug with: Phenothiazines, haloperidol
Increased CNS effects with: Alcohol

Nursing Considerations

- Alert: Expect to reduce dosage in hot weather and monitor client body temperature; drug interferes with sweating and ability of body to balance heat.
- Administer with meals if GI upset occurs; if client experiences dry mouth, give medication before meals; give after meals if drooling or nausea occurs.
- Monitor urinary output.
- Avoid the use of alcohol, sedatives, and over-the-counter drugs.
- Advise client to avoid activities requiring alertness until the effects of the drug are known.
- Suggest the use of sugarless candy and ice chips to combat dry mouth.

bromocriptine mesylate (Parlodel)

Drug Class

Antiparkinsonian agent; dopamine-receptor agonist

Indications and Dosage

Neuroleptic malignant syndrome (NMS)	*Adults*: 2.5 to 5 mg PO two to six times daily.

Half-life

15 hours

Common Adverse Effects
CNS: Dizziness, headache, fatigue, seizures, stroke
CV: Hypotension, acute myocardial infarction
GI: Nausea, abdominal cramps, constipation

Key Interactions
Decreased drug effectiveness with: Amitriptyline, haloperidol, imipramine, loxapine, monoamine oxidase inhibitors, methyldopa, metoclopramide, phenothiazines, reserpine, estrogens, hormonal contraceptives, progestins
Increased hypotensive effects with: Antihypertensives
Increased drug level with: Erythromycin
Risk for disulfiram-like reaction with: Alcohol

Nursing Considerations
- Administer drug in the evening with food to minimize adverse reactions.
- Monitor client for adverse reactions, which occur in many clients, particularly at start of therapy. Most reactions are mild to moderate; nausea is most common. Minimize adverse reactions by gradually adjusting dosages to effective levels.
- Obtain baseline and periodic evaluations of cardiac, hepatic, renal, and hematopoietic function if therapy is prolonged.
- Alert: Do not confuse bromocriptine with benztropine or bri-monidine, or Parlodel with pindolol.
- Instruct client to avoid dizziness and fainting by rising slowly to an upright position and avoiding sudden position changes.
- Advise client to avoid alcohol while taking drug.

disulfiram (Antabuse)
Drug Class
Aldehyde-dehydrogenase inhibitor

Indications and Dosage

Adjunct to management of alcohol abstinence	*Adults*: 250 to 500 mg PO as single dose in morning for 1 to 2 weeks or in evening if drowsiness occurs; maintenance dose of 125 to 500 mg PO daily (average 150 mg) until permanent self-control is established. Treatment may continue for months or years.

Half-life
Unknown

Common Adverse Reactions
CNS: Drowsiness, headache, fatigue
GI: Metallic or garlicky aftertaste
Skin: Skin eruptions
Other: Disulfiram reaction precipitated by alcohol use

Key Interactions
Increased duration of effect of co-administered drug with: Barbiturates
Increased CNS depression with: CNS depressants
Increased effect or level of co-administered drug with: Warfarin, midazolam, paraldehyde, phenytoin
Increased risk for behavior changes with: Isoniazid, TCAs
Risk for disulfiram reaction with: Alcohol, herbal preparations containing alcohol

Nursing Considerations
- Alert: Never give disulfiram until client has abstained from alcohol for at least 12 hours; ensure that client clearly understands consequences of drug and has given permission for use before administration.
- Use the drug only in cooperative, well-motivated clients who are receiving supportive psychiatric therapy.

- Before beginning therapy, perform a complete physical examination and laboratory studies, including complete blood count and chemistry and liver function studies; repeat regularly.
- Alert: Be aware of the drug reaction that may result from use with alcohol: flushing, throbbing headache, dyspnea, nausea, copious vomiting, diaphoresis, thirst, chest pain, palpitations, hyperventilation, hypotension, syncope, anxiety, weakness, blurred vision, confusion, and arthropathy. A severe drug reaction can cause respiratory depression, cardiovascular collapse, arrhythmias, myocardial infarction, acute heart failure, seizures, unconsciousness, and death.
- The longer the client remains on the drug, the more sensitive the client becomes to alcohol.
- Alert: Do not confuse Antabuse with Anturane.
- Alert: Caution family never to give this drug to clients without their knowledge; severe reaction or death could result if client drinks alcohol.
- Tell client to carry medical identification that identifies them as disulfiram users.
- Reassure client that drug-induced adverse reactions (unrelated to alcohol use), such as drowsiness, fatigue, impotence, headache, peripheral neuritis, and metallic or garlic taste, subside after approximately 2 weeks of therapy.
- Advise client not to drink alcoholic beverages or use products containing alcohol, including topical preparations and mouth-wash.
- Have client verify content of over-the-counter products with pharmacist before use.

Mental Health and Psychiatric Disorders

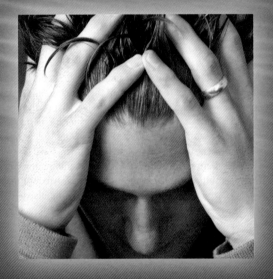

Anxiety Disorders

Anxiety disorders, which are conditions in which clients experience persistent anxiety that they cannot dismiss, are the most common psychiatric disorders for both adults and children. People with anxiety disorders feel that the foundations of their personalities are being threatened, even when no actual danger exists. That is, they perceive a threat, even if it is not real. Coping mechanisms are ineffective, and anxiety interferes with the activities of daily living.

Current research suggests that anxiety disorders have several possible origins and are most likely caused by a combination of neurobiologic vulnerabilities and psychosocial stress. Anxiety disorders include generalized anxiety disorder, obsessive-compulsive disorder, phobic disorders, panic attacks and panic disorder, acute stress disorder, and post-traumatic stress disorder.

Generalized Anxiety Disorder

In **generalized anxiety disorder** (GAD), clients experience chronic and excessive worry and anxiety most of the time. Such worry and anxiety interfere with daily life and relationships. Clients typically show signs of persistent, chronic, and severe anxiety.

Assessment

*Diagnostic and Statistical Manual of Mental Disorders,
Fourth Edition, Text Revision (DSM-IV-TR) Diagnostic
Criteria: GAD*

- Excessive anxiety and worry about several events or activities on most days for at least 6 months
- Difficulty controlling the worry
- Anxiety and worry associated with three or more of the following:
  1. Feeling restless, keyed up, or on edge
  2. Being easily fatigued
  3. Difficulty concentrating or mind going blank
  4. Irritability
  5. Muscle tension
  6. Sleep disturbance
- Anxiety and worry not confined to features of Axis I disorder
- Significant distress or impairment in social, occupational, or other important areas of function as a result of anxiety, worry, or physical symptoms
- Disturbance is not caused by substance or medical condition and does not occur exclusively during mood, psychotic, or pervasive developmental disorder

Adapted with permission from American Psychiatric Association. (2000). *Diagnostic and statistical manual of mental disorders (4th ed., text rev.).* Washington, DC: Author.

Common History and Physical Examination Findings
See also "Hamilton Rating Scale for Anxiety," p. 62.

- Worry related to everyday events, such as employment responsibilities, job or school performance, finances, family health, being late, household responsibilities
- Sweating, nausea, diarrhea
- Muscle tension, trembling, twitching, shakiness, muscle aches or soreness
- Exaggerated startle response
- Less prominent evidence of autonomic hyperarousal (eg, tachycardia, dyspnea, dizziness)
- Sleep disturbances
- Fatigue

Common Psychosocial Assessment Findings

- Anxiety level out of proportion to feared event or situation
- Difficulty controlling worrisome thoughts
- Worry shifts from one event or situation to another
- Interference with social, occupational, or other functioning
- No precipitating event or trigger for the worrying

Interdisciplinary Treatment Modalities

Psychopharmacology

▪ Antidepressants: selective serotonin reuptake inhibitors (SSRIs) (*see p. 186*)

▪ Anxiolytics: buspirone (*see p. 155*)

Cognitive-Behavioral Therapy (*see p. 116*)

▪ Cognitive therapy (*see p. 111*)

▪ Distraction

▪ Relaxation

▪ New breathing techniques

Nursing Care Planning

I NURSING DIAGNOSIS : Anxiety

Related to:	As Evidenced by:
Persistent chronic worry about multiple daily events or situations	Muscle tension
	Ease in startling
	Difficulty controlling worries
	Interference with functioning
	Sleep disturbances

Nursing Outcomes Classification (NOC): Anxiety Self-Control; Anxiety Level; Coping: Client will demonstrate measures to reduce anxious feelings and will verbalize decreased anxiety, with improved mood, sleep, and ability to function.

Nursing Interventions Classification (NIC): Anxiety Reduction

1. Use a calm and reassuring approach to create an atmosphere that facilitates trust. *Approaching clients calmly prevents overwhelming and startling them. Trust is essential to a therapeutic relationship.*
2. Assist clients to appraise situations objectively. *Objective appraisals enable clients to gain control over situations and make them more predictable.*
3. Help clients identify situations that precipitate anxiety and when the anxiety level changes. *Knowledge of anxiety-producing situations and indicators of increasing anxiety can assist clients to exert control over feelings.*
4. Support the use of appropriate defense mechanisms. *Appropriate defense mechanisms can assist in reducing anxiety.*
5. Administer prescribed medications as appropriate. *Drugs such as buspirone may help reduce or control anxiety in clients and promote feelings of safety.*

NIC: Anticipatory Guidance

1. Determine usual methods of problem solving. Help identify maladaptive strategies; provide suggestions for appropriate replacements. Encourage clients to refrain from using alcohol and to exercise regularly. *These interventions help clients determine the most beneficial strategies and substitute them for maladaptive ones. Lifestyle changes can help make clients more resilient to stress.*
2. Rehearse with clients various strategies to cope with anxiety. *Rehearsing enhances the chances for success when clients use these techniques.*
3. Refer clients to appropriate community agencies; suggest support groups. *Community agencies and support groups are tremendous resources for people who feel alone with their disorder.*

NURSING DIAGNOSIS: Sleep Deprivation

Related to:	As Evidenced by:
Prolonged chronic anxiety state	Fatigue
	Reports of difficulty sleeping
	Nervousness

NOC: Sleep; Rest: Client will report getting more sleep each night, with decreased fatigue.

NIC: Sleep Enhancement

1. Record sleep patterns and number of hours of sleep; encourage clients to monitor sleep patterns. *Information about current sleep patterns provides a baseline for planning appropriate interventions.*
2. Encourage clients to establish a bedtime routine. *Doing so facilitates the transition from wakefulness to sleep.*
3. Instruct clients to avoid foods and beverages that can interfere with sleep. For example, drinking coffee at night may contribute to insomnia, so clients should avoid caffeine after the late afternoon. *Caffeine, a stimulant, has a half-life of 8 to 14 hours; its effects vary.*
4. Encourage clients to discuss the anxiety and how it has affected sleep. Suggest participation in a support group. *Understanding anxiety can help clients develop adaptive strategies for dealing with it, thus improving sleep. Participation in a support group provides an outlet for sharing feelings and concerns.*

NIC: Environmental Management

1. Explain the need for a clean, comfortable bed and environment; encourage clients to avoid unnecessary exposures, drafts, overheating, or chilling. *Cleanliness and comfort promote relaxation and thereby facilitate the transition to sleep.*
2. Encourage clients to participate in relaxing and enjoyable activities before bed. Monitor their participation in fatigue-producing activities while awake. *Enjoyable and relaxing activities prepare the body for sleep. Overactivity can lead to being overtired.*
3. Urge clients to make their bedrooms as quiet and dark as possible and to use beds only for sleeping or sex. Assist them as possible to control or prevent undesirable or excessive noise. *A sleep-promoting environment helps reduce stimuli that contribute to nocturnal arousal. Even low levels of movement or noise may disturb sleep.*

| NURSING DIAGNOSIS: Powerlessness

Related to:	**As Evidenced by:**
Difficulty controlling anxiety and worry	Continued feelings of worry
	Interference with functional level
	Effect on sleeping

NOC: Depression Self-Control: Client will verbalize a gradual increase in control of anxieties, situations, and ability to function, with greater participation in outside activities.

NIC: Coping Enhancement

1. Encourage clients to discuss feelings. To help them adopt more realistic appraisals, help them identify evidence for and against their feelings. Assist clients to develop objective appraisals of events. Discuss the consequences of not dealing with anxiety. *Emotional responses are understandable, but ultimately irrational and self-defeating. Rational examination of feelings can help clients restructure faulty thought patterns.*

2. Listen to clients' verbalizations of feelings, perceptions, and fears. Provide an accepting, calm, and reassuring atmosphere. *Avoidance behaviors are attempts to reduce stress. Fear levels will remain high, however, until clients confront fears often enough for them to dissipate.*

3. Assist clients to identify their strengths and abilities and to break complex tasks and goals into small, manageable steps. Encourage gradual mastery of situations. *Focusing on strengths promotes feelings of self-worth. Using small manageable steps prevents overwhelming clients and increases the chances for success. Mastery promotes feelings of control.*

4. Appraise clients' needs and desires for social support; assist in identifying support systems. *Resources for support help minimize feelings of isolation and aloneness.*

Obsessive-Compulsive Disorder

Obsessive-compulsive disorder (OCD) is an anxiety disorder in which clients experience recurrent **obsessions** (intrusive and persistent ideas, thoughts, images, or impulses), compulsions (ritualistic behaviors performed either in accord with a specific set of rules or in a routine manner), or both. Obsessions and compulsions are time consuming and cause significant impairment, distress, or both. People with OCD do not voluntarily produce obsessions but feel cognitively invaded by them, usually finding them repugnant or meaningless. Clients engage in compulsions to prevent or reduce anxiety, not to increase pleasure or satisfaction. In fact, they can resist the compulsion for a short period, but this delay creates a tremendous anxious tension relieved only by performing the compulsive act.

Assessment

DSM-IV-TR Diagnostic Criteria: OCD

- Obsessions or compulsions:

  1. Obsessions as recurrent thoughts, impulses, or images that are intrusive or inappropriate and cause marked distress, not excessive worries about real problems; attempts by client to ignore, suppress, or neutralize these thoughts with some other action or thought; recognition of obsession as product of own mind

  2. Compulsions as repetitive behaviors or mental acts that client feels driven to perform in response to obsession or according to rigidly applied rules; unconnected realistically with what they are designed to neutralize or prevent; clearly excessive

- Recognition by client of excessiveness or unreasonableness of obsessions or compulsions

- Obsessions or compulsions causing marked distress, consuming time, or significantly interfering with normal routines, occupation, usual social activities, or relationships

- Obsessions or compulsions not restricted to another mental disorder if present

- Disturbance not caused by a substance or medical condition

Adapted with permission from American Psychiatric Association. (2000). *Diagnostic and statistical manual of mental disorders (4th ed., text rev.).* Washington, DC: Author.

Common History and Physical Examination Findings
See also "Yale-Brown Obsessive-Compulsive Scale," *p. 64.*

- Behavioral or verbal demonstration of compulsion or obsession taking more than 1 hour per day

- Difficulty with concentration because of distracting intrusions
- Sleep disturbance
- Skin breakdown, irritation (from excessive handwashing)

Common Psychosocial Assessment Findings

- Significant distress
- Guilt
- Impaired functioning
- Avoidance of situations involving the content of the obsession
- Possible alcohol or substance use

Interdisciplinary Treatment Modalities

Cognitive-Behavioral Therapy *(see p. 116)*

- Cognitive therapy *(see p. 111)*
  - Thought stopping
  - Distraction
- Relaxation
- Guided imagery
- Cue cards

Psychopharmacology

- Antidepressants: SSRIs, TCAs *(see p. 185)*

Nursing Care Planning

I NURSING DIAGNOSIS: Anxiety

Related to:	As Evidenced by:
Perceived stress or threat	Obsessions, compulsions, or both
	Inability to control obsessions or compulsions
	Awareness of behaviors as excessive or unreasonable
	Difficulty maintaining functional level

NOC: Anxiety Control: Client will verbalize decreased anxiety and obsessions, and demonstrate fewer compulsions.

NIC: Anxiety Reduction

1. Use a calm and reassuring approach to create an atmosphere that facilitates trust. Avoid calling attention to obsessions or compulsions or arguing with clients about them initially. *Approaching clients calmly prevents overwhelming and startling them. Trust is essential to a therapeutic relationship. Preventing, arguing, or calling attention to compulsions or obsessions can increase anxiety.*

2. Encourage clients to verbalize comfortable feelings. Acknowledge their feelings and perceptions. *Use of comforting methods prevents increasing anxiety. Acknowledging feelings promotes trust and allows clients to begin to identify possible cues and triggers for anxiety.*

3. Help clients identify situations that precipitate anxiety and when anxiety level changes. *Knowledge of anxiety-producing situations and indicators of increasing anxiety can help clients exert control over feelings.*

4. Support use of appropriate defense mechanisms while attempting to refocus clients on reality. *Support and refocusing can assist in reducing anxiety.*

5. Assist clients to appraise situations objectively. *Objective appraisals enable clients to gain control over situations and make them more predictable.*

6. Administer prescribed medications as appropriate. *Anxiolytics or antidepressants may help reduce or control anxiety initially and promote feelings of safety.*

NIC: Anticipatory Guidance

1. Determine usual methods of problem solving. Help identify maladaptive strategies; provide suggestions for appropriate replacements. Encourage clients to refrain from using alcohol and to exercise regularly. *These interventions help clients determine the most beneficial strategies and substitute them for maladaptive ones. Lifestyle changes can help make clients more resilient to stress.*

2. Encourage clients to keep a diary or log of the behaviors/rituals, along with their frequency, duration, and surrounding circumstances. Review information for possible triggers or precipitating factors. *A diary or log provides information for developing individualized strategies to reduce engagement in rituals.*

3. Initially, allot ample time within clients' usual routine for ritualistic behavior; help clients adapt schedules accordingly. *Allowing time initially for completion of ritualistic behaviors prevents increasing the client's anxiety.*

4. Work with clients to develop a schedule for gradually limiting time allotted to obsessions or compulsions. Encourage clients to engage in other activities or to focus on other feelings during the rest of the period. *Setting limits provides clients time to engage in behaviors to alleviate anxiety. It also demonstrates understanding of the significance of the behaviors without allowing them to overtake life.*

5. Teach clients appropriate techniques and strategies to manage and tolerate anxiety. Rehearse with them various strategies to begin to limit compulsions or obsessions. *Teaching strategies provides clients with ways to control anxiety. Rehearsing enhances the chances for success when clients use these strategies.*

6. Describe relaxation interventions. Teach controlled-breathing and guided-imagery techniques. Individualize content according to clients' preferences and demonstrate appealing techniques. *Controlled breathing and relaxation techniques decrease the sympathetic arousal that accompanies high anxiety. These techniques also help improve sleep.*

7. Assist clients to identify situations when use of relaxation techniques would help. *Appropriate use of techniques enhances the chances for a successful outcome.*

8. Encourage frequent repetition and practice of techniques. *Practice increases the chances that clients will use techniques correctly when needed.*

| NURSING DIAGNOSIS: Ineffective Coping

Related to:	*As Evidenced by:*
Obsessions or compulsions	Repeated engagement in time-consuming rituals
	Interference in usual level of functioning
	Inability to control them
	Feelings of guilt
	Recognition that obsessions or compulsions are excessive

NOC: Coping: Client will demonstrate fewer ritualistic behaviors and increased ability to function independently.

NIC: Coping Enhancement

1. Encourage clients to discuss feelings; validate them. To help clients adopt more realistic appraisals of events, identify evidence for and against their feelings. Assist them to develop objective appraisals. Discuss the consequences of not dealing with guilt. *Feelings are real to clients but ultimately irrational and self-defeating; validation promotes trust. Rational examination of feelings can help clients identify possible sources of anxiety and restructure faulty thought patterns and behaviors.*

2. Discuss ritualistic behaviors with clients. Listen to verbalizations of feelings, perceptions, and fears. Provide an accepting, calm, and reassuring atmosphere. *Ritualistic behaviors are attempts to reduce stress. Anxiety levels will remain high, however, until clients learn ways of confronting stress.*

3. Provide clients with opportunities to participate in activities that they can accomplish easily or enjoy. Give positive feedback for accomplishments. *Complex activities may be difficult for clients. Participating in easy or enjoyable activities can foster self-esteem.*

4. Encourage and assist clients gradually to limit time spent in rituals. Teach methods to control rituals and to reduce anxiety. Assist clients to break complex goals into small, manageable steps. Encourage gradual mastery of the situation. *Gradual, controlled limit setting helps clients gain control over anxiety, eliminating or reducing it to a manageable level that does not interfere with functional ability. Small manageable steps prevent overwhelming clients and increase the chances for success.*

| NURSING DIAGNOSIS: Impaired Skin Integrity

Related to:	*As Evidenced by:*
Compulsion involving frequent and excessive skin cleaning	Redness and irritation from rubbing
	Cracks, fissures, breaks in skin
	Excess dryness and flaking

NOC: Tissue Integrity: Skin and Mucous Membranes: Client will exhibit clean, dry, and intact skin without evidence of irritation or breakdown.

NIC: Skin Surveillance

1. Inspect the skin's condition, including color, warmth, turgor, texture, intactness, and edema. *Inspection helps nurses to determine the extent of impairment and to individualize interventions.*
2. Monitor areas for redness, breakdown, discoloration, bruising, rashes, or abrasions. Assess for excessive dryness. *Rituals involving skin cleaning can lead to skin breakdown.*
3. Assist clients to gradually reduce skin-cleaning rituals. *Doing so helps remove the underlying source of the impaired skin integrity.*

NIC: Skin Care, Topical Treatments

1. Encourage clients to wear nonrestrictive clothing. *Restrictive clothing provides an additional source for irritation and subsequent breakdown of the skin.*
2. Avoid use of alkaline soaps on the skin. *They can be irritating.*
3. Apply topical lotions and emollients as ordered. *They add moisture to the skin.*
4. Encourage clients to drink adequate fluids, including water. *Fluids help hydrate the skin.*

Panic Disorder

Panic disorder is characterized by recurrent, unpredictable **panic attacks**, which involve discrete periods of intense discomfort or fear and peak within 10 minutes. Clients experience extreme physiologic discomfort along with severe emotional distress. Panic disorder can occur with or without **agoraphobia**, a marked fear of being alone or in a public place from which escape would be difficult or help would be unavailable in the event of becoming disabled.

Assessment

DSM-IV-TR Diagnostic Criteria: Panic Disorder

- Recurrent unexpected panic attacks: Discrete periods of intense fear or discomfort with four or more of the following that develop abruptly and peak within 10 minutes:
  1. Palpitations, pounding heart, or accelerated heart rate
  2. Sweating

3. Trembling or shaking
4. Smothering or shortness of breath
5. Feeling of choking
6. Chest pain or discomfort
7. Abdominal distress or nausea
8. Dizziness, unsteadiness, light-headedness, or faintness
9. Derealization or depersonalization
10. Fear of losing control or going crazy
11. Fear of dying
12. Paresthesias (numbness or tingling)
13. Chills or hot flushes

- After at least one attack, 1 month (or more) of concern about more attacks, worry about the implications of the attack or its consequences, significant related behavior change, or a combination of all of these
- Panic attacks not caused by substance use, a medical condition, or another psychiatric disorder
- With agoraphobia
  - Anxiety related to being in places or situations from which escape might be difficult or embarrassing or in which help may not be available in the event of having an unexpected or situationally predisposed panic attack or panic-like symptoms
  - Situations avoided or endured with marked distress or with anxiety
  - Not better accounted for by another mental disorder
- Without agoraphobia

Adapted with permission from American Psychiatric Association. (2000). *Diagnostic and statistical manual of mental disorders (4th ed., text rev.)*. Washington, DC: Author.

Common History and Physical Examination Findings
See also "Hamilton Rating Scale for Anxiety," *p. 62.*

- Apprehension
- Increased rate, pitch, and volume of speech
- Automatisms: tapping fingers, jingling coins or keys, twisting hair
- Palpitations
- Sweating
- Tremors
- Shortness of breath
- Feelings of being suffocated
- Chest pain

- Nausea
- Abdominal distress
- Dizziness
- Paresthesias
- Chills or hot flushes
- Tachycardia
- Hypertension
- Confusion, inability to focus

Common Psychosocial Assessment Findings

- Excessive apprehension, feeling as if "on edge"
- Agoraphobia
- Disruption in social functioning
- Feelings of embarrassment, shame
- Feelings of losing control
- Fear of dying or going crazy
- Demoralization
- Possible depression

Common Laboratory and Diagnostic Test Findings

- **Arterial blood gases:** Compensated respiratory alkalosis (decreased carbon dioxide and bicarbonate levels, near normal pH)

Interdisciplinary Treatment Modalities

Cognitive-Behavioral Therapy (*see p. 116*)

- Cognitive therapy (*see p. 111*)
- Behavioral therapy (*see p. 108*)
- Relaxation
- Breathing techniques

Psychopharmacology

- Antidepressants: SSRIs, TCAs (*see p. 185*)
- Anxiolytics: benzodiazepines (*see p. 150*)

Nursing Care Planning

| NURSING DIAGNOSIS: Anxiety

Related to:	As Evidenced by:
Recurrent, unexpected panic attacks	Feelings of intense fear or discomfort
	Sweating, trembling
	Sensations of shortness of breath, choking
	Complaints of light-headedness, dizziness
	Fear of losing control, dying, going crazy
	Extreme worry about outcome of everyday activities

NOC: Anxiety Self-Control; Anxiety Level; Coping: Client will demonstrate measures to reduce anxious feelings and will verbalize decreased anxiety and fewer panic episodes.

NIC: Anxiety Reduction

1. Use a calm and reassuring approach to create an atmosphere that facilitates trust. Stay with clients and be direct, using as few words as possible. Avoid touching clients. *Approaching calmly prevents overwhelming and startling clients. Trust is essential to a therapeutic relationship. Staying with clients ensures safety. Direct and short verbal exchanges prevent overwhelming and confusing clients. Touching invades interpersonal space, which could exacerbate anxiety level.*

2. Administer prescribed medications as appropriate. *Anxiolytics or antidepressants may help reduce or control anxiety initially and promote feelings of safety.*

3. Once the panic episode subsides, help clients identify situations that precipitate anxiety and when anxiety level changes. Assist clients to identify early signs of panic episodes. *Knowledge of anxiety-producing situations and indicators of increasing anxiety can assist clients to exert control over feelings.*

4. Support use of appropriate defense mechanisms. *They can assist in reducing anxiety.*

5. Help clients appraise situations objectively. *Objective appraisals enable clients to gain control over situations and make them more predictable.*

6. Determine usual methods of problem solving by clients. Help them identify maladaptive strategies; provide suggestions for appropriate replacements. Encourage clients to refrain from using alcohol and to exercise regularly. *These interventions help clients determine the most beneficial strategies and substitute them for maladaptive ones. Lifestyle changes can help make clients more resilient to stress.*

7. Teach controlled breathing methods. Describe relaxation interventions. Individualize content according to the preferences of clients; demonstrate appealing techniques. *Controlled breathing and relaxation techniques decrease the sympathetic arousal that accompanies high anxiety. They also help to improve sleep.*

8. Assist clients to identify situations when use of relaxation techniques would help. *Appropriate use of techniques enhances the chances for a successful outcome.*

9. Rehearse with clients various strategies to cope with anxiety. Encourage frequent repetition and practice. *Rehearsing and practice enhance the chances for correct use of and success with techniques.*

NIC: Coping Enhancement

1. Encourage clients to discuss feelings of powerlessness, helplessness, and fear. Discuss panic episodes with clients. Listen to verbalizations of feelings, perceptions, and fears. Provide an accepting, calm, and reassuring atmosphere. *Anxiety levels will remain high until clients confront the feelings or triggers often enough for fear to dissipate. Discussing the event or feeling is a form of exposure therapy.*

2. To help clients adopt more realistic appraisals of events, help them identify evidence for and against their feelings. Assist them to develop objective appraisals. Discuss the consequences of not dealing with feelings. *Rational examination of feelings can help clients restructure faulty thought patterns.*

3. Implement as ordered appropriate therapies such as distraction, positive self-talk, exposure therapy, systematic desensitization, or

implosive therapy. Encourage and assist clients to expose themselves gradually to the environment or situation associated with the panic episode. Assist clients to break complex goals into small, manageable steps. Encourage gradual mastery of situations. *Avoiding situations associated with panic episodes is impractical and an ineffective response to stress. Gradual, controlled exposure eventually will desensitize clients to triggers. Small manageable steps prevent overwhelming clients and increase the chances for success.*

NIC: Counseling

1. Provide facts as necessary and appropriate; assist clients to identify the problem causing distress. Point out discrepancies between feelings and behaviors. *Facts are necessary to help dispel irrational and self-defeating responses.*

2. Assist clients to identify strengths; encourage new skill development; reinforce new skills and use of appropriate techniques for panic control. *New strategies and appropriate panic-control techniques enhance the ability of clients to deal with stress; drawing on strengths promotes feelings of control.*

| NURSING DIAGNOSIS: Ineffective Tissue Perfusion

Related to:	As Evidenced by:
Physiologic effects of panic	Hyperventilation
	Tachycardia, palpitations
	Shortness of breath
	Feelings of suffocation
	Dizziness, light-headedness
	Paresthesias

NOC: Circulation Status; Respiratory Status: Gas Exchange; Vital Signs: Client will demonstrate signs and symptoms of adequate tissue perfusion and vital signs within acceptable parameters.

NIC: Hemodynamic Regulation

1. Assess heart rate and blood pressure as indicated. Assist with measures, such as breathing techniques, relaxation, and distraction

to promote decreases in pulse rate and blood pressure. *Stimulation of the sympathetic nervous system secondary to panic episodes results in elevations of pulse and blood pressure. Although temporary, these manifestations can add to an already heightened level of anxiety.*

2. Attempt to minimize or reduce environmental stressors. *They exacerbate anxiety.*

3. Administer anxiolytics or antidepressants as ordered. *These drugs are effective in treating panic disorder.*

NIC: Respiratory Monitoring

1. Assess respiratory rate, depth, and effort. Observe chest movement, including use of accessory muscles. *Clients with panic disorder commonly exhibit hyperventilation.*

2. Have clients assume a safe, comfortable position, usually sitting up in a chair or bed. *A comfortable position eases the work of breathing and reduces oxygen demand; an upright position allows for adequate lung expansion. Use of a chair or bed reduces risk of injury.*

3. Assist clients to concentrate on their breathing. Work with them to perform the necessary steps to slow breathing. *Slow, rhythmic breathing enhances oxygen consumption and reduces excess carbon dioxide removal.*

4. Monitor oxygen saturation levels as indicated. Anticipate the need for oxygen therapy if oxygen saturation falls below acceptable parameters. Prepare clients for procedures and for being touched before initiating any procedures. *Hyperventilation increases oxygen demand. Invading personal space (eg, during treatments or procedures) can compound an already severe panic level. Supplemental oxygen may be necessary to meet the increased demand until the panic episode subsides.*

5. Institute measures to relieve severe anxiety. *The anxiety level associated with panic is severe and the underlying cause of manifestations. Relieving panic facilitates a return to pre-panic status.*

| NURSING DIAGNOSIS: Risk for Injury; Risk for Self-directed Violence

Related to:	As evidenced by:
Recurrent, unexpected panic attacks	Extreme anxiety
	Loss of control
	Confusion, disorientation
	Impaired judgment and thinking
	Feelings of depersonalization
	Feelings of derealization

NOC: Personal Safety Behavior: Client will remain free from injury and self-harm.

NIC: Security Enhancement

1. Provide a nonthreatening environment and demonstrate a calm approach; stay with clients until panic subsides. *A nonthreatening environment and calm approach minimize the risk of exposing clients to additional stressors. Staying with clients fosters trust and ensures safety.*
2. Listen to and acknowledge the feelings and fears of clients. *These are very real to clients.*
3. If changes will occur, discuss them in advance and introduce them gradually. *Gradual exposure to changes prevents overwhelming clients and further increasing their anxiety. It also helps clients prepare for and learn to adapt to the change, thereby enhancing their control.*

NIC: Behavior Management: Self-Harm

1. Develop appropriate expectations with clients; contract with them as appropriate for "no self-harm." *Joint development of expectations fosters a sense of control over the situation; a no self-harm contract may reduce the risk for self-harm.*
2. Work with clients to develop positive coping strategies as appropriate and how to identify possible triggers to panic attacks. *Positive coping strategies and early identification of possible triggers can help clients prevent or minimize future panic attacks.*

3. Provide positive reinforcement for use of appropriate coping behaviors and expression of feelings. *Positive reinforcement promotes continued participation with these activities, enhances the chances for success, and fosters self-esteem.*

4. Assist clients to identify triggers and feelings that prompted self-harm behavior; help clients identify more appropriate coping strategies for use and their consequences. *Working with clients to identify triggers and more appropriate coping strategies promotes effective problem-solving skills.*

Acute Stress Disorder

Acute stress disorder (ASD) occurs within the first month of exposure to extreme trauma: combat, rape, physical assault, near-death experience, or witnessing a murder, with symptoms beginning during or shortly after the event. **Dissociation**, a state of detachment in which people experience the world as dream like and unreal, is a primary feature and may be accompanied by poor memory of specific events surrounding the trauma (dissociative amnesia). Usually, ASD resolves within 2 to 28 days after exposure to the trauma.

Assessment

DSM-IV-TR Diagnostic Criteria: ASD

- Exposure to a traumatic event with both of the following: experiencing, witnessing, or being confronted with an event involving actual or potential death, serious injury, or a threat to the physical integrity of self or others; response involved intense fear, helplessness, or horror
- During or after event, clients have at least three of the following:
  1. Numbing, detachment, no emotion
  2. Reduced awareness (eg, "being in a daze")
  3. Derealization
  4. Depersonalization
  5. Dissociative amnesia (eg, cannot recall an important aspect of the trauma)
- Persistent re-experiencing of trauma through recurrent images, thoughts, dreams, illusions, flashbacks, or a sense of reliving the experience; or clients are distressed when exposed to reminders

- Marked avoidance of stimuli that remind clients of the trauma
- Marked symptoms of anxiety or increased arousal
- Significant distress or impairment of social, occupational, or other important areas of functioning or ability to pursue a necessary task
- Duration of at least 2 days but no more than 4 weeks, occurring within 4 weeks of the traumatic event
- Disturbance is not the *direct* physiologic result of a substance or a medical condition, is not better accounted for by brief psychotic disorder, and is not merely an exacerbation of a pre-existing disorder

Adapted with permission from American Psychiatric Association. (2000). *Diagnostic and statistical manual of mental disorders (4th ed., text rev.).* Washington, DC: Author.

Common History and Physical Examination Findings

See also "Hamilton Rating Scale for Anxiety," *p. 62.*

- Feelings of hopelessness, despair, guilt
- Reports of feeling detached from the body or being in a dream-like state
- Difficulty sleeping
- Poor concentration
- Exaggerated startle response
- Motor restlessness, nervousness
- Hypertension, tachycardia, tachypnea

Common Psychosocial Assessment Findings

- Dissociative amnesia
- Avoidance of the event, situation, or anything that evokes remembering the trauma
- Interference with ability to function (social, occupational, or other important areas)

Interdisciplinary Treatment Modalities

Cognitive-Behavioral Therapy *(see p. 116)*

- Cognitive therapy *(see p. 111)*
- Systematic desensitization *(see p. 137)*

- Exposure therapy (*see p. 121*)
- Relaxation
- Breathing retraining

Psychopharmacology

- Antidepressants: SSRIs, TCAs (*see p. 150*)
- Anxiolytics: benzodiazepines (*see p. 185*), buspirone (*see p. 155*)
- β-Blockers

Nursing Care Planning

See also "Post-traumatic Stress Disorder," *p. 324.*

NURSING DIAGNOSIS: Anxiety

Related to:	As Evidenced by:
Recent exposure to traumatic event	Feelings of guilt
	Dissociation
	Difficulty sleeping
	Poor concentration
	Reports of recurrent thoughts and dreams of event
	Distress with reminders of trauma
	Poor concentration
	Nervousness
	Hypervigilance
	Avoidance of situations associated with event
	Difficulty with daily functioning

NOC: Anxiety Self-Control; Anxiety Level: Client will demonstrate measures to reduce anxiety and verbalize decreased anxiety level, with improved mood, sleep, concentration, and function.

NIC: Anxiety Reduction

1. Use a calm and reassuring approach to create an atmosphere that facilitates trust. *A calm approach prevents overwhelming and startling clients. Trust is essential to a therapeutic relationship.*

2. Help clients identify situations that precipitate anxiety and when the anxiety level changes. *Knowledge of anxiety-producing situations and indicators of increasing anxiety can assist clients to exert control over feelings.*

3. Support use of appropriate defense mechanisms. *They can assist in reducing anxiety.*

4. Assist clients to appraise situations objectively. *Objective appraisals enable clients to gain control over and make situations more predictable.*

5. Administer prescribed medications as appropriate. *Anxiolytics or antidepressants may help to reduce or control anxiety initially and promote feelings of safety.*

NIC: Anticipatory Guidance

1. Determine the client's usual methods of problem solving. Help identify maladaptive strategies; suggest appropriate replacements. Encourage clients to refrain from using alcohol and to exercise regularly. *These interventions help clients determine and substitute the most beneficial strategies for maladaptive ones. Lifestyle changes can make clients more resilient.*

2. Rehearse with clients various strategies to cope with anxiety. *Rehearsing enhances the chances for success when clients use these techniques.*

3. Refer clients to appropriate community agencies. Suggest joining a support group. *Community agencies and support groups are tremendous resources for people who feel alone with their disorder.*

NIC: Simple Relaxation Therapy

1. Teach controlled breathing methods. Describe relaxation interventions. Individualize content according to client preferences; demonstrate appealing techniques. *Controlled breathing and relaxation techniques decrease the sympathetic arousal that accompanies high anxiety. They also help improve sleep.*

2. Assist clients to identify situations when use of relaxation techniques would help. *Appropriate use of techniques enhances the chances for a successful outcome.*

3. Encourage frequent repetition and practice of techniques. *Practice increases the chances that clients will use techniques correctly when needed.*

NURSING DIAGNOSIS: Ineffective Coping

Related to:	As Evidenced by:
Significantly heightened anxiety level secondary to recent trauma	Hypervigilance
	Nervousness
	Avoidance of situations involving reminders of trauma
	Difficulty concentrating
	Recurrent thoughts and dreams
	Difficulty in functioning

NOC: Coping: Client will demonstrate appropriate coping strategies to manage anxiety and return to previous level of functioning.

NIC: Coping Enhancement

1. Encourage clients to discuss feelings. To help them adopt more realistic appraisals of the event, assist them to identify evidence for and against feelings. Help them develop objective appraisals. Discuss the consequences of not dealing with guilt. *The emotional responses of clients are understandable but ultimately irrational and self-defeating. Rational examination of feelings can help clients restructure faulty thought patterns.*

2. Discuss the event with clients. Listen to verbalizations of feelings, perceptions, and fears. Provide an accepting, calm, and reassuring atmosphere. *Avoidance behaviors are attempts to reduce stress. Fear levels will remain high, however, until clients confront fears often enough for them to dissipate. Discussing the event is a form of exposure therapy.*

3. Encourage and assist clients gradually to expose themselves to the environment in which the event occurred. Assist clients to break complex goals into small, manageable steps. Encourage gradual mastery of the situation. *Avoiding situations involving the trauma may be impractical and is an ineffective response to stress. Gradual, controlled exposure eventually will desensitize clients to the trigger. Small, manageable steps prevent overwhelming clients and increase the chances for success.*

NIC: Counseling

1. Provide facts as necessary and appropriate; assist clients to identify the problem causing distress. Point out discrepancies between feelings and behaviors. *Facts are necessary to help dispel irrational and self-defeating responses.*

2. Assist clients to identify strengths; encourage new skill development; reinforce new skills. *Development of new strategies enhances clients' ability to deal with stress; drawing on strengths promotes feelings of control.*

Post-traumatic Stress Disorder

When symptoms of ASD continue for more than 1 month and are accompanied by functional impairment or stress, the diagnosis changes to acute **post-traumatic stress disorder** (PTSD). The traumatic event associated with PTSD may be from natural causes (eg, earthquakes) or human activity (eg, terrorist attacks, violent crimes, combat).

Assessment

DSM-IV-TR Diagnostic Criteria: PTSD

- Exposure to traumatic event: experiencing, witnessing, or being confronted with actual or potential death, serious injury, or threatened physical integrity of self or others; response involved intense fear, helplessness, or horror. **Note:** Children may display disorganized or agitated behavior.

- Persistent re-experiencing of trauma in one (or more) of the following ways:

  1. Recurrent and intrusive distressing recollections, including images, thoughts, or perceptions. **Note:** Young children may engage in repetitive play that uses themes or aspects of the trauma.

  2. Recurrent distressing dreams of the event. **Note:** Children may have frightening dreams without recognizable content.

  3. Acting or feeling as if the trauma were recurring (eg, reliving the event, illusions, hallucinations, and "flashbacks," including those on awakening or when intoxicated).

  4. Intense psychological distress at exposure to cues that resemble the trauma.

  5. Physical reactivity when exposed to cues that resemble the trauma.

■ Persistent avoidance of stimuli associated with the trauma. General responsiveness is numb (not present before the trauma), as indicated by at least three of the following:

1. Efforts to avoid thinking, feeling, or talking about the trauma
2. Efforts to avoid activities, places, or people that remind client of the trauma
3. Inability to recall an important aspect of the trauma
4. Greatly diminished interest or participation in significant activities
5. Feeling detached or estranged from others
6. Restricted range of affect
7. Sense of a short future (eg, does not expect to have a career, normal lifespan)

■ Persistent symptoms of increased arousal (not present before the trauma), as indicated by at least two of the following:

1. Difficulty falling or staying asleep
2. Irritability or anger
3. Difficulty concentrating
4. Hypervigilance
5. Exaggerated startle response

■ Symptoms for more than 1 month
■ Disturbance causing significant distress or impairment of social, occupational, or other important areas of functioning

Adapted with permission from American Psychiatric Association. (2000). *Diagnostic and statistical manual of mental disorders (4th ed., text rev.)*. Washington, DC: Author.

Common History and Physical Examination Findings

- Exposure to traumatic event
- Sleep disturbances
- Nightmares or recurrent dreams
- Decreased concentration
- Physical injuries
- Substance use
- Sexual difficulties

Common Psychosocial Assessment Findings

- Flashbacks, re-experiencing of trauma
- Depression
- Emotional numbness
- Anger, guilt, remorse

- Low self-esteem
- Anxiety, panic
- Difficulty expressing love, empathy
- Problems experiencing pleasure
- Difficulties in interpersonal relationships
- Occupational problems

Interdisciplinary Treatment Modalities

Cognitive-Behavioral Therapy (*see p. 116*)

- Cognitive therapy (*see p. 111*)
- Systematic desensitization (*see p. 137*)
- Exposure therapy (*see p. 121*)
- Relaxation
- Breathing retraining

Family Therapy (*see p. 122*)

Group Therapy (*see p. 123*)

Psychopharmacology

- Antidepressants: SSRIs, TCAs (*see p. 185*)
- Anxiolytics (*see p. 150*)

Nursing Care Planning

NURSING DIAGNOSIS: Post-trauma Syndrome

Related to:	As Evidenced by:
Exposure to traumatic event	Re-experiencing the trauma
	Sleep difficulties
	Nightmares/flashbacks
	Psychic numbing
	Decreased concentration
	Hypervigilance

NOC: Coping; Fear Control: Client will demonstrate recovery from the intense emotional trauma, with fewer and eventual resolution of symptoms.

NIC: Coping Enhancement

1. Encourage clients to discuss feelings. To help them adopt more realistic appraisals of the event, assist clients to identify evidence for and against feelings. Assist clients to develop objective appraisals. Discuss the consequences of not dealing with feelings. *Emotional responses are understandable but ultimately irrational and self-defeating. Rational examination of feelings can help clients to restructure faulty thought patterns.*

2. Discuss the traumatic event with clients. Listen to verbalizations of feelings, perceptions, and fears. Provide an accepting, calm, and reassuring atmosphere. *Avoidance behaviors are attempts to reduce stress. Fear levels will remain high, however, until clients confront the fear often enough for it to dissipate. Discussing the event is a form of exposure therapy.*

3. If possible, encourage and assist clients gradually to expose themselves to the environment in which the event occurred. *Avoiding stimuli associated with the trauma may be impractical and ineffective. Gradual, controlled exposure eventually will desensitize clients to triggers.*

NIC: Counseling

1. Provide facts as necessary and appropriate; assist clients to identify the problem causing distress. Point out discrepancies between feelings and behaviors. *Facts are necessary to help dispel irrational and self-defeating responses.*

2. Assist clients to identify strengths; encourage new skill development; reinforce new skills. *Development of new strategies enhances the ability of clients to deal with stress; drawing on strengths promotes feelings of control.*

NURSING DIAGNOSIS: Anxiety

Related to:	As Evidenced by:
Post-traumatic stress response	Poor sleep
	Irritability
	Cognitive impairment
	Guilt/remorse

NOC: Anxiety Control: Client will verbalize a decreased anxiety level and improved mood, sleep, and cognition.

NIC: Anxiety Reduction

1. Help clients identify situations that precipitate anxiety and when anxiety level changes. *Knowledge of anxiety-producing situations and indicators of increasing anxiety can assist clients to exert control over the feelings.*
2. Support the use of appropriate defense mechanisms. *They can assist in reducing anxiety.*
3. Assist clients to appraise situations objectively. *Objective appraisals enable clients to gain control over and make situations more predictable.*

NIC: Anticipatory Guidance

1. Determine usual methods of problem solving. Help clients identify maladaptive strategies; provide suggestions for replacing them with appropriate ones. Encourage clients to refrain from using alcohol and to exercise regularly. *These interventions help clients determine the most beneficial strategies and substitute them for those that are maladaptive. Lifestyle changes can help make clients more resilient to stress.*
2. Rehearse with clients various strategies to cope with anxiety. *Rehearsing enhances the chances for success when clients use these techniques.*
3. Refer clients to appropriate community agencies. Suggest that they consider joining a support group. *Community agencies and support groups are tremendous resources for people who feel alone with their disorder.*

NIC: Simple Relaxation Therapy

1. Teach controlled breathing methods. Describe relaxation interventions. Individualize content according to preferences of clients; demonstrate appealing techniques. *Controlled breathing and relaxation techniques decrease the sympathetic arousal that accompanies high anxiety. They also help to improve sleep.*
2. Assist clients to identify situations when use of relaxation techniques would help. *Appropriate use of techniques enhances the chances for a successful outcome.*

3. Encourage frequent repetition and practice of techniques. *Practice increases the chances that clients will use techniques correctly when needed.*

NIC: Therapy Group

1. Encourage self-disclosure and discussion of the past only as related to the function and goals of the group. Encourage clients to share with the group such commonalities as anger, sadness, humor, mistrust, and other feelings. *Self-disclosure and discussion in conjunction with sharing promotes group cohesiveness and effectiveness.*

2. Provide social reinforcement, structured group exercises, role playing, and problem solving as appropriate. *Specific therapeutic activities within a group promote group function and help clients gain insight into their behaviors and responses.*

| NURSING DIAGNOSIS: Compromised Family Coping

Related to:	As Evidenced by:
Temporary family disorganization	Client's hypervigilance and fears
	Family frustration/irritability
	Interpersonal relationship problems
	Marital problems

NOC: Family Coping; Family Normalization: Family will provide appropriate support to client with a return to previous level of family function prior to traumatic event.

NIC: Family Involvement Promotion

1. Identify family expectations for client, family structure, and family roles. Meet with the family to educate them about PTSD. *Knowledge of this family enhances effectiveness when planning specific interventions. Increasing the family's understanding of PTSD will help them view the client's behavior differently, thereby fostering support for the client.*

2. Listen to the family's concerns; accept coping styles without judgment. *Hearing family members without judgment promotes a feeling of being understood and valued as well.*

3. Engage client's partner or significant other and family in treatment plan. Teach them how to listen reflectively. *Partnering with family members and encouraging family decision making increase the likelihood of successful treatment.*

NIC: Family Support

1. Listen to family concerns, feelings, and questions; facilitate communication among all. *Such communication is necessary to facilitate trust and promote a positive outcome.*

2. Respect and support adaptive coping mechanisms; provide feedback regarding the family's coping. *Supporting adaptive coping and providing feedback promote the use of the most effective methods for the situation.*

3. Refer to family therapy as appropriate. *Family therapy helps to modify family behavior to promote family functioning.*

Cognitive Disorders

C **ognitive disorders** involve a disruption of or deficit in cognitive function, which encompasses orientation, attention, memory, vocabulary, calculation ability, and abstract thinking. With most cognitive disorders, the brain itself is temporarily or permanently compromised. Common manifestations include disturbed perceptions, delusions, paranoia, and aggressive and disruptive behaviors. Clients may sense that their thinking is impaired and become frustrated, anxious, frightened, or distraught. High emotion may compound an already disordered state.

The American Psychiatric Association lists the following categories under cognitive disorders:

- Delirium, dementia, and amnestic and other cognitive disorders
- Mental disorders resulting from a general medical condition
- Substance-related disorders (*see Chapter 24*)

Delirium

Delirium usually results from an acute disruption in the homeostasis of the brain. When the cause of disruption subsides or is eliminated, related cognitive deficits generally resolve within days or weeks.

Any process, disorder, or agent that disrupts integrity of the central nervous system and diffusely impairs its cellular functioning can induce delirium. Delirium may be the result of primary brain disease, such as head injury or tumors; systemic diseases, such as acid-base or electrolyte imbalances, hypoperfusion, or hypoxia; postsurgical response; trauma; substance withdrawal; or specific drug toxicities. Medications are the primary exogenous offenders, especially in older adults. Nevertheless, multiple factors often play a role.

Assessment

Diagnostic and Statistical Manual of Mental Disorders, Fourth Edition, Text Revision (DSM-IV-TR) Diagnostic Criteria: Delirium

---

- Disturbed consciousness (reduced environmental awareness) and decreased capacity to focus, sustain, or shift attention
- Cognition changes (eg, memory deficit, disorientation, language disturbance) or perceptual disturbances not better explained by a pre-existing, established, or evolving dementia
- Rapid development of change or disturbance (usually hours to days) with fluctuation
- Evidence from client history, physical examination, or laboratory tests supporting disturbance caused by:
  - General medical condition
  - Substance withdrawal
  - Substance intoxication
  - More than one etiology (eg, a medical condition and substance intoxication)

Delirium Not Otherwise Specified: Condition lacking criteria for any specific type of delirium; evidence to establish a specific etiology is insufficient

Adapted with permission from American Psychiatric Association. (2000). *Diagnostic and statistical manual of mental disorders (4th ed., text rev.).* Washington, DC: Author.

Common History and Physical Examination Findings
See also "Mental Status Examination," *p. 53.*

- Abrupt onset of changes
- History revealing underlying medical condition or substance use
- Confusion, disorientation

- Disturbed memory, especially recent memory
- Language disturbances
- Daytime sleepiness/nighttime agitation
- Difficulty falling asleep
- Restlessness, hyperactivity
- Picking at clothes, attempting to get out of bed when unsafe or inappropriate, pulling out tubes, wandering

Common Psychosocial Assessment Findings

- Recent changes in memory
- Anxiety, fear
- Depression
- Anger
- Euphoria
- Apathy
- Inattention, inability to focus
- Rapid shifts in emotional states
- Calling out, screaming, muttering, moaning
- Impaired judgment
- Misinterpretations
- Hallucinations, delusions

Common Laboratory and Diagnostic Test Findings

- Evidence of underlying medical condition or substance
- Electroencephalogram: abnormal, showing generalized slowing

Interdisciplinary Treatment Modalities

Elimination or correction of underlying cause

Safety measures/environmental control

Client reorientation

Psychopharmacology

- Typical antipsychotics (haloperidol [*see p. 248*])
- Atypical antipsychotics (quetiapine, risperidone, olanzapine, aripiprazole, and ziprasidone [*see p. 238*])

Nursing Care Planning

| NURSING DIAGNOSIS: Acute Confusion

Related to:	As Evidenced by:
Delirium of known or unknown etiology	Disorganized thinking
	Speech disturbance
	Perceptual disturbances
	Impaired memory
	Difficulty focusing
	Inattention
	Agitation

Nursing Outcomes Classification (NOC): Cognitive Orientation: Client will return to baseline cognitive functioning.

Nursing Interventions Classification (NIC): Delirium Management

1. Identify underlying etiology for delirium; initiate measures to reduce or eliminate factors associated with the condition. *The underlying cause of delirium must be reduced or eliminated for the condition to resolve.*

2. Approach clients calmly from the front, calling them by name and introducing yourself. *A calm approach prevents overwhelming clients. Calling clients by name and introducing oneself help clients to focus and interpret events correctly.*

3. Eliminate stimuli that invite misinterpretation, such as abstract pictures or excessive noise. Use cues such as clocks, recognizable photos, and calendars. Ensure a well-lit environment. *Removing excess stimuli reduces the risk for worsening confusion and agitation. Using cues helps clients re-orient to time and place. The key is to remove difficult-to-interpret cues and replace them with simple, easy-to-recognize ones. A well-lit room minimizes the risk for misinterpretation of the environment.*

4. Implement consistent routines. Reinforce their predictability by telling clients what they are doing, what to expect, time of day, and other relevant data as activities proceed. *Even though clients may be disoriented, they often recognize and feel reassured by the*

presence of familiar and supportive staff and relatives. Consistency is stabilizing.

5. Provide directed activity, such as psychomotor tasks (eg, bags with familiar items to "pack" and "unpack," Velcro to fasten and unfasten, and zippers to open and close). *Directed activities help distract clients from anxiety and provide sensory stimulation at a level adjusted to compromised function.*

6. Assist with needs for safety, hydration, nutrition, comfort, and pain management. *Meeting the clients' needs provides reassurance and comfort.*

7. Avoid situations that require clients to think abstractly. Focus on concrete thinking. *Clients with delirium lack the attention and focus to think abstractly; attempts to think abstractly can add to fear, anxiety level, and frustration.*

8. Never assume clients do not need or will not understand explanations. Accept behavior nonjudgmentally and recognize fears. *Clouded consciousness waxes and wanes. Acceptance is important to avoid demeaning clients for actions that they cannot control.*

9. Administer medication as ordered; monitor clients closely. *Agitation may be severe enough to warrant medication, such as when a client's behavior threatens the safety of self, family, or staff. Close monitoring is necessary to prevent adverse effects.*

NIC: Reality Orientation

1. Speak to clients in a calm, unhurried, and distinct manner, repeating information as necessary. Use gestures or objects when communicating. *A calm and unhurried approach prevents overwhelming clients. Repetition is important to help clients regain or maintain focus. Gestures or objects help increase comprehension of verbal communication.*

2. Inform clients of person, place, and time as often as necessary. Use objects to aid in refocusing. Encourage use of aids, such as glasses, hearing aids, or dentures. *Reorientation is necessary to ensure a focus on reality and to promote recognition. Cues aid in stimulating memory and promoting appropriate behavior. The use of aids fosters appropriate interpretation of sensory input.*

3. Ask questions and give simple directions one at a time. *Limiting questions and directions prevents overwhelming clients and adding to frustration and anxiety levels.*

4. Provide realistic reassurance, giving clients explanations that they can comprehend. Allow time for clients to process information and to respond to questions. *Realistic reassurance validates feelings. Allowing adequate time for understanding and answering prevents overwhelming clients and increasing their anxiety.*

5. Correct misperceptions in a matter-of-fact manner. *Validating feelings about misperceptions is important, but correction is necessary to avoid reinforcing misperceptions.*

| NURSING DIAGNOSIS: Risk for Injury

Related to:	*As Evidenced by:*
Confusion and disorientation	Difficulty focusing
	Impaired judgment
	Inattention, reduced awareness
	Hallucinations, delusions
	Wandering
	Pulling out tubes, attempts to get out of bed
	Sleep disturbance

NOC: Risk Control; Personal Safety Behavior: Client will remain physically safe and free from harm.

NIC: Environmental Management: Safety

1. Identify safety hazards in the environment. *Doing so creates a baseline from which to develop appropriate safety measures.*

2. Place personal and familiar items (eg, call light, water pitcher, eyeglasses) close at hand. *Placing necessary objects within reach minimizes the risk of injury associated with the client's attempts at getting them.*

3. Alert staff and family to the possibility that clients may wander; arrange for continuous observation if indicated. *Clients with delirium have sustained significant injuries by wandering, falling down stairs, or getting lost. Alerting others and arranging for continuous observation helps prevent accidental injury.*

4. Keep beds in the lowest position with rails down, unless policy demands otherwise. Assist with toileting; ensure adequate lighting of environment. *Many clients with delirium, especially*

older adults, are injured climbing over raised bed rails. Regular toileting may help prevent clients from attempting to get out of bed alone. Lighting needs to be bright enough so clients can see clearly.

5. Avoid the use of restraints. *Physical limitation may cause clients to become agitated and fearful, which increases stress and risk for injury.*

NIC: Fall Prevention

1. Provide assistive devices as indicated. *They aid in stabilizing gait and mobility.*
2. Instruct clients to call for assistance with movement, transfer, and ambulation as indicated. *Assistance with mobility reduces the risk of falling.*
3. Implement fall prevention programs, as dictated by agency policy. *They aid in reducing injuries.*

NURSING DIAGNOSIS: Bathing/Hygiene, Toileting, Feeding, and Dressing/Grooming Self-Care Deficit

Related to:	As Evidenced by:
Cognitive impairment	Inability to attend to needs
	Inattention and difficulty focusing

NOC: Self-Care; Activities of Daily Living: Client will participate in meeting basic needs as much as possible within the limits of the disorder, gradually resuming self-care as condition resolves.

NIC: Self-Care Assistance

1. Support clients' efforts to carry out whatever activities of daily living they can. *Doing so increases clients' participation, independence, and self-esteem and provides opportunities to enhance their focus and attention.*
2. Provide assistance; assume responsibility for those necessary activities that clients cannot manage. *Assistance when necessary reduces frustration and anxiety.*
3. Establish a routine to carry out activities, including regular toileting, offering fluids and food, and providing an opportunity for passive or active exercise. *A consistent routine stabilizes and helps re-establish order for clients.*

| NURSING DIAGNOSIS: Deficient Knowledge

Related to:	*As Evidenced by:*
Family's lack of understanding of diagnosis, progression, and prognosis	Abrupt onset of condition Changes in the client's cognition

NOC: Knowledge: Disease Process; Knowledge: Fall Prevention; Knowledge: Treatment Regimen

NIC: Teaching: Disease Process; Teaching: Individual

1. Explain the nature of delirium. Assist client and family to realize that associated confusion and behavior have a biological basis and are transient. *Clients who realize that their thinking is disordered and their families may be frightened. Understanding that the condition is transient may help reduce anxiety levels.*

2. Describe the process, progress, and prognosis of delirium. Teach family about measures being used to control or minimize symptoms. Provide continual updates to client and family as to the state of the underlying problem and the progress being made to resolve it. *This information helps alleviate some anxiety and apprehension.*

Dementia

Dementia is the term used for a syndrome characterized by several cognitive deficits that result from a general medical condition, use of a substance, or multiple biological etiologies. Although there are several types, all forms of dementia affect memory and cognition. Approximately seven million people in the U.S. have chronic cognitive impairment related to dementia; in some communities 50% of people 85 years or older have dementia.

Various disorders are included in the category of dementia:

- Dementia of the Alzheimer's type (with early onset or with late onset)
- Vascular dementia
- Dementia due to HIV disease
- Dementia due to head trauma
- Dementia due to Parkinson's disease
- Dementia due to Huntington's disease

- Dementia due to Pick's disease
- Dementia due to Creutzfeldt-Jakob disease
- Dementia due to general medical condition
- Substance-induced persisting dementia
- Dementia due to multiple etiologies
- Dementia not otherwise specified

Regardless of the category, all dementias are characterized by ongoing multiple cognitive deficits, memory impairment, and a decline from previous level of function that are severe enough to impair social or occupational function. Problems typically include the following:

- Impaired learning
- Compromised ability for complex tasks
- Impaired reasoning
- Compromised spatial ability and orientation
- Language deficits
- Behavior problems

Alzheimer's disease is the most prevalent form of dementia. Its incidence and prevalence directly correlate with increased age. The information that follows relates to dementia of the Alzheimer's type. It can be applied, however, to any form of dementia.

Assessment

DSM-IV-TR Diagnostic Criteria: Dementia

■ Multiple cognitive deficits manifested by both:

1. Impaired memory (either for new or previously learned information)
2. One (or more) of the following: aphasia, apraxia, agnosia, disturbed executive functioning

■ Significant impairment in social or occupational function from cognitive deficits, representing a decline from previous levels

■ Gradual onset with continuing cognitive decline

■ Cognitive deficits not from other central nervous system conditions that cause progressive deficits in memory and cognition, systemic conditions known to cause dementia, or substance-induced conditions

■ Deficits not occurring exclusively during delirium

■ Disturbance not better explained by another Axis I disorder (eg, schizophrenia)

■ Early onset if age 65 or less; late onset if older than age 65

Adapted with permission from American Psychiatric Association. (2000). *Diagnostic and statistical manual of mental disorders (4th ed., text rev.)*. Washington, DC: Author.

Common History and Physical Examination Findings

See "Questionnaire for Dementia," *p. 72* and "Functional Dementia Scale," *p. 74.*

- Cognitive changes
- Aphasia, language difficulties
- Apraxia
- Agnosia
- Problems with executive functions
- Impaired memory
- Gait disturbances
- Possible seizure
- Neglect of personal hygiene
- Incontinence (severe, late stage)

Common Psychosocial Assessment Findings

- Spatial disorientation
- Poor judgment/insight
- Apathy
- Personality changes
- Mood swings
- Lack of awareness of memory loss or change in cognition
- Disinhibited behavior (inappropriate joking, undue familiarity with strangers)
- Delusions
- Superimposed delirium
- Wandering, agitation, aggression

Common Laboratory and Diagnostic Test Findings

- **Computed tomography/magnetic resonance imaging**: brain atrophy; widened cortical sulci and enlarged cerebral ventricles
- **Microscopic examination**: senile plaques, neurofibrillary tangles, granulovascular degeneration, neuronal loss, astrocytic gliosis, amyloid angiopathy; possible Lewy bodies in cortical neurons

Interdisciplinary Treatment Modalities

Psychopharmacology
- Cognitive enhancers (donepezil, galantamine, rivastigmine [*see p. 269*])
- Antipsychotics (*see p. 237*)
- Antidepressants (*see p. 185*)
- Mood stabilizers (*see p. 224*)
- Anxiolytics (*see p. 150*)

Safety Measures/Environmental Management

Cognitive Reorientation

Behavior Management

Family Support/Caregiver Support

Nursing Care Planning

I NURSING DIAGNOSIS: Chronic Confusion

Related to:	As Evidenced by:
Diagnosis of Alzheimer's disease	Memory impairment
	Forgetfulness
	Lack of awareness of changes
	Apraxia
	Agnosia

NOC: Cognition: Client will exhibit adequate mental functioning with assistance.

NIC: Dementia Management

1. Control environmental stimulation. Help establish a calming atmosphere. Encourage the family to remove household clutter and to provide adequate lighting without glare. Create predictability and simplify choices. Assist the family to establish a daily routine for grooming, meals, and activities; teach them to ask relatives and friends to visit, but to do so one or two at time. *Controlled stimulation will help clients feel secure at home. Simple choices and tasks that they can complete successfully*

prevent frustration and loss of self-esteem. Nonglare lighting is less disruptive and helps decrease perceptual difficulties. Limiting visitors allows clients to continue socializing in a controlled way.

2. Introduce yourself when initiating contact with clients; address them distinctly by name. Speak slowly in a clear, low, warm, and respectful tone of voice. *These measures prevent startling clients. Using a client's name helps reorient him or her as needed.*

3. Use distraction, not confrontation, to manage behavioral problems. *Confrontation increases frustration and stress.*

4. Provide space for clients to pace or wander safely; provide finger foods if they cannot sit and eat. *Space minimizes the risk of injury; finger foods can help promote adequate nutrition.*

5. Encourage one-to-one and group activities geared to the client's cognitive abilities and interests. When giving directions, do so one at a time. *Limitations minimize overstimulation, which can increase anxiety. Individual simple directions prevent overwhelming clients.*

6. Use symbols to locate areas or important items. *Symbols may be easier for clients to comprehend than written words.*

NIC: Cognitive Stimulation

1. Orient clients to person, place, and time. Provide environmental memory cues. Cut out pictures from magazines and place them on cabinets and drawers to illustrate contents. Provide a large-print calendar in a conspicuous spot and record all appointments there. Encourage clients to review the calendar daily. *Environmental cues will help jog memory and keep clients as independent as possible for as long as possible.*

2. Reinforce and repeat information. *Repetition promotes awareness.*

NURSING DIAGNOSIS: Risk for Injury

Related to:	As Evidenced by:
Cognitive impairment	Progressive changes in memory and executive function
	Impaired judgment
	Memory loss
	Disinhibited behavior

NOC: Personal Safety Behavior; Safe Home Environment:
Client will remain free from injury. The family will adjust the home as necessary to ensure it is in optimal condition to maintain safe and independent living for client.

NIC: Environmental Management: Safety

1. Identify danger areas and safety hazards in the home. Instruct the family to make garages and basements unavailable to clients, because dangerous items often are stored there. Teach them to lock medications, poisons, cleaning agents, and other toxic fluids in secure containers or rooms. Ensure that doors leading outside are locked or have alarms installed. Instruct the family to secure windows and any doors on the upper floors of the home. *Decreasing cognitive skills increase clients' risk for injury. Keeping certain areas off-limits and the rest of the house safe and secure maximizes freedom at home while protecting clients.*

2. Modify the environment to minimize hazards and risks. Use safety covers on electrical outlets and remove electrical items that pose hazards. Move the thermostat on the hot water heater to a low setting. Remove all electrical appliances from counters and control knobs from the stove and oven. *Making the home safer should give the family some peace of mind about the safety of clients. Monitoring the home is the best intervention for maintaining safety. Interventions will help prevent accidental bums or fires.*

3. Recommend appropriate protective and adaptive devices. *Protective devices limit mobility or access to harm; adaptive devices increase environmental safety.*

4. Provide emergency phone numbers; have the family keep them readily available. *Quick access is crucial during a crisis.*

NURSING DIAGNOSIS: Interrupted Family Processes

Related to:	As Evidenced by:
Changes in client's health status	Progressive cognitive changes
	Changes in role performance
	Deterioration in self-care abilities
	Increasing dependency needs
	Agitation, aggression

NOC: Family Coping: The family will demonstrate positive coping measures to deal with changes.

NIC: Family Process Maintenance

1. Identify effects of role changes on family processes. Promote family cohesion. Help family members, including clients, identify their feelings about role and health status changes. Help them resolve any guilt feelings. Identify effective coping mechanisms; encourage their use as family adjusts to changes. Discuss strategies for normalizing family life. *Open communication about the effects of Alzheimer's disease will help family members. Clients may feel guilty about not being able to help more or about becoming a burden on the family; caregivers may have resentment about increased responsibilities.*

2. Minimize disruptions by facilitating family routines and rituals. *Encouraging normal activities reduces feelings of guilt or anxiety related to the client's current condition.*

3. Discuss existing social support mechanisms; assist the family to use them. Help them resolve any conflicts; suggest attending an Alzheimer's support group. Identify home care needs and how the family might incorporate them into their lifestyle. *Helping the family resolve feelings and identify appropriate coping behaviors will decrease stress. Support groups are a tremendous resource for sharing feelings and gaining insight and help. Incorporating home care needs minimizes disruptions.*

| NURSING DIAGNOSIS: Risk for Caregiver Role Strain

Related to:	*As Evidenced by:*
Continued progression of disease	Increased requirements for care
	Inability to perform self-care activities
	Increased dependency on caregiver
	Increasing safety issues with cognitive deterioration

NOC: Caregiver Stressors; Caregiver Emotional Health; Caregiver Physical Health: Caregiver will identify need for assistance, obtaining essential respite and support to maintain own functioning.

NIC: Caregiver Support

1. Determine the caregiver's level of knowledge and acceptance of role. Provide practical support. Explore reaction and help identify stressors, tasks, or behaviors that are most frustrating or anxiety producing. Help caregiver develop a plan for managing them. Provide support for decisions. Give information about the disease and local support groups. *Helping caregivers become aware of their feelings, strengths, the progressive nature of Alzheimer's disease, and available supports empowers them to manage the increasing demands while protecting their emotional state. Thinking through and planning ahead will help them manage responsibilities.*

2. Teach techniques to improve the security of clients. *Doing so reduces the risk of injury to clients and caregivers.*

3. Explore with caregivers how they are coping; teach stress management techniques and health maintenance strategies to sustain physical and mental health. *Determining coping strategies and providing instruction about stress management and health maintenance strategies enhance the ability of caregivers to provide necessary care.*

4. Give encouragement to caregivers during setbacks for clients. *Setbacks can promote guilt, frustration, and anxiety. Encouragement helps preserve self-esteem.*

NIC: Emotional Support

1. Provide emotional support. Make supportive or empathetic statements. *Emotional support helps reduce feelings of anxiety in stressful situations.*

2. Encourage caregivers to get adequate rest and to maintain own physical, emotional, and spiritual health. Help caregivers recognize that caregiving is stressful. Encourage them to express feelings of anxiety, anger, or sadness. Encourage them not to feel ashamed or guilty if they experience impatience, frustration, sadness, or anger. *Deep breathing, meditation, and visualization, as well as physical exercise and adequate rest, can help caregivers manage anxiety and stress. Finding sources for personal comfort and happiness will help them maintain an identity separate from the caregiving role. They then can come to understand that these emotions are natural when caring for someone who may be unhappy, ungrateful, or difficult.*

NIC: Respite Care

1. Monitor endurance of caregivers. Establish a plan for respite care. Encourage caregivers to set realistic limits on how much they can do. Counsel them to avoid becoming isolated and to accept help from others. *Caregivers cannot perform total full-time care alone.*

2. Coordinate volunteers for in-home services. Arrange for substitute caregivers. Identify community resources for respite care or other family members or friends who can regularly relieve the caregiver for a few hours at a time. *Respite is essential to prevent burnout, which is common among full-time caregivers, especially those who are socially isolated or have no relief from their duties.*

| NURSING DIAGNOSIS: Decisional Conflict

Related to:	**As Evidenced by:**
Progressive nature of disease and uncertainty about future health and resources	Continuing cognitive decline
	Loss of ability to plan and think
	Increasing dependency

NOC: Decision Making; Participation in Healthcare

Decisions: Family will verbalize appropriate future plans, identifying available support for achieving outcomes.

NIC: Decision-Making Support

1. Establish communication; facilitate articulation for goals of care. *Communication is important for the therapeutic relationship; knowledge of goals facilitates an individualized plan of care.*

2. Provide information as requested. Describe options available for care, including full-time nursing at home, adult daycare centers, nursing homes, and other long-term facilities. Help the family explore the advantages and disadvantages of each option. Supply all information as requested, but avoid portraying a hopeless prognosis. Respect the clients' right to receive or not receive information. *Family members need information so they can plan for the future. The current plan of caregiving may not be feasible*

if clients need more than resources allow. Clients still may be in denial; the healthcare team needs to respect the right of clients to not receive information.

3. Help clients clarify values and make important decisions while cognitive function is high. Encourage them to provide advance directives. *Facilitating decisions now helps ensure that others can carry out the wishes of clients if they cannot make necessary legal decisions.*

NURSING DIAGNOSIS: Grieving

Related to:	As Evidenced by:
New diagnosis of dementia	Changes in current status
	Denial of problems
	Reaction to diagnosis
	Progressive nature of condition
	Potential impairment of functional ability

NOC: Grief Resolution; Psychosocial Adjustment: Life Change: Client will verbalize feelings about diagnosis and potential decline in functional ability. Family will set realistic goals, maintain productivity, and use effective coping.

NIC: Grief Work Facilitation

1. Assist clients to identify and to express fears and feelings. Help them deal with their initial reaction. Listen carefully and empathetically. Communicate acceptance. Include significant others. *Encouraging clients to express feelings and listening empathetically help them release sadness and fear. They also help clients to feel that others care.*

2. Instruct the family about the phases of grieving; support progression through them. *Loss of cognitive function is one of the most frightening changes a person can face. The family needs time to process their feelings.*

3. Help clients identify existing coping strategies and consider new ones. Examples include living in the present, meditating, praying, and practicing deep breathing or relaxation. *Establishing a plan for stress management can help clients during times of fear and*

anxiety. Stress reduction techniques also may increase feelings of well-being.

NIC: Anticipatory Guidance

1. Assist the family to identify available resources. *Doing so reveals additional support. Options allow the family to find solutions for problems, which enhances feelings of control.*
2. Rehearse techniques needed to cope with upcoming crises as appropriate. *Practicing techniques facilitates their use when needed.*

16

Dissociative Disorders

D issociative disorders involve alterations in self-awareness in an effort to escape an upsetting event or feeling. This normal method of self-preservation against emotionally overloaded situations happens when neither resistance nor escape is possible. It can include actively pretending to be somewhere or someone else, experiencing amnesia, or being able to "cut off" pain perception from body regions. The cognitive outcome is fragmented memory, which can lead to patchy or disorganized recall, seemingly illogical associations, and extreme affective reactions (eg, rage in response to relatively minor interpersonal "offenses"). Dissociation leading to impaired functioning requires treatment. The degree of disruption of the self and the intensity and types of interventions vary.

Currently, there are four types of dissociative disorders:

1. **Depersonalization disorder**: characterized by a recurring or persistent feeling that one is detached from one's own thinking; affected clients feel that they are outside their mind or body, much like an observer
2. **Dissociative amnesia**: characterized by loss of memory that is not organic and involves an inability to recall events or facts too extensive to be labeled as mere forgetfulness
3. **Dissociative fugue**: sudden travel away from home coupled with an inability to remember the past and confusion about identity or the adoption of a new identity

4. **Dissociative identity disorder**: acquisition of two or more identities or personality states (**alters**) who take control over their behavior

Dissociative Identity Disorder

Dissociative identity disorder (DID), formerly known as multiple personality disorder, involves the acquisition of alters, which are two or more identities or personalities. Each alter has its own traits, behavior patterns, memories, and ways of engaging in interpersonal relationships. Clients usually have a primary personality, but alters can emerge (usually during times of great stress) with wildly different characteristics. DID involves an inability to recall important personal information that is too extensive to be labeled as forgetfulness. During periods of "altered" personality, clients may not be able to remember objective events or things that happened to them. Most clients with DID also experience severe depression, panic attacks, and psychotic symptoms.

Assessment

Diagnostic and Statistical Manual of Mental Disorders, Fourth Edition, Text Revision (DSM-IV-TR) Diagnostic Criteria: DID

- Evidence of two or more distinct identities or personalities, each with its own consistent pattern of perceiving, relating to, and thinking about environment and self
- At least two identities or personalities recurrently controlling client's behavior
- Inability to recall important personal information; lack of recall too extensive to be described as ordinary forgetfulness
- Disturbance not caused by a substance or medical condition. **Note:** In children, symptoms not attributed to "imaginary friends" or other fantasy play.

Adapted with permission from American Psychiatric Association. (2000). *Diagnostic and statistical manual of mental disorders (4th ed., text rev.).* Washington, DC: Author.

Common History and Physical Examination Findings

- Memory/recall impairment
- Fatigue
- Severe anxiety level

- Self-inflicted injuries
- Headaches

Common Psychosocial Assessment Findings

- Two or more identities or personality states
- Inability to function
- Depression
- Suicidal ideas
- Feelings of being overwhelmed
- Feelings of being detached
- Depersonalization
- Low self-esteem
- Possible history of abuse or trauma

Interdisciplinary Treatment Modalities

Psychotherapy

- Individual psychotherapy (*see p. 126*)

Group Therapy (*see p. 123*)

Art Therapy

Milieu Therapy (*see p. 130*)

Psychopharmacology

- Anxiolytics (lorazepam [*see p. 169*])
- Antidepressants (SSRIs [*see p. 185*])

Nursing Care Planning

NURSING DIAGNOSIS: Disturbed Personal Identity

Related to:	As Evidenced by:
Overwhelming stress and anxiety	Development of "alters"
	Depersonalization
	Significant memory loss
	Inability to function
	History of abuse or trauma

Nursing Outcomes Classification (NOC): Identity; Distorted Thought Self-Control: Client will verbalize diminished feelings of depersonalization and dissociation.

Nursing Interventions Classification (NIC): Reality Orientation

1. Approach clients slowly and from the front. Speak in a slow, distinct manner with appropriate volume. *A calm approach from the front prevents startling clients and increasing anxiety level.*

2. Orient clients to the "here and now" using physical grounding techniques such as lighting areas if dark; asking clients to keep their eyes open, stand up, or hold the hands of a staff member; having clients maintain eye contact or walk around and look at present surroundings; or suggesting clients chew on ice chips. *Orientation measures can break the dissociative state by focusing clients on physical reality. Experiencing stimuli through the senses connects clients to the "here and now."*

3. Orient clients to the "here and now" using verbal grounding techniques, such as stating the place, day, time, and date; calling them by their legal names, not an "alter" name; identifying yourself and validating the adult status of clients by having them look at their size in relation to yours. *Verbal grounding techniques will remind clients that they are in the present, safe, and adults.*

4. Assist clients to learn grounding techniques. *Teaching about grounding techniques helps clients to use them appropriately, bringing them into the present and reminding them that they are safe.*

5. Assist clients to understand the existence of alters and to identify the role of each. *Clients may be unaware of the presence of alters. Identifying the role of each helps to determine the need being met by the alter.*

NIC: Self-Esteem Enhancement

1. Assist clients to acknowledge the relationship between anxiety, feelings of being overwhelmed, and the development of alters. Explore previous achievements and reasons for feelings. Encourage clients to identify strengths and resources. Reinforce identified strengths. *Realistic self-expectations, positive reinforcement, and continued feedback aid in increasing sense of self.*

2. Determine locus of control for clients and their self-confidence in their own judgment. Assist in setting realistic goals. Provide clients with experiences to increase autonomy as appropriate. Convey confidence in their ability to handle situations. *Opportunities to practice independent functioning will help clients develop self-confidence, thereby enhancing self-esteem.*

3. Discuss fears and perceptions about assuming responsibility for behavior. Encourage clients to assume more responsibility for behavior gradually. Encourage independence, but be available for help and assistance when needed. Facilitate family support and provide positive feedback for behavior changes. *Assuming responsibility for their own behavior will help clients gain control over their emotional state, diminish reliance on dissociation and other maladaptive coping mechanisms, and foster feelings of self-esteem.*

| NURSING DIAGNOSIS: Risk for Self-Mutilation

Related to:	As Evidenced by:
Overwhelming feelings of stress and being threatened, along with use of maladaptive coping mechanisms	Memory loss Evidence of injuries, cuts Anxiety/panic

NOC: Impulse Self-Control; Self-Mutilation Restraint: Client will exhibit no further evidence of self-injury and demonstrate appropriate coping strategies to deal with anxiety.

NIC: Behavior Management: Self-Harm

1. Determine the appropriate level of self-harm precautions for clients; explain the precautions fully to clients. *Physical safety of clients is a priority.*

2. Assess suicide or self-harm potential, and evaluate the needed level of precautions at least daily. *Potential for self-harm can vary; risk may increase or decrease at any time.*

3. Be alert to sharp objects and other potentially dangerous items (eg, glass containers, lighters); these should not be in the possession of clients who are not feeling safe. *Clients can use many common objects self-destructively. If clients lack effective impulse control, they might use these objects if they are available.*

4. If clients are at risk for serious self-harm, use restraint or seclusion with no access to objects that can be used for self-harm. If this is necessary, begin to talk to clients about regaining internal control over their behavior as soon as possible. *Use of restraints or seclusion is a last resort. If used, it is especially important for clients to think about reassuming control of themselves at the onset of restraint or seclusion.*

5. Openly and directly discuss the ability of clients to be safe, in a matter-of-fact manner. *An open and nonjudgmental approach avoids conveying the message that clients are unworthy or bad, yet addresses safety issues.*

6. Negotiate a "no self-harm" contract, both verbally and in writing, and identify situations that trigger self-harm impulses. *Agreeing to the "no self-harm" contract increases safety and helps clients gain control over their behavior. Identifying triggers also will help clients recognize risky situations so that they can act before becoming overwhelmed by emotions.*

7. Help clients to identify at least one "safe" person per shift that they can go to for support and problem solving during a self-harm crisis. *Identifying one safe person promotes a sense of security and safety and gives clients responsibility for seeking out this person during a crisis.*

NIC: Impulse Control Training

1. Discuss the concept of having self-harm ideas as distinct from acting on those ideas. *Many clients do not recognize the difference between having urges and acting on them.*

2. Convey belief that clients can gain control over self-harm behavior, even if the urge for self-harm persists. *Clients will benefit from knowing that the nurse believes they can gain control over self-harm behaviors.*

3. Explore activities or behaviors that clients might use when self-harm urges are more intense. Work with clients to develop steps that they can take when the urge to harm self occurs. Suggest activities such as deep breathing, seeking out a staff member to talk to, drawing pictures of what is bothering them, writing in a journal, or engaging in sports to overcome the urge. Recognize that clients can use any appealing activity that is not harmful to

replace self-injurious behavior. *Clients are less likely to act out self-harm ideas if they are otherwise occupied. Replacing maladaptive coping mechanisms with positive actions teaches clients that alternatives to self-harm exist.*

4. Provide positive reinforcement for successful outcomes; encourage clients to reward themselves for successful outcomes. *Positive reinforcement enhances self-esteem and reinforces use of appropriate coping mechanisms.*

NURSING DIAGNOSIS: Ineffective Coping

Related to:	As Evidenced by:
Perception of inability to control stressors and traumatic events	Use of maladaptive coping methods
	Development of alters
	Detachment and depersonalization
	Feelings of being overwhelmed

NOC: Coping: Client will demonstrate appropriate positive coping strategies for emotional control.

NIC: Coping Enhancement

1. Provide a safe, nonjudgmental environment that is simple and structured. Reduce stimuli that clients may misinterpret as threatening. *A calm, simple, structured environment reduces anxiety and encourages clients to diminish defensive responses.*

2. Assess clients for indications of stress and appearance of alters. Assist them to appraise the situation objectively and to identify possible triggers for each altered state. *Objective evaluation and information about stress and triggers can aid in developing appropriate and adaptive methods to respond.*

3. Involve clients as much as possible in planning their own treatment. *Participation in their own plans of care can help to increase a sense of responsibility and control in clients.*

4. Maintain the focus of care on the "here-and-now." *Keeping clients focused on reality is important to reduce the risk for dissociation.*

5. Encourage clients to identify and express their feelings and fears; convey acceptance of clients' feelings. Help clients identify situations in which they are more comfortable expressing feelings. *Discussion of current feelings can help clients work through them and begin to distinguish between current and past feelings.*

6. Provide opportunities for clients to express emotions and release tension in a safe, nondestructive way, such as group discussion, activities, and physical exercise. Use role-playing to practice expressing emotions. *Expressing feelings can be helpful even if the feelings are uncomfortable for clients. Role-playing allows clients to try out new behaviors in a supportive environment.*

7. As appropriate, monitor the pace of clients in uncovering memories. *Manifestations that therapy is moving too fast may include attempts at self-mutilation, psychotic symptoms, and increased episodes of dissociation.*

8. Help clients recognize early signs of anxiety and identify times when strong emotions begin to be overwhelming. *Keeping a journal of antecedents and developing a concrete plan for managing emotions are useful coping strategies. The sooner clients recognize the onset of anxiety, the more quickly they will be able to alter their responses.*

9. Educate clients about the recovery process. *Clients may have idealistic fantasies of a "quick fix." They need to know that treatment may involve uncovering painful feelings and memories.*

Eating Disorders

C ollectively, **eating disorders** involve eating consistently below or above a person's caloric needs to maintain a healthy weight, are accompanied by anxiety and guilt, occur without hunger or fail to produce satiety, and result in physiologic imbalances or medical complications. The two most serious eating disorders are anorexia nervosa and bulimia nervosa.

Anorexia Nervosa

Anorexia nervosa is a life-threatening condition that involves a disturbed body image, emaciation, and an intense fear of becoming obese. Historically, anorexia has been diagnosed most frequently in white, affluent, well-educated adolescent and young-adult women. This disorder is becoming more widely distributed among social classes and cultures.

Assessment

Diagnostic and Statistical Manual of Mental Disorders, Fourth Edition, Text Revision (DSM-IV-TR) Diagnostic Criteria: Anorexia Nervosa

- Refusal to maintain weight at or above normal for age and height
- Weight loss or failure to gain expected weight during growth period causing body weight to be less than 85% of expected
- Intense fear of gaining weight or becoming fat
- Disturbance of body weight or shape with undue influence of same on self-evaluation or denial of seriousness of current low body weight
- Amenorrhea (at least three consecutive menstrual cycles)
- *Restricting type*: limitation of food intake without regularly engaging in binge eating or purging
- *Binge eating and purging type*: regular participation in binge eating or purging behaviors (self-induced vomiting or misuse of laxatives, diuretics, or enemas) with limitation of intake

Adapted with permission from American Psychiatric Association. (2000). *Diagnostic and statistical manual of mental disorders* (4th ed., text rev.). Washington, DC: Author.

Common History and Physical Examination Findings

See also "Criteria for Hospitalization: Eating Disorders," *p. 76,* and "Inventory for Clients with Eating Problems," *p. 80.*

- Emaciated appearance, skeletal muscle atrophy, loss of fatty tissue
- Breast tissue atrophy
- Blotchy or sallow skin
- Lanugo (a covering of soft, fine hair) on the trunk
- Dryness or loss of scalp hair
- Hypotension, bradycardia
- Painless salivary gland enlargement
- Fatigue
- Sleep difficulties
- Cold intolerance and hypothermia
- Peripheral edema
- Constipation
- Bowel distention
- Slow reflexes

- Loss of libido
- Wearing oversized clothing in an effort to disguise body size
- Layering clothing or wearing unseasonably warm clothing to compensate for cold intolerance and loss of adipose tissue

Common Psychosocial Assessment Findings

- Preoccupation with body size
- Distorted body image
- Descriptions of self as "fat" or dissatisfaction with a particular aspect of appearance
- Low self-esteem
- Social regression, isolation
- Perfectionism
- Ritualism
- Inflexible thinking, all-or-none reasoning, intellectualization, overgeneralization
- Paradoxical obsession with food, such as preparing elaborate meals for others (*see* "Eating Attitudes Test," *p. 77.*)
- Feelings of despair, hopelessness, and worthlessness
- Suicidal thoughts

Common Laboratory and Diagnostic Test Findings

- **Complete blood count**: anemia, leukopenia, thrombocytopenia
- **Serum electrolyte levels**: decreased chloride, calcium, potassium, magnesium, and phosphate
- **Blood urea nitrogen level**: elevated
- **Hepatic enzyme levels**: elevated
- **Serum eholesterol**: elevated
- **Hormone levels**: decreased T3; decreased follicle-stimulating hormone, luteinizing hormone, and estrogen and progesterone; depressed insulin; increased glucagons, cortisone, epinephrine, and growth hormones (long-term starvation)
- **ECG**:
  - Low-voltage ST segment depression
  - T-wave flattening
  - Prolonged QT interval
  - QT interval prolongation or U waves (from hypokalemia)

Interdisciplinary Treatment Modalities

Psychotherapy

■ Individual psychotherapy (*see p. 126*)

Behavioral Therapy (*see p. 108*)

■ Cognitive-behavioral therapy (*see p. 116*)

Group Therapy (*see p. 123*)

Family Therapy (*see p. 122*)

Psychopharmacology

■ Antidepressants: SSRIs (fluoxetine [Prozac]; *see p. 201*)

Nursing Care Planning

NURSING DIAGNOSIS: Imbalanced Nutrition, Less Than Body Requirements

Related to:	As Evidenced by:
Refusal to ingest or retain ingested food	Emaciated appearance
	Weight less than 85% of expected
	Hypotension, bradycardia
	Fatigue
	Anemia
	Laboratory test abnormalities
Physical exertion in excess of caloric intake	Loss of fatty tissue
	Skeletal muscle atrophy

Nursing Outcomes Classification (NOC): Nutritional Status; Nutritional Status: Food and Fluid Intake; Nutritional Status: Nutrient Intake: Client will demonstrate an adequate dietary intake to meet body requirements and maintain weight that is appropriate for age and height, with vital signs and electrolyte levels that are within acceptable parameters.

Nursing Interventions Classification (NIC): Eating Disorder Management

1. Teach and reinforce concepts of healthy nutrition with clients. *Doing so helps ensure understanding of nutritional requirements and fosters compliance to achieve positive outcomes.*

2. Establish the amount of desired daily weight gain. Use behavior modification techniques to promote behaviors that contribute to weight gain and to limit weight loss behaviors as appropriate. Develop a behavior modification contract for gradual weight gain that includes the number of calories per day, amount of exercise with limitations, and a system of rewards for compliance with the contract (or restrictions for noncompliance). *A well-defined behavioral modification program that specifies desired weight gain will provide consistency, decrease power struggles, and enhance compliance.*

3. Develop meal plans with clients. Establish expectations for appropriate eating behaviors, intake of food/fluid, and amount of physical activity. *Including clients in meal planning and expectations enhances their sense of control.*

4. Monitor vital signs, food and fluid intake and output, and weight. Weigh clients daily at the same time and under the same conditions. *Hypotension and bradycardia may result from starvation. Monitoring intake, output, and weight aids in evaluating effectiveness of interventions*

5. Arrange for one-to-one supervision during meals and remain with clients up to 1 hour after eating, observing clients during and after meals and snacks. *Direct observation will diminish opportunities to avoid eating, to hoard or hide food, or to vomit.*

6. Discuss with clients the need to avoid excessive exercise. Discuss the importance of exercise for physical and mental fitness, but acknowledge that clients must stop relying on exercise for weight reduction. *Clients with eating disorders may engage in excessive exercise to burn calories. By focusing on physical fitness, clients may begin to associate exercise with health promotion instead of weight loss.*

7. Use a supportive, firm, nonjudgmental, and matter-of-fact approach in regulating eating behavior. *Clients should not view a matter-of-fact approach as punishment. This approach also helps alleviate guilt, leading clients to experience feelings of acceptance.*

8. Encourage clients to use daily logs to record feelings as well as circumstances surrounding urges to vomit or exercise to excess. *Participation from clients promotes feelings of control. Record keeping provides clients with insight into their behaviors.*

9. Provide support as clients begin to integrate new eating behaviors, changes in body image, and lifestyle alterations. *Support helps clients progress toward goal achievement and provides reinforcement for positive behaviors, increasing the chances for successful outcomes.*

NIC: Nutrition Management

1. Ascertain clients' preferences; collaborate with a dietitian with regard to calories and type of nutrients needed to meet requirements. *Incorporating preferences along with necessary nutrients promotes compliance from clients to achieve adequate nutrition.*

2. Provide a liquid diet using supplements or through nasogastric or nasoduodenal tube as necessary to maintain an adequate oral intake. *A liquid diet will provide adequate nutrition and fluid if clients are unwilling to eat and drink.*

NIC: Nutritional Monitoring

1. Monitor trends in weight loss or gain and type and amount of usual exercise. *Monitoring for changes provides direct evidence of compliance with the dietary plan.*

2. Assess clients for manifestations of poor nutrition in each body system. Note any changes in manifestations from the initial assessment, including the development of new manifestations. *Inadequate nutrition affects all body systems. Resolution of initial manifestations indicates improved nutritional status. The development of new manifestations may suggest a worsening of the client's status.*

NIC: Fluid/Electrolyte Management

1. Monitor serum electrolyte levels. Evaluate results of additional laboratory tests, including serum albumin, total protein, hemoglobin, and hematocrit. Assess for signs and symptoms of fluid and electrolyte imbalance. *Results of laboratory tests provide objective evidence of nutritional status. Signs and symptoms of imbalances can provide additional evidence of abnormalities.*

2. Keep an accurate record of intake and output. Give fluids as appropriate. *Intake and output monitoring is a valuable indicator of fluid balance. Fluid intake is necessary to correct possible dehydration.*
3. Administer prescribed supplemental electrolytes as appropriate; monitor for side effects and for response to therapy. *Electrolyte deficiencies are commonly associated with eating disorders and impaired nutrition. Supplements provide a means for replacing decreased electrolytes, thereby reducing the risk for complications.*

| NURSING DIAGNOSIS: Disturbed Body Image

Related to:	As Evidenced by:
Fears of gaining weight	Low body fat percentage
	Preoccupation with body size
	Wearing of oversized clothing to disguise body size
	View of self as "fat"
	Overgeneralizations

NOC: Body Image; Self-Esteem: Client will verbalize a realistic and positive view of self, appearance, and self-worth.

NIC: Body Image Enhancement

1. Use cognitive restructuring techniques; assist clients to review own and others' bodies realistically. *Clients can confront and substitute irrational beliefs with more realistic ones. External, objective feedback will help clients attain a healthier, more realistic body image.*
2. Monitor frequency of statements of self-criticism. Assist clients to identify aspects of their physical appearance about which they feel positive. Help clients separate physical appearance from personal worth. *Self-criticism and negative self-perceptions promote an unrealistic body image. Evaluating changes in self-comments and self-descriptions, verbalizations of self-acceptance, and willingness to focus on positive attributes provide measures to evaluate progress toward goal achievement.*

NIC: Self-Esteem Enhancement

1. Assist clients to acknowledge the relationship between overly high self-expectations and feelings of inadequacy. Explore previous achievements and reasons for self-criticism or guilt. Encourage clients to identify strengths and resources. Reinforce identified strengths. *Realistic self-expectations, positive reinforcement, and ongoing feedback will increase self-esteem.*
2. Determine locus of control and self-confidence in judgment for clients. Encourage them to make decisions and choices independently. Convey confidence in the ability of clients to handle situations. *Opportunities to practice independent functioning will enhance self-confidence and self-esteem.*
3. Enhance communication and socialization skills by promoting information, role-playing, and participation in group activities with peers. *Enhanced social skills will improve peer relationships and contribute to improving clients' self-esteem.*

| NURSING DIAGNOSIS: Disturbed Thought Processes

Related to:	*As Evidenced by:*
Distorted body image	Descriptions of self as "fat"
	Preoccupation with body size
	Desire for perfectionism
	Inflexible thinking

NOC: Disordered Thought Self-Control: Client will demonstrate a realistic thinking process and body perception.

NIC: Cognitive Restructuring

1. Assist clients to identify patterns of dysfunctional thinking; anticipate need for therapy. *Identification of dysfunctional thinking must occur first so that clients can then work to change it. Therapy helps to uncover and correct dysfunctional patterns.*
2. Encourage clients to try new behaviors. *Doing so provides opportunities for clients to practice the most effective yet comfortable behaviors and helps foster confidence in choices.*

❘ N U R S I N G   D I A G N O S I S : Interrupted Family Processes

Related to:	As Evidenced by:
Family conflicts and control issues	Overcontrolling parent
	Family's inability to handle conflicts

NOC: Family Coping; Family Functioning: Client and family will demonstrate ability to communicate directly and manage conflicts constructively.

NIC: Family Therapy

1. Determine usual roles of clients within family systems and areas of dissatisfaction or conflict. *Families are highly individualized; knowledge of the specific roles of these family members provides a basis for intervention.*
2. Progress discussion from least to most emotionally laden material. *Starting with the least emotionally laden material helps establish rapport and trust.*
3. Facilitate family discussion; help family members clarify what they need and expect from one another. *Clarification promotes sharing and awareness.*
4. Assist family members to change by changing self as they relate to other family members; facilitate restructuring family subsystems as appropriate. *Families are systems in which a change in one member ultimately affects all other members. Restructuring of family subsystems may be necessary to relieve conflict and improve communication.*
5. Refer the client and family to local support groups. Suggest contact with Anorexia Nervosa and Related Eating Disorders, Inc. (www.anred.com), a national organization created to help clients and families understand what anorexia nervosa is and convince them that they need help.
6. Reinforce concepts of family therapy (*see p. xx*).

NIC: Family Integrity Promotion

1. Determine typical family relationships; identify typical family coping mechanisms and conflicting priorities among family members. *Identification of coping mechanisms provides opportunities to promote use of effective strategies while eliminating*

ineffective ones. Identification of conflicts aids in communicating and planning appropriate strategies to resolve them.

2. Explore ways for each member to increase autonomy. Role-play direct, constructive communication patterns for family members. *Children have more power to make decisions and accept responsibility for own behavior. Role-play of open communication provides an example and gives family members permission to express their thoughts and feelings openly.*

3. Encourage family members to identify and express conflicts openly. Encourage family members to speak for themselves by making "I," rather than "we," statements. *Communicating assertively fosters individuality and personal efficacy among family members. Family members need to learn to distinguish and be responsible for their own feelings, words, and actions.*

Bulimia Nervosa

Bulimia nervosa is a recurrent pattern of uncontrollable consumption of large amounts of food (**binge eating**), followed by attempts to eliminate the body of the excess calories (**purging**). Bulimia nervosa may occur alone or in conjunction with the food restriction of anorexia. Clients with bulimia nervosa compensate for excessive food intake by self-induced vomiting, obsessive exercise, use of laxatives and diuretics, or all of these behaviors. They may consume an incredible number of calories (an average of 3415 calories per binge) in a short period, induce vomiting, and perhaps repeat this behavior several times a day.

Assessment

DSM-IV-TR Diagnostic Criteria: Bulimia Nervosa

- Recurrent binge eating (amount greater than what most would eat during similar period under similar circumstances) in a discrete period; client experiencing no sense of control
- Recurrent inappropriate behavior to compensate for weight gain, such as misuse of laxatives, diuretics, enemas, or other medications; self-induced vomiting; excessive exercise; or fasting

- Episodes of binge eating and inappropriate compensatory behaviors persisting at least twice a week for 3 months
- Undue influence of body shape and weight on self-evaluation
- Disturbance not exclusive to episodes of anorexia nervosa
- *Purging type*: regular use of self-induced vomiting or misuse of laxatives, diuretics, or enemas during current episode
- *Nonpurging type*: use of other inappropriate compensatory behaviors (eg, fasting) without regular use of purging behaviors during the current episode

Adapted with permission from American Psychiatric Association. (2000). *Diagnostic and statistical manual of mental disorders (4th ed., text rev.).* Washington, DC: Author.

Common History and Physical Examination Findings

- Weight within normal range or slightly overweight or underweight
- Dental caries; chipping of teeth
- Scars on dorsum of hand
- Parotid gland enlargement
- Esophagitis
- Gastric dilation
- Menstrual irregularity
- Dependency on laxatives

Common Psychosocial Assessment Findings

- Signs of depression, anxiety, or both
- Possible substance abuse or dependence involving alcohol or stimulants
- Dissatisfaction with body, desire to lose weight, fear of gaining weight
- Passivity, dependency, and lack of assertiveness
- Possible family disorganization, lack of cohesion, or conflict

Common Laboratory and Diagnostic Test Findings

- **Serum electrolyte levels**: hypokalemia, hyponatremia, hypochloremia
- **Serum bicarbonate level**: elevated (metabolic acidosis [from vomiting]); decreased (metabolic acidosis [from laxative abuse])
- **Serum amylase level**: slightly elevated
- **ECG**: abnormalities and changes

Interdisciplinary Treatment Modalities

Psychotherapy

- Individual psychotherapy (*see p. 126*)

Behavioral Therapy (*see p. 108*)

- Cognitive-behavioral therapy (*see p. 116*)

Group therapy (*see p. 123*)

Psychopharmacology

- Antidepressants: SSRIs (fluoxetine [Prozac]; *see p. 201*); TCAs (*see p. 185*)

Nursing Care Planning

I N U R S I N G D I A G N O S I S : Imbalanced Nutrition, Less than Body Requirements

Related to:	As Evidenced by:
Binge eating with inappropriate compensatory behaviors	Overeating
	Overuse of laxatives, diuretics, enemas
	Self-induced vomiting
	Excessive exercise
	Fasting
	Below normal weight
	Dental caries
	Dental enamel erosion
	Fluid and electrolyte imbalances
	Distorted body image

| NURSING DIAGNOSIS: Imbalanced Nutrition, More than Body Requirements

Related to:	As Evidenced by:
Binge eating	Overeating
	Weight slightly above normal
	Feelings of being out of control

NOC: Nutritional Status; Nutritional Status: Food and Fluid Intake; Nutritional Status: Nutrient Intake: Client will demonstrate an adequate dietary intake to meet body requirements and maintain weight that is appropriate to age and height.

NIC: Eating Disorder Management

1. Teach and reinforce concepts of healthy nutrition with clients. *Doing so ensures their understanding of nutritional requirements and fosters compliance to achieve positive outcomes.*
2. Establish the amount of desired daily weight gain in consultation with nutritionist or dietitian. Use behavior modification techniques to promote behaviors that contribute to weight gain or maintenance and to limit weight loss behaviors as appropriate. Develop a behavior modification contract for gradual weight stabilization (if appropriate) that includes number of calories per day, amount of exercise with limitations, and a system of rewards for compliance with contract (or restrictions for noncompliance). *A well-defined behavioral modification program that specifies desired weight goals will provide consistency, decrease power struggles, and enhance compliance.*
3. Develop meal plans with clients. Establish expectations for appropriate eating behaviors, food/fluid intake, amount of physical activity, and avoidance of purging behaviors, if appropriate. *Including clients will enhance their sense of control.*
4. Ensure adequate consumption of foods high in fiber. *Adequate fiber is necessary to promote normal bowel elimination without the use of laxatives and prevent constipation.*
5. Restrict food availability to scheduled, pre-served meals and snacks. *Doing so minimizes the risk of hoarding food to facilitate binge eating.*
6. Monitor vital signs, food and fluid intake and output, and weight. Weigh clients daily at the same time and under the same conditions.

Hypotension and bradycardia may result from starvation. Monitoring intake, output, and weight ensures health and provides evidence for determining the effectiveness of the plan.

7. Arrange for one-to-one supervision during meals and remain with clients up to 1 hour after eating, observing clients during and after meals and snacks. *Direct observation will diminish opportunities to avoid eating, to hoard or hide food, or to engage in purging activities.*

8. Discuss with clients the need to avoid excessive exercise. Discuss the importance of exercise for physical and mental fitness, but that clients must stop relying on exercise for weight reduction. Provide a supervised exercise program when appropriate. *Clients with eating disorders may engage in excessive exercise to burn calories. By focusing on physical fitness, they may begin to associate exercise with health promotion instead of weight loss.*

9. Use a supportive, firm, nonjudgmental, and matter-of-fact approach in regulating eating behavior. *Clients should not view a matter-of-fact approach as punishment. This approach also helps alleviate guilt, leading clients to experience feelings of acceptance.*

10. Encourage clients to use daily logs to record feelings, as well as circumstances surrounding overeating, or urges to vomit or exercise to excess. *Participation from clients promotes feelings of control. Record keeping provides clients with insight into their behaviors.*

11. Provide support as clients begin to integrate new eating behaviors, changes in body image, and lifestyle alterations. *Support helps clients progress toward goal achievement and provides reinforcement for positive behaviors, increasing the chances for successful outcomes.*

NIC: Nutrition Management

1. Ascertain preferences of clients; collaborate with the dietitian with regard to calories and type of nutrients needed to meet requirements. Encourage calorie intake appropriate for body type and lifestyle. *Incorporating preferences along with necessary nutrients promotes compliance from clients to achieve adequate nutrition.*

2. Allow initial avoidance of some foods that clients identify as bad or problematic, ensuring that they get adequate nutrition. Gradually begin including foods that clients have avoided. *Allowing clients to avoid some foods helps minimize their anxiety about dietary changes. Gradually introducing avoided foods reduces anxiety related to these foods and helps clients learn that these foods are not detrimental.*

3. Urge client's family and friends to refrain from bringing in food or other items used by clients for purging, such as laxatives, diuretics, or enemas. *Lack of access to foods and purging items reduces the risk for overeating and purging and avoids reinforcement of problem behaviors.*

NIC: Nutritional Monitoring

1. Assess weight daily, monitoring trends in weight and type and amount of usual exercise. *Monitoring for changes provides direct evidence of compliance by clients with the dietary plan.*

2. Avoid letting clients weigh themselves more than once daily or to skip daily weighing. *Weighing more than once a day or skipping daily weights helps reinforce fears or beliefs of being overweight, which may promote the need to binge or purge.*

3. Assess clients for manifestations of poor nutrition in each body system. Note any changes in manifestations from initial assessment, including the development of new manifestations. *Inadequate nutrition affects all body systems. Resolution of initial manifestations indicates improved nutritional status. Development of new manifestations may suggest worsening of status.*

NIC: Fluid/Electrolyte Management

1. Monitor for abnormal serum electrolyte levels. Evaluate results of additional laboratory tests including serum albumin, total protein, hemoglobin, and hematocrit. Assess for signs and symptoms of fluid and electrolyte imbalance. *Results of laboratory tests provide objective evidence of nutritional status. Signs and symptoms of imbalances can provide additional evidence of abnormalities.*

2. Keep an accurate record of intake and output. Give fluids as appropriate. *Intake and output monitoring is a valuable indicator of fluid balance. Fluid intake is necessary to correct possible dehydration.*

3. Administer prescribed supplemental electrolytes as appropriate; monitor for side effects and for response of clients to therapy. *Electrolyte deficiencies are commonly associated with eating disorders and impaired nutrition. Supplements provide a means for replacing decreased electrolytes, thereby reducing risk for complications.*

| NURSING DIAGNOSIS: Disturbed Body Image

Related to:	As Evidenced by:
Feelings of being fat and fears of gaining weight	Dissatisfaction with body; preoccupation with others' view of appearance
	Unrealistic expectations
	Body weight within normal parameters or slightly underweight/overweight
	Use of purging behaviors

NOC: Body Image: Client will verbalize a realistic and positive view of self.

NIC: Body Image Enhancement

1. Assist clients to review own and others' bodies realistically. *Clients can confront and substitute irrational beliefs with more realistic ones. External, objective feedback will help clients attain a healthier, more realistic body image.*
2. Monitor frequency of self-critical statements. Assist clients to identify aspects of physical appearance that they identify as positive. Help clients separate physical appearance from personal worth. *Self-criticism and negative self-perceptions promote an unrealistic body image. Evaluating changes in self-comments and self-descriptions, verbalizations of self-acceptance, and willingness to focus on positive attributes provide measures to evaluate progress toward goal achievement.*
3. Work with clients to describe and discuss feelings related to body image. Help clients identify and separate these feelings from eating or purging behaviors in a nonjudgmental manner. *Identifying feelings can assist clients to make the connection between feelings and food.*

| NURSING DIAGNOSIS: Chronic Low Self-Esteem

Related to:	As Evidenced by:
Negative view of self as being fat	Distorted body image
	Dissatisfaction with body
	Dependency, passivity, high self-expectations

NOC: Self-Esteem: Client will verbalize positive feelings of self-worth.

NIC: Self-Esteem Enhancement

1. Assist clients to acknowledge the relationship between high self-expectations and feelings of inadequacy. Explore previous achievements and reasons for self-criticism or guilt. Encourage clients to identify strengths and resources. Reinforce identified strengths. *Realistic self-expectations, positive reinforcement, and ongoing feedback will increase self-esteem.*

2. Determine locus of control for clients and confidence in their own judgment. Encourage them to make decisions and choices independently. Convey confidence in their ability to handle situations. *Opportunities to practice independent functioning will help clients improve self-confidence and self-esteem.*

3. Provide teaching about assertiveness; refer clients to appropriate resources for assertiveness training. *Assertiveness training helps reduce the passivity of clients and may foster increased self-confidence.*

4. Enhance communication and socialization skills by promoting information, role-playing, and participation in group activities with peers. *Enhanced social skills will improve peer relationships and contribute to improving self-esteem.*

| NURSING DIAGNOSIS: Powerlessness

Related to:	As Evidenced by:
Uncontrolled episodes of binge eating in secret	Excessive intake of calories within a short period
	Use of purging or nonpurging behaviors after binging
	Low self-esteem
	Guilt associated with binge episodes
	Passivity, dependency

NOC: Health Beliefs; Personal Autonomy: Client will demonstrate measures to control and avoid binge eating behaviors.

NIC: Self-Responsibility Facilitation

1. Set limits on client's behavior related to eating. *Limit setting reduces the risk for binge-eating behavior.*
2. Encourage clients to verbalize feelings related to eating, including anxiety and guilt about binging. *Verbalization of feelings aids in decreasing anxiety related to behaviors and provides information for clients about the emotional aspects of binge eating.*
3. Assist clients to identify their usual responses to anxiety and guilt. Discuss with clients the types of foods that they commonly use for binge eating. *Identifying the types of food eaten helps clients recognize the use of food as a means of coping with feelings.*
4. Work with clients to determine ways to relieve anxiety and cope with feelings that do not involve food or eating. *Separating feelings from food is important to achieve control over the situation.*
5. Provide positive reinforcement for participation from clients in identifying and openly expressing feelings. Teach clients about appropriate methods for problem solving. *Positive feedback and appropriate problem-solving methods promote self-worth and confidence.*

Impulse-Control Disorders

Impulse-control disorders are characterized by irresistible impulsivity and are viewed as symptoms of an underlying brain disorder or a pervasive personality trait. They include actions performed with little or no regard for consequences. Impulsive characteristics include unpredictable behavior, hypervigilance that results in threats toward others for mild offenses, irresponsibility, low tolerance for frustration, poor problem-solving ability, disturbed relationships, restlessness, and general disregard for social rules and customs.

Impulse-control disorders involve discrete episodes of failure to resist aggressive impulses, which results in serious injury to self, assaults on others, or destruction of property. The person experiences increased tension before committing the act and then relief, excitement, or gratification when the act is committed. Regret or remorse may follow.

Impulse-control disorders are commonly classified as:

- Intermittent explosive disorder
- Kleptomania (stealing)
- Pyromania (fire-setting)
- Pathologic gambling
- Trichotillomania (hair pulling)

Intermittent Explosive Disorder

Intermittent explosive disorder involves discrete episodes of acting on aggressive impulses and causing serious injury or property damage. The person experiences aggression considerably out of proportion to any potentiating or triggering factor. This disorder is commonly found in men with dependent personality traits who respond with violence when feeling useless or ineffective.

Assessment

Diagnostic and Statistical Manual of Mental Disorders, Fourth Edition, Text Revision (DSM-IV-TR) Diagnostic Criteria

- Failure to resist aggressive impulses resulting in serious assaultive acts or property destruction
- Degree of aggressiveness grossly out of proportion to any precipitating psychosocial stressors
- Not better accounted for by another mental disorder or general medical condition; not caused by direct physiologic effects of a substance

Adapted with permission from American Psychiatric Association. (2000). *Diagnostic and statistical manual of mental disorders (4th ed., text rev.)*. Washington, DC: Author.

Common History and Physical Examination Findings

See also "Violence Danger Assessment," *p. 70.*

- Tingling, tremors, palpitations, chest tightness, or head pressure prior to aggressive episode
- Irritability
- Rage
- Increased energy
- Asymmetric reflexes

Common Psychosocial Assessment Findings

- Extreme distress
- Racing thoughts
- Rapid depressed mood and fatigue (after act)
- Job loss
- School suspension

- Difficulties in marriage, interpersonal relationships
- Social or occupational impairment
- Legal problems

Interdisciplinary Treatment Modalities

Communication

Limit Setting (*see p. 127*)

Cognitive-Behavioral Therapy (*see p. 116*)
- Guided discovery
- Anger management

Behavior Therapy (*see p. 108*)
- Token economy

Group Therapy (*see p. 123*)

Family Therapy (*see p. 122*)

Psychopharmacology
- Antipsychotics (*see Chapter 10*)
- Sedative-hypnotics (*see Chapter 7*)
- Antidepressants (*see Chapter 8*)
- Mood stabilizers (*see Chapter 9*)
- Anticonvulsants

Restraint/Seclusion (*see p. 134*)

Nursing Care Planning

I **NURSING DIAGNOSIS**: Risk for Other-Directed Violence

Related to:	*As Evidenced by:*
Episodes of impulsivity	Anger
	Violent behavior/outbursts
	Irritability
	Rage

Nursing Outcomes Classification (NOC): Aggression Self-Control; Impulse Self-Control: Client will demonstrate ability to control behavior, refraining from harming others or destroying property.

Nursing Interventions Classification (NIC): Anger Control Assistance

1. Develop rapport and trust with clients. Appear calm and in control. Speak in a normal, nonprovocative, and nonjudgmental tone. Demonstrate an accepting attitude. *Speaking therapeutically can help defuse anger and foster insight for clients. An accepting attitude helps promote feelings of worthiness.*

2. Be alert to verbal and nonverbal behavior that indicates the feelings of clients. Ask what they are feeling. State observations of what you see (what clients are doing behaviorally) and how clients may be feeling. *Clients may be unaware of behaviors. Verbalization of feelings helps validate observations and assists clients to connect feelings with behaviors.*

3. Be alert for possible triggers or factors that may precipitate anger. Monitor potential for inappropriate anger and aggression in clients; intervene before they occur. *Typically, tension building and signs of increasing agitation occur before clients act. Prompt recognition allows for early intervention should behavior begin to escalate.*

4. Assist clients to identify the source of anger and concerns. Encourage clients to describe and clarify the experience to increase awareness of and triggers for problematic feelings. Use open-ended questions. Avoid "why" questions. Listen and paraphrase the responses of clients. *Verbalization of experience helps clients increase their awareness of and triggers for problematic feelings. Using open-ended questions provides meaningful descriptions. Clients may interpret "yes-or-no" questions as interrogation. They may interpret "why" questions as accusatory, which can cause defensive feelings in the client. Listening and paraphrasing aid in validating observations.*

5. Minimize exposure of clients to stimulation. *They may interpret any stimulus as a potential threat, which may lead to explosive behavior.*

6. Provide clients with appropriate outlets for anger or tension. Assist them to develop ways to express feelings in a nondestructive manner. Teach clients about calming measures, such as taking deep breaths or time-outs. Talk with clients about their ideas for a plan of action that would help deal with the situation. Explain the benefits of expressing anger adaptively and nonviolently. *Clients need to learn measures to control anger; doing so in a nonthreatening environment reduces fears and promotes adaptive coping. Getting input from clients affirms their competence and provides information for further problem solving.*

7. Administer medications as ordered. If the situation escalates, call for assistance. If absolutely necessary, anticipate the need for seclusion and restraints. *Quick action is necessary if the situation continues to escalate. Efforts are aimed at ensuring the safety of all parties involved. Clients must be maintained in the least restrictive environment.*

NIC: Impulse Control Training

1. Assist clients to identify the problem or situation and to determine possible actions. Help clients determine the benefits and limitations of possible actions. *Identifying the underlying problem and possible courses of action provides clients with positive methods to deal with feelings rather than using aggression or violence.*

2. Help clients replace anger-stimulating self-talk with more suitable self-talk. Teach thought-stopping techniques. *Self-talk is powerful and self-fulfilling. Cognitive restructuring promotes behavior changes.*

3. Provide opportunities for clients to practice or role-play actions within the therapeutic environment. Provide positive reinforcement for behavior changes. *Practicing appropriate responses and actions promotes compliance. Positive reinforcement fosters self-esteem in clients and enhances the chances for future use of these actions or responses.*

NIC: Limit Setting

1. Establish firm, reasonable expectations for behavior; communicate them clearly to clients. Identify, with input from clients as appropriate, undesirable behavior. Have all staff members

enforce limits consistently. *Consistently implementing limits helps prevent clients from trying to manipulate staff and will help them gain control of behavior.*

2. Avoid power struggles or trying to dissuade clients from grandiose, delusional ideas. Refrain from arguing or bargaining about established expectations and consequences. Accept acting-out behavior neutrally; do not respond with irritation or anger. Avoid feeding into emotions; maintain a professional demeanor. Redirect clients into productive or more appropriate activities. *Power struggles and arguments may contribute to increased tension. Not participating in emotions and thwarting attempts to upset staff help prevent escalation of behavior. Clients need positive outlets for feelings.*

3. Modify behavioral expectations and consequences as needed. Decrease limit setting as the behavior of clients approximates that which is desired. *Modification is necessary to accommodate for reasonable changes in situations.*

NURSING DIAGNOSIS: Ineffective Coping

Related to:	As Evidenced by:
Episodes of destructive or violent behavior	Anger
	Aggressiveness
	Racing thoughts
	Property destruction
	Legal problems
	Problems with marriage and interpersonal relationships

NOC: Coping: Client will verbalize awareness of typical appraisals of precipitating events, ways to reframe thoughts and behavioral responses more constructively, and awareness of personal competencies in problem solving and coping.

NIC: Coping Enhancement

1. Suggest that clients keep a journal about angry feelings and identify situations that trigger anger. *Journaling helps clients gain*

insight into patterns of behavior and provides a means to consciously identify precursors to feeling out of control or enraged. The ability to identify situations that trigger anger helps empower clients to implement other strategies that will modulate angry responses before acting on them.

2. Assist clients to recognize anger-stimulating self-talk and help clients replace this type of self-talk with more positive self-talk. *Self-talk is powerful and self-fulfilling; appropriate use facilitates changes in behavior.*

3. Role-play appropriate respect for the feelings of others. Teach the use of "I" statements and taking responsibility for one's own feelings. *Role-playing respect provides clients with opportunities to learn to value the dignity of others and show respect. Using "I" statements minimizes the risk for arguments and power struggles.*

4. Teach assertiveness skills. *Assertiveness training provides clients with appropriate tools for meeting own needs without infringing on the rights of others.*

5. Instruct clients in methods for problem solving, including problem identification, identification of possible solutions, implementation of a solution, and evaluation. Allow clients to participate in opportunities for problem solving. *Clients may be unaware or may never have learned an effective and appropriate method for approaching problems. Participating in problem solving helps reinforce appropriate techniques.*

6. Work with clients to develop goals for behavior and coping. Provide positive feedback for goal achievement. *Goal achievement promotes feelings of self-worth and self-esteem.*

19

Mood Disorders

ood refers to a pervasive and sustained emotional coloring of experience or overall emotional feeling. **Mood disorders** involve a disturbance in mood, with wide-ranging signs and symptoms that affect the person's physiologic, psychological, and social functioning. Signs and symptoms include problems with sleep, appetite, weight, or libido; problems with cognition such as distorted attention, memory, or thinking; impulse-control problems; behavioral difficulties, such as withdrawal or fatigue; and somatic manifestations, such as headache, upset stomach, or muscle tension. Because of the myriad signs and symptoms and the inability to assess mood objectively, mood disorders often go undetected.

Generally, mood disorders are classified into two groups:

- Depressive disorders
  - Major depressive disorder
  - Dysthymic disorder
- Bipolar disorders
  - Bipolar I disorder
  - Bipolar II disorder
  - Cyclothymic disorder

Other mood disorders include those caused by a general medical condition as well as substance-induced mood disorders.

Major Depressive Disorder

Major depression is one of the most common illnesses of any type (medical or psychiatric) and affects people of all ages and backgrounds. It is currently the leading cause of disability in clients 15 to 44 years old in the United States, and it is projected to be the second leading cause of disability among all age groups in approximately 10 to 12 years. Major depression can develop at any age, with average onset age of 32 years. Depression in older adults may be difficult to diagnose because many older people suffer from comorbid physical diseases (eg, heart disease, diabetes). Because depression often accompanies these diseases, and because older adults face physical, psychological, and social losses, healthcare professionals may conclude incorrectly that depression is a normal consequence. In fact, clients themselves may share this attitude, leading them to fail to report concerning symptoms.

Depression, like all psychiatric illnesses, results from a combination or interaction of genes, environment, individual life history, development, and neurobiological makeup. Definitive causes have not yet been discovered.

Assessment

Diagnostic and Statistical Manual of Mental Disorders, Fourth Edition, Text Revision (DSM-IV-TR) Diagnostic Criteria: Major Depression

- Over 2 weeks, a change from client's previous functioning with depressed mood or decreased interest or pleasure and at least four of the following:
  1. Significant weight loss without dieting or weight gain or markedly decreased or increased appetite
  2. Hypersomnia or insomnia
  3. Psychomotor agitation or slowness
  4. Fatigue or energy loss
  5. Feelings of worthlessness or guilt
  6. Difficulty concentrating or indecisiveness
  7. Recurrent thoughts of death, either with or without suicide ideation
- Symptoms causing significant distress or impairment of social, occupational, or other functioning
- Symptoms not caused by a substance or a general medical condition

Adapted with permission from American Psychiatric Association. (2000). *Diagnostic and statistical manual of mental disorders (4th ed., text rev.).* Washington, DC: Author.

Common History and Physical Examination Findings

See also "Beck Depression Inventory," *p. 82,* "Hamilton Rating Scale for Depression," *p. 86,* and "Mood Disorder Questionnaire," *p. 89.*

- Weight changes
- Increased or decreased appetite
- Increased sleeping or insomnia
- Fatigue
- Slow body movements
- Difficulties with sexual functioning
- Occupational problems
- Marriage/relationship problems
- Substance use/abuse
- Pacing

Common Psychosocial Assessment Findings

- Sad, depressed, or flat affect
- Tearfulness, irritability
- Obsessive rumination
- Possible panic attacks
- Feelings of guilt, worthlessness, failure
- Loss of pleasure in activities (anhedonia)
- Withdrawal
- Suicidal thoughts, suicide ideation, suicide attempts

Interdisciplinary Treatment Modalities

Psychotherapy

■ Individual psychotherapy (*see p. 126*)

Group Therapy (*see p. 123*)

Family Therapy (*see p. 122*)

Marital Therapy

Electroconvulsive Therapy (*see p. 146*)

Phototherapy (*see p. 147*)

Cognitive Therapy (*see p. 111*)

Behavior Therapy (*see p. 108*)

Milieu Therapy (*see p. 130*)

Psychopharmacology

■ Antidepressants: SSRIs, TCAs, MAOIs (*see p. 185*)

Nursing Care Planning

NURSING DIAGNOSIS: Risk for Suicide

Related to:	As Evidenced by:
Depression	Suicidal thoughts, ideation, or attempts
	Feelings of worthlessness, failure, guilt
	Flat affect
	Anhedonia
	Inability to function in usual role

Nursing Outcomes Classification (NOC): Suicide Self-Restraint: Client will refrain from attempting suicide and harming self.

Nursing Interventions Classification (NIC): Suicide Prevention

1. Observe clients closely and continually. Remove all dangerous objects. *These measures help maintain safety.*
2. Discuss with clients the reasons for such monitoring. *Giving this information can help ensure the cooperation of clients and also foster their understanding of the close observation.*
3. Engage clients in a "no self-harm" contract. *Such a contract reinforces limits and can encourage clients to assume self-control. Feedback helps clients differentiate inappropriate from appropriate responses, as well as possible triggers and causes associated with behavior.*
4. Spend regularly scheduled time with clients during the day. *Such interaction helps clients feel worthwhile and enables them to discuss issues of concern and any brewing problems.*

NURSING DIAGNOSIS: Hopelessness

Related to:	As Evidenced by:
Intense feelings of guilt, worthlessness	Obsessive rumination
	Tearfulness
	Loss of pleasure in activities
	Flat, depressed affect

	Lack of interest in self-care
	Insomnia
	Loss of appetite

NOC: Depression Self-Control; Will to Live: Client will verbalize reasons to continue participation in daily life and positive aspects.

NIC: Mood Management

1. Discuss both positive and negative aspects of the situation with clients. *Clients may not be able to recognize positive elements of their situation. Objective support from others can be useful to this process.*
2. Assist clients to identify helpful support people. *Having resources to draw on may help clients recognize people they can turn to in difficult moments and provide validation of worth and meaning to others.*
3. Assist clients to consider other coping strategies when stress, emotions, or feelings are intense, or when life circumstances are becoming overwhelming. Possibilities include exercise, relaxation techniques, discussion with trusted friends or healthcare providers, and cognitive restructuring. *Alternative coping techniques must be available before clients can abandon self-destructive strategies.*
4. Discuss with a physician the possible need for medication, dosage adjustments, or a new pharmacologic approach. *Depressive symptoms may benefit from pharmacologic therapy or more intensive or stronger medications.*

| NURSING DIAGNOSIS: Self-Care Deficit, Bathing/ Hygiene, Dressing/Grooming, Feeding, Toileting

Related to:	As Evidenced by:
Depression	Lack of interest in self and personal care
	Weight loss
	Fatigue
	Loss of appetite
	Slowed body movements

NOC: Self-Care: Activities of Daily Living: Client will demonstrate ability to perform personal care activities with minimal to no assistance.

NIC: Self-Care Assistance

1. Monitor clients' ability to provide self-care; provide assistance as necessary. *Clients with depression may not be aware of or exhibit interest in self-care.*
2. Provide clients with their own clothes and personal grooming and hygiene supplies if possible. *Having familiar items helps lessen fears and anxieties, aiding in the completion of tasks.*
3. Establish a routine for dressing, grooming, and hygiene, preferably initiating these tasks in the morning and setting limits as to how long clients spend on these tasks. If necessary, break the tasks into simple steps. *Establishing a routine reduces the need for clients to make decisions about self-care. Performing tasks in the morning may be more effective because clients typically have the most energy at this time. Time limits provide clients with concrete expectations for task completion. Breaking the task into simple steps prevents overwhelming clients and fosters achievement.*
4. Assess intake of food and fluids; record intake and daily weight. Offer clients nutritious finger foods and fortified liquids. *Depression may lead to a lack of interest in eating. Nutritious finger foods and fortified liquids help meet nutritional needs without clients expending effort.*
5. Establish a routine for sleep at night and provide comfort measures. Avoid letting clients sleep for long periods during the day. *A routine for sleep including comfort measures establishes expectations for sleep and promotes relaxation. Sleeping for long periods during the day interferes with the need and ability to sleep at night.*
6. Encourage client participation in activities based on ability. Provide assistance as necessary, gradually encouraging independence. *Participation in self-care promotes self-confidence and fosters self-esteem.*

Bipolar Disorders

Bipolar disorders, like depressive disorders, are marked by a disturbance in mood. The difference is that clients with bipolar disorders experience mood swings ranging from profound depression to extreme euphoria, termed **mania**. Symptoms during depressive episodes are consistent with those of major depression. Symptoms during manic episodes include grandiosity; rapid thoughts, actions, and speech; sleep disturbances; and spending sprees. Episodes of bipolar mood disturbances alternate with periods of normal mood and associated behaviors.

Bipolar disorders typically include bipolar I and bipolar II disorders. Bipolar I disorder affects men and women equally; bipolar II disorder is more common in women.

Assessment

DSM-IV-TR Diagnostic Criteria: Bipolar Disorders

- One or more manic or mixed episodes and often one or more major depressive episodes; not better explained by other psychiatric disorders and not the direct result of a substance or other medical condition
- *Manic episode*: Mood abnormally and persistently elevated and expansive or irritable for at least 1 week; three or more of the following exhibited to a significant degree for at least 1 week:
  1. Excessive participation in pleasurable activities with a high potential for painful results
  2. Decreased need for sleep
  3. Inflated self-esteem or grandiosity
  4. Increased goal-oriented activity or agitation
  5. Easy distractibility, excessive speech, or racing thoughts
  6. Markedly impaired functioning in several areas
- *Major depressive episode*:
  1. Depressed mood most of the day
  2. Markedly decreased interest in nearly all activities
  3. Weight gain, decreased/increased appetite, or significant weight loss without dieting
  4. Hypersomnia or insomnia
  5. Psychomotor agitation or slowness
  6. Fatigue or energy loss

> 7. Feelings of worthlessness or guilt
> 8. Difficulty concentrating or indecisiveness
> 9. Recurrent thoughts of death with or without suicide ideation
>
> ■ *Mixed Episode:* Client with criteria for both manic and major depressive episodes nearly every day for 1 week or longer; markedly impaired occupational or social functioning; hospitalization necessary to prevent harm to self or others; or psychotic features; symptoms not the direct effects of a substance or general medical condition
>
> Adapted with permission from American Psychiatric Association. (2000). *Diagnostic and statistical manual of mental disorders (4th ed., text rev.).* Washington, DC: Author.

Common History and Physical Examination Findings

See also "Mood Disorder Questionnaire," *p. 89,* "Hamilton Rating Scale for Depression," *p. 86, and* "Suicide Assessment," *p. 91.*

ASSOCIATED DEPRESSIVE FINDINGS

- Weight changes
- Increased or decreased appetite
- Increased sleeping or insomnia
- Fatigue
- Slow body movements
- Difficulties with sexual functioning
- Occupational problems
- Marriage/relationship problems
- Substance use/abuse
- Pacing

ASSOCIATED MANIC FINDINGS

- Flamboyant exaggerated dress
- Pressured speech
- Sleep disturbances
- Spending sprees
- Promiscuous sexual behavior
- Excessive and illogical rhyming, punning, and word associations
- Excessive talking or laughing

Common Psychosocial Assessment Findings

ASSOCIATED DEPRESSIVE FINDINGS

- Sad, depressed, or flat affect
- Tearfulness, irritability

- Obsessive rumination
- Possible panic attacks
- Feelings of guilt, worthlessness, failure
- Loss of pleasure in activities (anhedonia)
- Withdrawal
- Inability to function in usual role

ASSOCIATED MANIC FINDINGS
- Extreme mood swings
- Irritability or sudden outbursts of misplaced rage
- Distractibility, restlessness
- Hyperactivity, intrusiveness
- Exaggerated self-esteem
- Delusions of grandeur, elation, and other forms of excessive activity
- Rapid "flights of ideas"
- Ignorance of environmental boundaries; invasion of others' personal space
- Little or no concept of inappropriate behaviors
- Risk-taking behaviors

Interdisciplinary Treatment Modalities

Psychotherapy
- Individual psychotherapy (*see p. 126*)

Cognitive-Behavioral Therapy (*see p. 116*)

Family Therapy (*see p. 122*)

Interpersonal and Social Rhythm Therapy (IPSRT)

Psychopharmacology
- Lithium (*see p. 231*)
- Anticonvulsants (Divalproex sodium [*see p. 227*]; carbamazepine [*see p. 225*])
- Atypical antipsychotics (*see p. 238*)

Nursing Care Planning

I N U R S I N G   D I A G N O S I S : Risk for Self- or Other-Directed Violence

Related to:	As Evidenced by:
Impulsivity and impaired judgment	Risk-taking behaviors
	Irritability
	Anger, aggressiveness
	Belligerence
	Invasiveness, lack of boundaries

NOC: Impulse Self-Control; Suicide Self-Restraint; Aggression Self-Control: Client will demonstrate appropriate self-control behaviors to refrain from harming self and others.

NIC: Mood Management

1. Evaluate mood initially and then at regular intervals; determine whether clients pose a safety risk to self or others. Assess level of risk for violence. Interact with clients regularly. Assist clients to consciously monitor mood, such as with a rating scale or journal. Help identify thoughts and feelings underlying the dysfunctional mood. *Assessing mood and risk for violence helps staff members establish appropriate guidelines and interventions. Regular interactions convey caring and provide a chance for clients to discuss feelings. Awareness of mood changes helps clients identify possible related stressors.*

2. Assist clients to express feelings appropriately; discuss anger management and determine appropriate behaviors when angry. Use limit-setting and behavior management strategies to help them refrain from intrusive and disruptive actions. Role play appropriate anger management; give clients feedback on behavior. *Providing limits and outlets for anger gives clients a concrete framework for managing impulses. Role playing and feedback reinforce constructive coping.*

3. Provide a consistent, structured environment. Use simple direct statements to inform clients about goals and expectations. *Consistency and structure provide clients with limits. Simple and direct statements prevent overwhelming clients with complex information.*

4. Use restrictive interventions. Limit the environment and remove dangerous objects. Use sedatives as needed. Use physical restraint or seclusion only as a last resort. *Limiting interactions with others is the best approach to prevent violence if anger and outbursts escalate. Medication can be effective. Seclusion and restraint should be used only if all other methods fail.*

5. Assist clients to identify precipitants of dysfunctional mood, differentiating what can and cannot be changed. Help identify available resources, personal strengths, and abilities to modify such precipitants. Teach new coping and problem-solving skills as necessary. *Knowledge of precipitants helps clients develop strategies to prevent mood changes. Using personal strengths and abilities enhances feelings of control.*

6. Administer prescribed mood stabilizer (eg, lithium) as indicated; monitor for side effects. Obtain serum lithium levels as appropriate. *Mood stabilizers are effective for bipolar disorders. Lithium has a narrow therapeutic window; thus, serum lithium levels need regular, close monitoring for signs of possible toxicity.*

NIC: Suicide Prevention; Environmental Management: Violence Prevention

1. Observe clients closely and continually. Place clients in a room near the nursing station. Remove all dangerous objects. Provide ongoing surveillance of all client access areas and therapeutically intervene as necessary. *These measures help maintain safety.*

2. Discuss with clients the reasons for such monitoring. *Sharing this information can help ensure clients' cooperation and also foster understanding of the close observation.*

3. Engage clients in a "no self-harm" contract. *Such a contract reinforces limits and can encourage clients to assume self-control. Feedback helps clients differentiate inappropriate and appropriate responses as well as possible triggers and causes associated with behavior.*

4. Spend regularly scheduled time with clients during the day. *Such interaction helps them feel worthwhile and enables them to discuss issues of concern and any brewing problems.*

NIC: Behavior Management: Overactivity/Inattention

1. Provide a structured and physically safe environment. Use a calm, matter-of-fact, reassuring approach. *A structured and safe*

environment and a calm, matter-of-fact approach help reduce exposure to stressors and promote a therapeutic relationship.

2. Develop a behavioral management plan that all care providers implement consistently. Communicate rules, expectations, and consequences in simple language. Set limits on intrusive, interruptive behaviors. Praise desired behaviors; provide consistent consequences for both desired and undesired behaviors. *Consistency and clear communication about rules and expectations reduce power struggles and promote feelings of security for clients. Positive feedback for desired behaviors helps reinforce them.*

3. Redirect or remove clients from sources of overstimulation. Monitor and regulate level of activity and environment. *Overstimulation increases stress, possibly leading to undesired behaviors.*

| NURSING DIAGNOSIS: Disturbed Thought Processes

Related to:	As Evidenced by:
Biochemical imbalances associated with psychiatric disorder	Episodes of depression and mania
	Delusions of grandeur
	Bizarre behaviors
	Inflated self-esteem
	Flight of ideas
	Feelings of worthlessness or excessive guilt

NOC: Distorted Thought Self-Control: Client will exhibit reality-based thinking and behavior that reflects appropriate thought content.

NIC: Reality Orientation

1. Use a calm, forthright approach; provide clear directions. Approach slowly and from the front; address clients by name when initiating interaction. *Providing structure and expectations communicates that staff members are effectively managing the milieu, which should diminish power struggles and increase feelings of security for clients.*

2. Interrupt confabulation by changing the subject or responding to the feeling or theme rather than the content. Engage clients in concrete, reality-oriented activities that focus on something outside the self. Involve clients in a reality-orientation group setting

when appropriate. *Focusing on the present and encouraging participation in a reality-orientation group promote logical thinking and reduce the possibility of distraction.*

NIC: Limit Setting

1. Establish firm, reasonable expectations for behavior; communicate them clearly to the client. Identify, with input from clients as appropriate, undesirable behavior. Have all staff members enforce limits consistently. *Consistently implementing limits helps prevent clients from trying to manipulate staff and will help clients gain control of behavior.*

2. Avoid power struggles or trying to dissuade clients from grandiose delusions. Refrain from arguing or bargaining about established expectations and consequences. Accept acting-out behavior neutrally; do not respond with irritation or anger. Avoid feeding into jokiness of clients; maintain a professional demeanor. Redirect clients into productive or more appropriate activities. *Power struggles and arguments may contribute to increased mania. Not participating in manic perceptions and thwarting clients' attempts to upset staff help prevent escalation of mania. These clients are highly distractible; staff members can use this factor to their advantage by redirecting energy when needed.*

3. Modify behavioral expectations and consequences as needed. Decrease limit setting as behavior of clients approximates that which is desired. *Modification is necessary to accommodate reasonable changes in situations.*

| NURSING DIAGNOSIS: Ineffective Health Maintenance

Related to:	As evidenced by:
Depression or mania	Limited food and fluid intake
	Inability to focus/maintain attention
	Lack of attention to self-care needs
	Sleep disturbances

NOC: Self-Care Status; Nutritional Status: Food and Fluid Intake; Fluid Balance: Client will maintain balanced rest, sleep, activity, personal care, and intake of adequate food and fluids.

NIC: Self-Care Assistance

1. Monitor ability to provide self-care; provide assistance as necessary. *Clients with bipolar disorder may not be aware of or exhibit interest in self-care.*

2. Provide clients with their own clothes and personal grooming and hygiene supplies if possible. *Having familiar items helps lessen fears and anxieties, aiding in the completion of tasks.*

3. Establish a routine for dressing, grooming, and hygiene, preferably initiating these tasks in the morning and setting limits as to how long clients spend on these tasks. If necessary, break the tasks into simple steps. *Establishing a routine reduces the need for clients to make decisions about self-care. Performing the tasks in the morning may be more effective because clients typically have the most energy then. Time limits provide concrete expectations for task completion. Breaking the task into simple steps prevents overwhelming clients and fosters achievement.*

4. Assess food and fluid intake; record intake and daily weight. Offer nutritious finger foods and fortified liquids. *Depression may lead to a lack of interest in eating. Nutritious finger foods and fortified liquids help meet nutritional needs without clients having to expend effort to eat.*

5. Establish a routine for sleep at night and provide comfort measures. Plan to have clients rest and calm down 1 hour before bedtime. Limit exposure to environmental stimuli, such as bright lights or loud music, before sleep; help clients identify activities that enhance relaxation. If needed, gently but firmly enforce schedules. Administer medications, as needed, for sleep and rest. *During manic phases, clients can go days without rest, which severely compromises physical health. Sleep is difficult because of hyperactivity. A routine for sleep including comfort measures establishes expectations for sleep and promotes relaxation.*

6. Encourage participation from clients in activities based on ability level. Provide assistance as necessary, gradually encouraging independence. *Participation in self-care promotes self-confidence and fosters self-esteem.*

NIC: Nutrition Management

1. Ascertain clients' food preferences. Monitor recorded nutritional intake for content and calories. *Offering foods that clients like increases the chances for success. Monitoring intake provides a basis for future interventions.*

2. Frequently offer foods that clients can eat "on the run" (eg, crackers, fruits, cheese, sandwiches). Provide high-protein, high-calorie nutritious finger foods that they can readily consume. *Clients may be too restless to sit for meals and too distracted to remember to eat. High-protein, high-calorie foods provide appropriate nutrients for energy needs.*

NIC: Nutritional Monitoring

1. Weigh clients at specified intervals; monitor trends in weight loss or gain. *Weight is an objective measure of nutritional status.*

2. Monitor vital signs, intake, and appropriate laboratory values, such as albumin, total protein, and hemoglobin and hematocrit levels. Assess for malnutrition. *Clients with mania are at risk for physical complications secondary to fluid, electrolyte, and nutrient depletion.*

NIC: Fluid Monitoring

1. Remind clients to drink frequently. Obtain a sports bottle so that clients can carry fluids with them. *Clients with mania may be too physically active to remember to drink. In addition, they are at high risk for dehydration, which is exacerbated with the use of lithium.*

2. Monitor intake and output of fluids, blood pressure, heart rate, and respiratory status. *These parameters provide objective evidence of fluid status.*

3. Evaluate results of laboratory tests, especially serum electrolyte levels. *Results provide information about body fluid components and chemical indicators of nutritional status.*

Personality Disorders

P ersonality comprises the sum of each person's unique biopsychosocial characteristics. It consistently influences the person's inner experience and behavior throughout life. Personality is as essential to self-identity as physical appearance. It may even be considered the psychological equivalent of physical appearance, because neither changes easily or quickly.

Personality disorders are collections of personality traits that have become so fixed and rigid that they cause inner distress and behavioral dysfunction. These disorders also can be explained as lifelong behavioral patterns that negatively affect many areas of life, cause problems, and are not produced by another disorder or illness. Symptoms of personality disorders are serious, and clients with these disorders are at risk for psychiatric comorbidities, such as mood, anxiety, and substance use disorders.

Personality disorders manifest with symptoms in two or more of the following areas: cognition (ways of perceiving and assigning meaning to self, others, and events); affectivity (the range, intensity, and appropriateness of emotionality); interpersonal behavior; and impulse control. Personality disorders are categorized into three clusters. Each cluster has descriptive similarities:

- Cluster A disorders, with odd or eccentric behavior as the core characteristic, include:
  - Paranoid personality disorder

- Schizoid personality disorder
- Schizotypal personality disorder
- Cluster B disorders, with dramatic, emotional, or erratic manifestations, include:
  - Antisocial personality disorder
  - Borderline personality disorder
  - Histrionic personality disorder
  - Narcissistic personality disorder
- Cluster C disorders, with anxious or fearful behaviors, include:
  - Avoidant personality disorder
  - Dependent personality disorder
  - Obsessive-compulsive personality disorder

Antisocial Personality Disorder

Antisocial personality disorder also includes psychopathic personality and sociopathic personality. Clients display aggression and irresponsibility that leads to frequent conflicts with society and subsequent involvement with the criminal justice system. Common associated behaviors include fighting, lying, stealing, domestic violence, substance abuse, and participation in confidence schemes. People with antisocial personality disorder are often superficially charming; however, they typically lack genuine warmth.

Assessment

Diagnostic and Statistical Manual of Mental Disorders, Fourth Edition, Text Revision (DSM-IV-TR) Diagnostic Criteria: Antisocial Personality Disorder

---

■ Pervasive pattern of disregard for and violation of the rights of others after age 15 years, as indicated by three (or more) of the following:

1. Failure to conform to social norms with respect to lawful behaviors, as indicated by repeatedly performing acts that are grounds for arrest
2. Deceitfulness, as indicated by repeated lying, use of aliases, or conning others for personal profit or pleasure
3. Impulsivity or failure to plan ahead

---

4. Irritability and aggressiveness, as indicated by repeated physical fights or assaults

5. Reckless disregard for safety of self or others

6. Consistent irresponsibility, as indicated by repeated failure to sustain consistent work behavior or honor financial obligations

7. Lack of remorse, as indicated by being indifferent to or rationalizing having hurt, mistreated, or stolen from others

■ Client at least 18 years of age with evidence of conduct disorder before age 15 years; behavior not occurring exclusively during schizophrenia or a manic episode

Adapted with permission from American Psychiatric Association. (2000). *Diagnostic and statistical manual of mental disorders (4th ed., text rev.).* Washington, DC: Author.

Common History and Physical Examination Findings

- Overt confidence
- Possible mild to moderate anxiety
- Poor work history
- Legal problems
- Injuries secondary to fights and assaults
- History of multiple sexual partners

Common Psychosocial Assessment Findings

- Distorted, narrow view of world
- Poor judgment
- Impulsivity, need for immediate gratification
- Absence of empathy
- Callous, cynical, and contemptuous of the feelings of others
- Excessively opinionated
- Self-assurance, cockiness
- Superficial charm
- Exploitive sexual relationships
- Dysphoria (tension, inability to tolerate boredom, depressed mood)

Interdisciplinary Treatment Modalities

Psychotherapy

■ Individual psychotherapy (see p. 126)

Behavioral Therapy (*see p. 108*)

■ Dialectical behavioral therapy (*see p. 119*)

Group Therapy (*see p. 123*)

Family Therapy (*see p. 122*)

Psychopharmacology

■ Atypical antipsychotics (*see p. 238*)

■ Antidepressants (*see p. 185*)

■ Mood stabilizers (*see p. 224*)

Nursing Care Planning

| NURSING DIAGNOSIS: Risk for Other-Directed Violence

Related to:	As Evidenced by:
Pervasive disregard for the rights of others	Impulsivity
	Inability to tolerate frustration; need for immediate gratification
	Contempt of others
	Conflict with authority
	Absence of empathy
	History of previous violence
	Assaultive behavior
	Lack of remorse

Nursing Outcomes Classification (NOC): Aggression Self-Control; Impulse Self-Control: Client will demonstrate self-restraint with others.

Nursing Interventions Classification (NIC): Anger Control Assistance

1. Develop rapport and trust with clients. Appear calm and in control. Speak in a normal, nonprovocative, and nonjudgmental tone. Demonstrate an accepting attitude. *Speaking in a therapeutic manner can help defuse anger and foster insight for clients. An accepting attitude helps promote feelings of worthiness.*

2. Be alert to verbal and nonverbal behavior that indicates the feelings of clients. Ask what they are feeling. State observations of what you see (what clients are doing behaviorally) and how clients may be feeling. *Clients may be unaware of behaviors. Verbalization of feelings helps validate observations and assists clients to connect feelings with behaviors.*

3. Be alert for possible triggers or factors that may precipitate anger. Monitor potential for inappropriate anger and aggression and intervene before it occurs. *Tension builds and signs of increasing agitation typically occur before clients act. Prompt recognition allows for early intervention should behavior begin to escalate.*

4. Assist clients to identify the source of anger and concerns. Encourage them to describe and clarify experiences to increase awareness of and triggers for problematic feelings. Use open-ended questions. Avoid "why" questions. Listen to clients' explanations, and paraphrase them when responding. *Verbalization of experiences helps clients increase their awareness of and triggers for problematic feelings. Using open-ended questions provides meaningful descriptions. Clients may interpret "yes-or-no" questions as interrogation and "why" questions as accusatory, leading to defensiveness. Listening and paraphrasing aid in validating observations.*

5. Minimize exposure of clients to stimulation. *Clients may interpret any stimulus as a potential threat, leading to explosive behavior.*

6. Provide clients with appropriate outlets to express anger or tension. Assist them to develop ways to express feelings nondestructively. Establish the expectation that clients can control their behavior. Teach calming measures, such as deep breathing or taking time-outs from stressful situations. Explain the benefits of expressing anger in adaptive, nonviolent ways. *Clients need to learn measures to control anger; doing so in a nonthreatening environment reduces fears and promotes adaptive coping. Getting input from clients affirms their competence and provides information for further problem solving.*

7. Administer medications as ordered. If a situation escalates, call for assistance. If absolutely necessary, anticipate the need for seclusion and restraints. *Quick action is necessary if a situation*

escalates. Aim efforts at ensuring the safety of all parties involved. Clients must be maintained in the least restrictive environment.

NIC: Limit Setting

1. Establish firm, reasonable expectations for behavior; communicate them clearly to clients. Identify, with input from clients as appropriate, undesirable behavior. Have all staff members enforce limits consistently. *Consistently implementing limits helps prevent clients from manipulating staff and helps clients gain control of their behavior.*

2. Avoid power struggles or trying to dissuade clients from grandiose delusions. Refrain from arguing or bargaining about established expectations and consequences. Accept acting-out behavior neutrally; do not respond with irritation or anger. Avoid feeding into emotions; maintain a professional demeanor. Redirect clients into productive or more appropriate activities. *Power struggles and arguments may contribute to increased tension. Not participating in emotions of clients and thwarting attempts to upset staff help prevent escalation of behavior. Clients need positive outlets for their feelings.*

3. Modify behavioral expectations and consequences as needed. Decrease limit setting as behavior of clients approximates that which is desired. *Modification is necessary to accommodate for reasonable changes in situations.*

NIC: Impulse Control Training

1. Assist clients to identify the problem or situation and to determine possible actions. Help them determine the benefits and limitations of possible actions. *Identifying the underlying problem and possible courses of action provides clients with methods other than aggression or violence to deal with feelings.*

2. Help clients replace anger-stimulating self-talk with more suitable self-talk. Teach thought-stopping techniques. *Self-talk is powerful and self-fulfilling. Cognitive restructuring promotes behavior changes.*

3. Provide opportunities for clients to practice or role-play actions within the therapeutic environment. Provide positive reinforcement for behavior changes. *Practicing appropriate responses and actions promotes compliance. Positive reinforcement fosters*

self-esteem and enhances the chances for future use of these actions or responses.

NIC: Environmental Management: Violence Prevention

1. Observe clients closely and continually. Place them in a room near the nursing station. Remove all dangerous objects. Provide ongoing surveillance of all client access areas and therapeutically intervene as necessary. *These measures help maintain safety.*
2. Discuss with clients the reasons for such monitoring. *Sharing this information can help ensure the cooperation of clients and foster understanding of the close observation.*
3. Spend regularly scheduled time with clients during the day. *Such interaction helps clients feel worthwhile and enables them to discuss issues of concern and any brewing problems.*

I NURSING DIAGNOSIS: Ineffective Coping

Related to:	As Evidenced by:
Antisocial behavior	Superficial, charming appearance
	Impulsive behavior
	Poor judgment
	Lying, manipulation of others
	Exploitive relationships
	Assaultive behavior
	Distorted view of world

NOC: Coping: Client will demonstrate appropriate behaviors to manage stress.

NIC: Coping Enhancement

1. Encourage clients to discuss feelings. To help them adopt more realistic appraisals of events, help clients identify evidence for and against their feelings. Assist them to develop objective appraisals. Discuss the consequences of not dealing with feelings. *Rational examination of feelings can help clients to restructure faulty thought patterns.*
2. Listen to verbalizations of feelings, perceptions, and fears. Provide an accepting, calm, and reassuring atmosphere. *Behaviors*

of clients are attempts to reduce stress. Anxiety and fear levels will remain high, however, until they confront the feelings.

3. Determine usual methods of problem solving. Help identify maladaptive strategies; suggest appropriate replacements. *These interventions help clients determine the most beneficial strategies and substitute them for maladaptive ones.*

4. Assist clients to break complex tasks into small, manageable steps. Encourage gradual mastery of the situation. *Using small manageable steps prevents overwhelming clients and increases the chances for success.*

5. Rehearse with clients various strategies to cope with anxiety and stressors. *Rehearsing enhances the chances for success when clients use these techniques.*

I NURSING DIAGNOSIS: Impaired Social Interaction

Related to:	As Evidenced by:
Antisocial behavior	Legal problems
	Exploitive relationships
	Contempt of others
	Superficial charm

NOC: Social Interaction Skills; Social Involvement: Client will demonstrate appropriate interaction with others.

NIC: Behavior Modification; Social Skills

1. Encourage clients to verbalize feelings associated with interpersonal problems. *Verbalization provides insight into underlying anxiety and fears.*

2. Assist clients to identify possible courses of action and their social/interpersonal consequences. *Such identification helps clients assume a beginning level of responsibility for thoughts, feelings, behaviors, and possible outcomes.*

3. Identify a specific social skill that will be the focus of training; assist clients to role-play it. Provide feedback about performance. *Targeting training on one social skill prevents overwhelming clients. Role-playing and providing feedback help to promote learning.*

NIC: Socialization Enhancement

1. Provide social skills training as necessary. Encourage patience in developing skills and relationships. *Social skills training is necessary to provide clients with the necessary tools to develop a relationship. Relationship development also takes time.*
2. Request and expect verbal communication. Help clients increase awareness of their strengths and limitations in communicating with others. *Use of appropriate communication skills is necessary for successful relationships.*
3. Encourage clients to form one social relationship. Consider group therapy as a forum for beginning social interaction. Encourage honesty in presenting oneself to others; encourage respect for the rights of others. *Initiating one relationship allows clients to focus on one thing at a time and avoid becoming overwhelmed. They may be able to experiment with social relationships within the safety of a group therapy setting. Honesty and respect for others facilitate trust.*

Borderline Personality Disorder

Borderline personality disorder (BPD) involves instability in mood, impulse control, and interpersonal relationships. Overall behavior is unpredictable and erratic. Clients tend to view people, circumstances, and overall life experience in terms of extremes— either all good or all bad. This tendency is referred to as splitting. Clients with BPD typically are described as demanding, self-destructive, contrary, and pessimistic.

Assessment

DSM-IV-TR Diagnostic Criteria: BPD

> ▪ Pervasive pattern of instability in interpersonal relationships, self-image, and affect and marked impulsivity in several contexts by early adulthood, as indicated by five (or more) of the following:
>
> 1. Frantic efforts to avoid real or imagined abandonment
> 2. Unstable and intense interpersonal relationships characterized by alternating extremes of idealization and devaluation

3. Identity disturbance (markedly and persistently unstable self-image or sense of self)

4. Impulsivity in at least two potentially self-damaging areas (eg, spending, sex, substance use)

5. Recurrent suicidal behavior, gestures, or threats, or self-mutilation

6. Affective instability from a marked reactivity of mood (intense episodic dysphoria, irritability, or anxiety usually lasting a few hours and only rarely more than a few days)

7. Chronic feelings of emptiness

Adapted with permission from American Psychiatric Association. (2000). *Diagnostic and statistical manual of mental disorders (4th ed., text rev.).* Washington, DC: Author.

Common History and Physical Examination Findings

- History of child abuse
- Use of transitional or favorite items for comfort and security
- Evidence of self-injury such as cuts or scratches on body
- Engagement in risky behaviors
- Occupational or school problems
- Substance abuse

Common Psychosocial Assessment Findings

- Self-undermining behaviors
- Psychotic-like symptoms during stress
- Fear of abandonment
- Inappropriate anger
- Labile mood
- Impulsivity
- Unstable, intense relationships
- Recurrent suicidal behavior, gestures, or threats
- Feelings of emptiness
- Dichotomous thinking
- Dissociation

Interdisciplinary Treatment Modalities

Psychotherapy

- Individual psychotherapy (*see p. 126*)

Cognitive Therapy (*see p. 111*)

Behavioral Therapy (*see p. 108*)

■ Dialectical behavioral therapy (*see p. 119*)

Family Therapy (*see p. 122*)

Psychopharmacology

■ Antidepressants (*see p. 195*)
■ Anticonvulsants (lamotrigine [*see p. 229*], gabapentin [*see p. 228*], topiramate [*see p. 235*], divalproex sodium [*see p. 227*])
■ Antipsychotics (*see p. 237*)
■ Anxiolytics (buspirone [*see p. 155*])

Nursing Care Planning

NURSING DIAGNOSIS: Risk for Self-Directed Violence; Risk for Self-Mutilation; Risk for Suicide

Related to:	As Evidenced by:
Unpredictable and erratic behavior	Engagement in risky behaviors
	Impulsivity
	Labile mood
	Recurrent suicidal behaviors, gestures, or threats
	Dichotomous thinking
	Cuts, scratches, or other injuries apparent on body

NOC: Impulse Self-Control; Self-Mutilation Restraint; Suicide Self-Restraint: Client will refrain from injuring self.

NIC: Impulse Control Training

1. Monitor clients for changes in behavior or mood. *Such observation optimizes safety and helps prevent clients from self-injury.*
2. Discuss with clients the reasons for such monitoring. *Giving this information can help ensure cooperation from clients and also foster their understanding of frequent observation.*

3. Engage clients in a "no self-harm" contract. *Such a contract reinforces limits and can encourage clients to assume self-control. Feedback helps clients differentiate inappropriate and appropriate responses as well as possible triggers and causes associated with behavior.*

NIC: Self-Mutilation Restraint

1. Identify with clients situations that lead to self-injury. *Knowledge of triggers helps clients determine appropriate methods to reduce their effects.*

2. Design a behavior modification plan; assist clients to identify positive alternatives to self-injury. *Planning fosters feelings of control over circumstances and impulses.*

3. Maintain consistency with clients; establish limits for behavior, responsibilities, and rules and maintain them. *Consistency and establishing and maintaining firm limits reduce the risk of negative behaviors.*

4. Provide information about emergency hotlines to call if the urge to harm self becomes overwhelming. *The team is obligated to put long-term measures in place to help ensure the safety of clients.*

NIC: Suicide Prevention

1. Assess presence and degree of suicide risk in clients; determine if they have the necessary means to follow through with the suicide plan. *Risk for suicide increases with a feasible or lethal plan, along with the means to complete the act.*

2. Conduct mouth checks after medication administration. *Clients may "cheek" the medication to use for a later suicide attempt.*

3. Reinforce use of a "no self-harm" contract; implement appropriate actions to reduce immediate distress in clients when negotiating the contract. *Although a "no self-harm" contract can reinforce limits and encourage clients to assume self-control, it can be overwhelming, leading to increased stress.*

4. Interact with clients at regular intervals, using a direct, nonjudgmental approach. *Frequent interaction conveys caring and openness and provides clients with an opportunity to discuss their feelings.*

5. Assist clients with measures to deal with future suicidal thoughts. *Planning appropriate measures to deal with future occurrences reduces the risk that clients will complete suicide.*

I N U R S I N G   D I A G N O S I S :   Risk for Other-Directed Violence

Related to:	As Evidenced by:
Marked impulsivity and identity disturbance	Dichotomous thinking
	Dissociation
	Feelings of emptiness
	Unstable, intensive relationships
	Inappropriate anger

NOC: Aggression Self-Control; Impulse Self-Control: Client will refrain from harming others.

NIC: Anger Control Assistance

1. Develop rapport and trust with clients. Appear calm and in control. Speak in a normal, nonprovocative, nonjudgmental tone. Demonstrate an accepting attitude. *Speaking therapeutically can help defuse anger and foster insight for clients. An accepting attitude helps promote feelings of worthiness.*

2. Be alert to verbal and nonverbal behavior that indicates the clients' feelings. Ask what clients are feeling. State observations of what you see (what clients are doing behaviorally) and how clients may be feeling. *Clients may be unaware of behaviors. Verbalization of feelings helps validate observations and assists clients to connect feelings with behaviors.*

3. Be alert for possible triggers or factors that may precipitate anger. Monitor potential for inappropriate anger and aggression in clients; intervene before they occur. *Signs of increasing tension and agitation typically occur before clients act. Prompt recognition allows for early intervention should behavior begin to escalate.*

4. Assist clients to identify the source of anger and concerns. Encourage clients to describe and clarify the experience to increase awareness of and triggers for problematic feelings. Use open-ended questions. Avoid "why" questions. Listen and paraphrase the responses of clients. *Verbalization of experience helps clients increase their awareness of and triggers for problematic feelings. Using open-ended questions provides meaningful descriptions. Clients may interpret "yes-or-no" questions as interrogation and*

"why" questions as accusatory, leading to defensiveness. Listening and paraphrasing aid in validating observations.

5. Minimize exposure of clients to stimulation. *Clients may interpret any stimulus as a potential threat, leading to explosive behavior.*

6. Provide clients with appropriate outlets to express anger or tension. Assist them to develop ways to express feelings in a nondestructive manner. Establish the expectation that clients can control their behavior. Teach clients about calming measures, such as deep breathing or taking time-outs. Explain the benefits of expressing anger adaptively and nonviolently. *Clients need to learn measures to control anger; doing so in a nonthreatening environment reduces their fears and promotes adaptive coping. Getting input from clients affirms their competence and provides information for further problem solving.*

7. Administer medications as ordered. If the situation escalates, call for assistance. If absolutely necessary, anticipate the need for seclusion and restraints. *Quick action is necessary if the situation escalates. Aim efforts at ensuring the safety of all parties involved. Clients must be maintained in the least restrictive environment.*

NIC: Limit Setting

1. Establish firm, reasonable expectations for behavior; communicate them clearly to clients. Identify, with input from clients as appropriate, undesirable behavior. Have all staff members enforce limits consistently. *Consistently implementing limits helps prevent clients from trying to manipulate staff and will help them gain control of behavior.*

2. Avoid power struggles or trying to dissuade clients. Refrain from arguing or bargaining about established expectations and consequences. Accept acting-out behavior neutrally; do not respond with irritation or anger. Avoid feeding into the emotions; maintain a professional demeanor. Redirect clients into productive or more appropriate activities. *Power struggles and arguments may contribute to increased tension. Not participating in emotions and thwarting attempts to upset staff help prevent escalation of behavior. Clients need positive outlets for feelings.*

3. Modify behavioral expectations and consequences as needed. Decrease limit setting as behavior approximates that which is

desired. *Modification is necessary to accommodate for reasonable changes in situations.*

NIC: Environmental Management: Violence Prevention

1. Observe clients closely and continuously. Place them in a room near nursing station. Remove all dangerous objects. Provide ongoing surveillance of all client access areas and therapeutically intervene as necessary. *These measures help maintain safety.*

2. Discuss with clients the reasons for such monitoring. *Giving this information can help ensure the cooperation of clients and also foster understanding of the close observation.*

3. Spend regularly scheduled time with clients during the day. *Such interaction helps clients feel worthwhile and enables them to discuss issues of concern and any brewing problems.*

| NURSING DIAGNOSIS: Chronic Low Self-Esteem

Related to:	As Evidenced by:
Identity disturbance	Labile mood
	Fear of abandonment
	Feelings of emptiness
	Inability to maintain interpersonal relationships

NOC: Self-Esteem: Client will verbalize positive statements of self-worth.

NIC: Self-Esteem Enhancement

1. Assist clients to acknowledge the relationship between self-image and feelings of inadequacy or abandonment. Explore previous achievements and reasons for self-criticism or guilt. Encourage clients to identify strengths and resources. Reinforce identified strengths. *Realistic self-expectations, positive reinforcement, and ongoing feedback will increase sense of self-esteem.*

2. Determine locus of control in clients and confidence in own judgment. Assist them to arrive at appropriate strategies for decision making and choices. Encourage clients to make decisions and choices independently. Convey confidence in their ability to handle situations. *Opportunities to practice independent functioning help clients improve self-confidence and self-esteem.*

3. Enhance communication and socialization skills by promoting information, role-playing, and interaction with staff. *Enhanced social skills will improve relationships for clients and contribute to improving self-esteem.*

| **N U R S I N G   D I A G N O S I S :** Ineffective Coping

Related to:	As Evidenced by:
Borderline personality	Demanding, self-destructive behavior
	Dichotomous thinking
	Poor impulse control
	Mood instability

NOC: Coping: Client will demonstrate use of adaptive coping skills.

NIC: Coping Enhancement

1. Encourage clients to verbalize feelings. If appropriate, suggest keeping a journal in which clients write about situations that cause emotional imbalance and subsequent feelings and behaviors. *Verbalizing feelings helps to identify feelings. Keeping a journal can provide insight about the responses of clients.*

2. Teach thought-stopping techniques. Foster constructive outlets for emotions. *Cognitive restructuring leads to behavior changes. Constructive emotional outlets reduce the risk for acting out.*

3. Assist clients to consider other coping strategies when stress, emotions, or feelings are intense, or when life circumstances are becoming overwhelming. Possibilities include exercise, relaxation techniques, discussion with trusted friends or healthcare providers, and cognitive restructuring. *Alternative coping technique must be available before clients can abandon former self-destructive strategies.*

4. Arrange for longer-term follow-up care for clients that focuses specifically on those with BPD. Consider programs that implement a dialectical behavioral approach. *BPD can be difficult to manage and requires specialized techniques with proven success. Dialectical behavioral approaches have evidence-based support.*

| NURSING DIAGNOSIS: Social Isolation

Related to:	As Evidenced by:
Intense and unstable interpersonal relationships	Dichotomous thinking
	Extreme idealization and devaluation
	Inappropriate anger
	Feelings of abandonment

NOC: Social Involvement; Social Interaction Skills: Client will demonstrate appropriate interaction with others.

NIC: Socialization Enhancement

1. Establish acceptable limits for relationships; assist clients if they cannot do so individually. *Limits for relationships are necessary until clients can control their own behavior.*
2. Assist clients to identify dichotomous thinking and manipulation as underlying problems with relationships. Provide social skills training, as necessary. Encourage patience in developing the skills and in relationships. *Social skills training is necessary to provide clients with the necessary tools to develop a relationship. Relationship development takes time.*
3. Request and expect verbal communication. Help clients increase awareness of strengths and limitations in communicating with others. Use role-playing to practice appropriate communication techniques. *Use of appropriate communication skills is necessary for successful relationships.*
4. Assist clients when interacting with others. Give positive feedback when clients interact appropriately. Encourage honesty in presenting self to others; encourage respect for the rights of others. *Positive feedback promotes continued use of appropriate techniques. Honesty and respect for others facilitate trust.*

NIC: Behavior Modification, Social Skills

1. Encourage clients to verbalize feelings associated with interpersonal problems. *Verbalization provides insight into underlying anxiety and fears.*
2. Assist clients to identify possible courses of action and their social/interpersonal consequences. *Such identification helps*

clients to assume a beginning level of responsibility for thoughts, feelings, and behaviors and possible outcomes.

3. Identify a specific social skill that will be the focus of training; assist clients to role-play the skill. Provide feedback about performance. *Targeting training on one social skill prevents overwhelming clients. Role-playing and providing feedback help to promote learning.*

Obsessive-Compulsive Personality Disorder

Obsessive-compulsive personality disorder is characterized by perfectionism, rigidity, controlling behavior, and extreme orderliness. These lifelong traits exist at the expense of efficiency, flexibility, and candor. Rigid perfectionism often results in indecisiveness, preoccupation with detail, and an insistence that others do things their way. Thus, clients may have difficulty being effective at work and socially and may have difficulty expressing affection, possibly appearing depressed. Clients with obsessive-compulsive personality disorder do not have actual obsessions or compulsions. Instead, their inner struggle is to gain self-control through the control of others and the environment.

Assessment

DSM-IV-TR Diagnostic Criteria: Obsessive-Compulsive Personality Disorder

▪ Pervasive pattern of preoccupation with orderliness, perfectionism, and mental and interpersonal control by early adulthood, at the expense of flexibility, openness, and efficiency, in several contexts, as indicated by four (or more) of the following:

1. Preoccupation with details, rules, lists, order, organization, or schedules to the extent that the primary point of the activity is lost

2. Perfectionism that interferes with task completion (eg, cannot complete a project because overly strict, self-imposed standards are not met)

3. Excessive devotion to work and productivity to the exclusion of leisure activities and friendships (not accounted for by obvious economic necessity)

4. Overconscientiousness, scrupulosity, and inflexibility about matters of morality, ethics, or values (not accounted for by cultural or religious identification)

5. Inability to discard worn-out or worthless objects even when they have no sentimental value

6. Reluctance to delegate tasks or to work with others unless they submit to exactly his or her way of doing things

7. A miserly spending style toward both self and others (viewing money as something to hoard for future catastrophes)

8. Rigidity and stubbornness

9. Inhibition in new interpersonal situations because of feelings of inadequacy

10. View of self as socially inept, personally unappealing, or inferior to others

11. Unusual reluctance to take personal risks or to engage in any new activities because they may prove embarrassing

Adapted with permission from American Psychiatric Association. (2000). *Diagnostic and statistical manual of mental disorders (4th ed., text rev.).* Washington, DC: Author.

Common History and Physical Examination Findings

- Formal, serious demeanor
- Reports of childhood perfectionism
- Precise, detailed responses to questions

Common Psychosocial Assessment Findings

- Perfectionism, rigidity
- Preoccupation with details, lists, rules
- Frugality
- Stubbornness
- Intense need for control
- Difficulty with decision making
- Limited insight
- Low self-esteem
- Critically judgmental of self
- Guilt, worthlessness related to inability to achieve goals
- Social isolation
- Inability to work collaboratively with others

Interdisciplinary Treatment Modalities

Psychotherapy

■ Individual psychotherapy (*see p. 126*)

Group Therapy (*see p. 123*)

Cognitive-Behavioral Therapy (*see p. 116*)

Psychopharmacology

- Antidepressants (*see p. 185*)
- Anxiolytics (*see p. 150*)

Nursing Care Planning

NURSING DIAGNOSIS: Anxiety

Related to:	As Evidenced by:
Pervasive preoccupation with control	Rigid perfectionism
	Inflexibility
	Excessive work
	Overconscientiousness
	Reluctance to take risks

NOC: Anxiety Self-Control: Client will demonstrate decreased anxiety with less need for control.

NIC: Anxiety Reduction

1. Use a calm, reassuring approach to create an atmosphere that facilitates trust. Avoid calling attention to the behavior of clients or arguing with them about behaviors initially. *Approaching clients calmly prevents overwhelming and startling them. Trust is essential to a therapeutic relationship. Preventing, arguing, or calling attention to behavior can increase anxiety level.*

2. Encourage clients to verbalize feelings in a manner comfortable for them. Acknowledge the feelings and perceptions of clients and their need for control. *Using comfortable methods prevents increasing anxiety level. Acknowledging the feelings of clients promotes trust.*

3. Support the use of appropriate defense mechanisms; assist clients to try new behaviors. *Intellectualization, rationalization, and reaction formation are defense mechanisms that clients with obsessive-compulsive personality disorder commonly use to exert control. Trying new behaviors creates a great deal of anxiety for these clients; assistance provides clients with support so that they can begin to change behavior.*

4. Assist clients to appraise situations objectively. *Objective appraisals enable clients to gain understanding and begin to associate the need for control with anxiety levels.*

5. Administer prescribed medications as appropriate. *Anxiolytics or antidepressants may be helpful in reducing or controlling anxiety initially and promote feelings of safety.*

| NURSING DIAGNOSIS: Impaired Social Interaction

Related to:	As Evidenced by:
Rigid perfectionism	Preoccupation with rules, details
	Reluctance to delegate
	Stubbornness
	Feelings of inadequacy in new situations
	Extreme focus on work to the exclusion of leisure activities

NOC: Social Interaction Skills; Social Involvement: Client will demonstrate appropriate interaction with others.

NIC: Behavior Modification: Social Skills

1. Encourage clients to verbalize feelings associated with interpersonal problems. *Verbalization provides insight into underlying anxiety and fears.*
2. Assist clients to identify possible courses of action and their social/interpersonal consequences. *Such identification helps clients assume a beginning level of responsibility for thoughts, feelings, and behaviors and possible outcomes.*
3. Determine usual methods of interaction. Help identify maladaptive strategies; provide suggestions for replacing them with appropriate ones. *These interventions help clients determine the most beneficial strategies and substitute them for those that are maladaptive.*
4. Assist clients in measures to relinquish control. Teach them appropriate techniques and strategies for delegating. Rehearse techniques. *Teaching strategies provides clients with the means to control anxiety. Rehearsing enhances the chances for success when clients use these strategies.*
5. Encourage frequent repetition and practice of techniques. *Practice increases the chances that clients will use the technique correctly when needed.*

Paranoid Personality Disorder

Paranoid personality disorder is characterized by suspiciousness, such that people are quick to take offense. Clients are quick to react with anger and counterattack in response to imagined attacks on their character or reputation. They usually cannot acknowledge their negative feelings toward others or that they project these negative feelings onto others. They may have few friends, look for hidden meaning in innocent remarks, be litigious and guarded, or bear grudges for imagined insults or slights. Marital or sexual difficulties are common and often involve issues related to fidelity. Despite their tendency to interpret the actions of others as deliberately threatening or demeaning, these people do not lose contact with reality.

Assessment

DSM-IV-TR Diagnostic Criteria: Paranoid Personality Disorder

- Pervasive distrust and suspiciousness of others by early adulthood, interpreting their motives as malevolent, in several contexts, as indicated by at least four of the following:
  1. Suspicion, without sufficient basis, that others are exploiting, harming, or deceiving
  2. Preoccupation with unjustified doubts about the loyalty or trustworthiness of friends
  3. Reluctance to confide in others because of unwarranted fear that they will maliciously use the information against the client
  4. Reading of hidden demeaning or threatening meanings into benign remarks or events
  5. Persistent grudges
  6. Perceived attacks on character or reputation that are not apparent to others and angry reactions or counterattacks
  7. Recurrent suspicions, without justification, about fidelity of spouse or partner
- Disorder not occurring exclusively during schizophrenia, a mood disorder with psychotic features, or another psychotic disorder; not the result of direct physiologic effects from a general medical condition

Adapted with permission from American Psychiatric Association. (2000). *Diagnostic and statistical manual of mental disorders (4th ed., text.rev.)*. Washington, DC: Author.

Common History and Physical Examination Findings

- Argumentativeness
- Recurrent complaining
- Problems with close relationships
- Highly critical of others
- Frequent involvement in legal disputes

Common Psychosocial Assessment Findings

- Guarded secretiveness
- Coldness
- Difficulty with interpersonal relationships
- Labile affect
- Stubbornness, sarcasm
- Combativeness
- Suspiciousness, feelings of being plotted against
- Blaming of others for shortcomings
- Rigidity, critical of others
- Difficulty accepting criticism
- Need for a high degree of control
- Hidden, unrealistic grandiose fantasies, usually associated with power and rank
- Negative stereotyping
- Brief psychotic episodes in response to stress
- Unwillingness to forgive
- Quick to counterattack

Interdisciplinary Treatment Modalities

Psychotherapy

- Individual psychotherapy (*see p. 126*)

Cognitive Therapy (*see p. 111*)

Behavioral Therapy (*see p. 108*)

Psychopharmacology

- Antipsychotics (*see p. 237*)

Nursing Care Planning

| NURSING DIAGNOSIS: Disturbed Thought Processes

Related to:	As Evidenced by:
Paranoid behavior	Suspiciousness
	Argumentativeness
	Guarded secretiveness
	Blaming of others
	Labile affect

NOC: Distorted Thought Self-Control: Client will demonstrate reality-based thoughts.

NIC: Reality Orientation

1. Use a calm, forthright approach; provide clear directions for clients. Approach slowly and from the front; address clients by name when initiating interaction. *Providing structure and expectations communicates that staff members are effectively managing the milieu, which should diminish power struggles and increase feelings of security for clients.*

2. Assist clients to identify patterns of dysfunctional thinking; anticipate need for therapy. *Identification of dysfunctional thinking must occur first so that clients can then work to change it. Therapy helps clients uncover and correct dysfunctional patterns.*

3. Interrupt paranoid thinking by changing the subject or responding to the feeling or theme rather than the content. Engage clients in concrete, reality-oriented activities that focus on something outside the self. *Focusing on the present promotes logical thinking and reduces the possibility of distraction or negative feelings.*

| NURSING DIAGNOSIS: Defensive Coping

Related to:	As Evidenced by:
Fears, distrust, and suspiciousness of others	Guarded secretiveness
	Feelings of being plotted against
	Criticism of others

	Negative stereotyping
	Quickness to counterattack
	Combativeness

NOC: Coping: Client will demonstrate appropriate coping strategies with reduced suspiciousness of others.

NIC: Coping Enhancement

1. Provide clients with clear information about the situation, safety, confidentiality, and care. Be open and direct. Avoid quietly talking to others while clients are nearby. *Clear information is necessary to help dispel suspiciousness in clients. Being open and direct may help to alleviate any suspicious beliefs on the part of clients. They may interpret the quiet talking as evidence of secretive behavior, which would reinforce suspiciousness.*

2. Encourage clients to discuss feelings. Listen to verbalizations of feelings, perceptions, and fears. Provide an accepting, calm, and reassuring atmosphere. *Anxiety levels and feelings of suspiciousness will remain high until clients confront the feelings.*

3. To help clients adopt more realistic appraisals of events, help them identify evidence for and against their feelings. Assist them to develop objective appraisals of their behavior. Discuss the consequences of not dealing with feelings. *Rational examination of feelings can help clients restructure faulty thought patterns.*

4. Encourage and support clients to participate in activities and interactions. Assist them to break down the activities into small manageable steps. Encourage gradual mastery of the situation. *Participation in activities and interactions fosters achievement. Using small manageable steps prevents overwhelming clients and increases the chances for success, providing positive feedback.*

I NURSING DIAGNOSIS: Impaired Social Interaction

Related to:	*As Evidenced by:*
Paranoid behavior	Distrust of others, suspiciousness Coldness
	Rigidity and criticism of others

NOC: Social Interaction Skills: Client will demonstrate measures for appropriate interaction with others.

NIC: Behavior Modification: Social Skills

1. Encourage clients to verbalize feelings associated with interpersonal problems. *Verbalization provides insight into underlying anxiety, fears, and suspiciousness.*

2. Request and expect verbal communication. Help clients increase awareness of strengths and limitations in communicating with others. *Use of appropriate communication skills is necessary for successful relationships.*

3. Assist clients to identify possible courses of action and their social/interpersonal consequences. *Such identification helps clients to assume a beginning level of responsibility for thoughts, feelings, behaviors, and possible outcomes.*

4. Provide social skills training, as necessary. Identify a specific social skill that will be the focus of training; assist clients to role-play the skill. Provide feedback about performance. *Social skills training is necessary to provide clients with the necessary tools to develop relationships. Targeting training on one social skill prevents overwhelming clients. Role-playing and providing feedback help promote learning.*

5. Encourage clients to form one social relationship. Consider group therapy as a forum for beginning social interaction. Encourage honesty in presenting self to others; encourage respect for the rights of others. *Initiating one relationship allows clients to focus on one thing at a time and avoid becoming overwhelmed. Clients may be able to experiment with social relationships within the safety of a group therapy setting. Honesty and respect for others facilitates trust.*

6. Encourage patience in developing skills and relationships. *Relationship development takes time.*

Schizoid Personality Disorder

Clients with **schizoid personality disorder** show an indifference to social relationships, flattened affectivity, and a cold, unsociable, and seclusive demeanor. They enjoy few, if any, activities. They usually never marry, have little interest in exploring their sexuality, and frequently live as adult children with parents or siblings. These lifelong loners often succeed at solitary jobs that others would find intolerable.

Assessment

DSM-IV-TR Diagnostic Criteria: Schizoid Personality Disorder

▪ Pervasive detachment from social relationships with a restricted range of emotional expression in interpersonal settings, beginning by early adulthood; seen in various contexts, as indicated by four (or more) of the following:

1. No desire for or enjoyment of close relationships (including family)
2. Consistent selection of solitary activities
3. Little to no interest in sexual experiences with others
4. Pleasure in few, if any, activities
5. No close friends or confidants other than first-degree relatives
6. Indifference to praise or criticism
7. Emotional coldness, detachment, or flattened affect

▪ Condition not occurring exclusively during schizophrenia, a mood disorder with psychotic features, another psychotic disorder, or a pervasive developmental disorder; not a direct physiologic effect of a general medical condition

Adapted with permission from American Psychiatric Association. (2000). *Diagnostic and statistical manual of mental disorders (4th ed., text rev.).* Washington, DC: Author.

Common History and Physical Examination Findings

- Lack of close relationships
- Engagement in solitary activities or hobbies
- Lack of goals or aspirations
- Occupation involving little contact with others
- Unmarried, little or no sexual contact

Common Psychosocial Assessment Findings

- Constricted affect
- Emotionally aloof and indifferent
- Difficulty expressing emotions
- Indecisiveness
- Little involvement in decision making
- No engagement with other people
- Indifference to praise or criticism
- Limited to no social skills

Interdisciplinary Treatment Modalities

Psychotherapy

- Individual psychotherapy (*see p. 126*)

Social Skills Training

Cognitive-Behavioral Therapy (*see p. 116*)

Group Therapy (*see p. 123*)

Psychopharmacology

- Anxiolytics (*see p. 150*)
- Antidepressants (*see p. 185*)
- Antipsychotics (*see p. 237*)

Nursing Care Planning

I **NURSING DIAGNOSIS**: Chronic Low Self-Esteem

Related to:	As Evidenced by:
Schizoid personality disorder	Constricted affect
	Lack of goals
	Indecisiveness
	Difficulty expressing emotions
	Indifference

NOC: Self-Esteem; Quality of Life: Client will verbalize positive statements about self and life.

NIC: Coping Enhancement

1. Establish a therapeutic relationship. Proceed slowly and emphasize the technical aspects of treatment in the beginning. Do not confront clients about their need for distance within the therapeutic relationship. Be consistent and stable. Provide calm reassurance and an atmosphere of acceptance. *Fear of others also includes a fear of the nurse. The outlined approach will help clients sense the nurse's concern but will not press them beyond comfortable*

limits. The nurse can model safety and security in social relationships first within the therapeutic relationship.

2. Seek to understand clients' perceptions of their fears. Assist them to develop objective appraisals of events. Explore fears about others; use cognitive-restructuring techniques to address irrational thought patterns. *Thought patterns predict behavior. Cognitive restructuring can replace faulty cognitions that lead to negative behaviors.*

3. Encourage clients to examine unrealistic aspects of fears. Explore previous methods of dealing with problems; support the use of appropriate defense mechanisms and approaches. Encourage verbalization of feelings, perceptions, and fears. *Many clients with schizoid personality disorder fear unbearable dependency and have unrealistic fantasies about friendships. Examining these fears and fantasies is the first step toward helping clients to abandon them.*

| NURSING DIAGNOSIS : Impaired Social Interaction

Related to:	As Evidenced by:
Pervasive detachment from social relationships	Cold appearance
	Lack of close friends or confidants
	Preference for being alone
	Engagement in solitary activities
	Emotional aloofness and indifference
	Limited to no social skills

NOC: Social Involvement: Client will begin to participate in social relationships and activities.

NIC: Behavior Modification: Social Skills

1. Encourage clients to verbalize feelings associated with interpersonal problems. *Verbalization provides insight into underlying fears.*

2. Assist clients to identify possible courses of action and their social/interpersonal consequences. *Such identification helps clients to begin to assume responsibility for thoughts, feelings, and behaviors and possible outcomes.*

3. Provide appropriate social skills training. *Such training promotes behavioral change that facilitates effective relationships.*

4. Identify a specific social skill that will be the focus of training; assist clients to role-play the skill. Provide feedback about performance. *Targeting training on one social skill prevents overwhelming clients. Role-playing and providing feedback help to promote learning.*

NIC: Socialization Enhancement

1. Encourage clients to form one social relationship. Provide social skills training, as necessary. Encourage patience in developing relationships. *Initiating one relationship allows clients to focus on one thing at a time and avoid becoming overwhelmed. Relationship development takes time.*

2. Consider group therapy as a forum for beginning social interaction. Encourage honesty in presenting self to others; encourage respect for the rights of others. *Clients may be able to experiment with social relationships within the safety of a group therapy setting. The therapist will need to protect clients from confrontation or criticism by others about their inability to participate or share. Honesty and respect for others facilitate trust.*

3. Request and expect verbal communication. Help clients increase awareness of strengths and limitations in communicating with others. *Use of appropriate communication skills is necessary for successful relationships.*

4. As therapy progresses, encourage clients to find an outside activity or job that allows some limited social interaction. *Even moderate social interaction can overwhelm clients. The desire for an outside activity can become an important motivating force to continue therapy.*

Sexual and Gender Disorders

D isorders related to sexuality and gender identity are among the most intimate concerns any human can have. This category includes sexual disorders, paraphilias, and gender identity disorders. All these problems can have significant consequences for self-concept, self-esteem, and overall quality of life.

Sexual dysfunction refers to a disruption of any of the phases of human sexual response. Sexual dysfunction is subdivided into four major categories:

- Desire disorders
  - Hypoactive sexual desire disorder
  - Sexual aversion disorder
- Arousal disorders
  - Female sexual arousal disorder
  - Male erectile dysfunction
- Orgasmic disorders
  - Female orgasmic disorder
  - Male orgasmic disorder
  - Premature ejaculation
- Pain disorders
  - Dyspareunia (male or female)
  - Vaginismus

In addition, these disorders can be classified as lifelong or acquired, generalized or situational, or psychological or combined.

Paraphilias refer to sexual expressions involving recurrent, intensely sexually arousing fantasies as well as sexual urges or behaviors. The expressions can involve nonhuman objects, suffering or humiliation of oneself or partner, or children or other nonconsenting people. To be considered paraphilias, the urges, fantasies, and behaviors also must cause clinically significant distress or impair social, occupational, or other important areas of functioning. Paraphilias include the following:

- Exhibitionism
- Fetishism
- Frotteurism
- Pedophilia
- Sexual masochism
- Sexual sadism
- Transvestic fetishism
- Voyeurism
- Others such as telephone scatologia, necrophilia, partialism, zoophilia, coprophilia, klismaphilia, and urophilia

Gender identity disorders are characterized by a strong identification with the opposite gender and persistent discomfort with one's assigned sex.

Erectile Dysfunction

Erectile dysfunction (ED) involves a persistent or recurrent inability to attain or to maintain an erection sufficient for satisfactory sexual performance. ED has different patterns. Some men report an inability to obtain any erection. Others complain of an adequate erection but losing tumescence during penetration. Others report erections sufficient for penetration that lose tumescence before or during thrusting. ED is a common problem that increases with aging. One in 10 men is thought to have ED, but many are reluctant to discuss it. ED has no cure, but effective drug treatment usually is well tolerated.

Assessment

Diagnostic and Statistical Manual of Mental Disorders, Fourth Edition, Text Revision (DSM-IV-TR) Diagnostic Criteria: ED

- Persistent or recurrent inability to attain or to maintain until completion of sexual activity an adequate erection
- Marked distress or interpersonal difficulty due to dysfunction
- Not better accounted for by another Axis I disorder
- Not from direct physiologic effects of a substance or medical condition
- Types: lifelong, acquired; generalized, situational; due to psychological or combined factors

Adapted with permission from American Psychiatric Association. (2000). *Diagnostic and statistical manual of mental disorders (4th ed., text rev.)*. Washington, DC: Author.

Common History and Physical Examination Findings

- Reports of difficulty attaining or maintaining erection
- Medication as treatment for other disorders

Common Psychosocial Assessment Findings

- Sexual anxiety
- Fear of failure
- Concerns about sexual performance
- Shame, guilt
- Decreased subjective sense of sexual excitement and pleasure
- Disruption of marital or sexual relationships

Interdisciplinary Treatment Modalities

Pharmacologic Agents
Mechanical Methods (vacuum pump)
Surgery (penile prosthesis)
Sexual Counseling

Nursing Care Planning

I N U R S I N G   D I A G N O S I S :   Sexual Dysfunction

Related to:	As Evidenced by:
ED	Reports of inability to attain or maintain erection
	Concerns about sexual performance
	Decreased sense of pleasure with sexual activity

Nursing Outcomes Classification (NOC): Sexual Functioning: Client will verbalize increased ability to engage in sexual activity with increased pleasure.

Nursing Interventions Classification (NIC): Sexual Counseling

1. Establish rapport with clients; provide privacy and confidentiality. *Sexual information is a very private and personal matter.*
2. Provide information about sexual functioning as appropriate. When questioning clients, start by explaining that many people experience sexual difficulties. *Sharing intimate information is difficult.*
3. Begin the discussion with the least sensitive topics and gradually proceed to more sensitive or intimate topics. *Initiating the discussion with less sensitive areas allows clients to become comfortable with the discussion.*
4. Provide facts and answer any questions that clients may have. If appropriate, use humor and encourage clients to use humor. *Facts are important to clarify any sexual myths or misconceptions that clients may have that are contributing to current feelings. Humor can help relieve anxiety and embarrassment.*
5. Discuss alternative forms of sexual expression that are acceptable to clients as appropriate. Include clients' spouses or sexual partners in the discussion. Encourage open communication. *Alternative forms of sexual expression can promote feelings of intimacy and closeness. Partner or spousal participation promotes sharing. Improved communication enhances feelings of emotional intimacy and satisfaction.*
6. If necessary, refer couples to a sex therapist for counseling as appropriate. *A sex therapist has the expertise to facilitate sexual functioning.*

| NURSING DIAGNOSIS: Disturbed Body Image

Related to:	As Evidenced by:
ED	Feelings of shame, guilt
	Sexual anxiety
	Relationship distress

NOC: Body Image; Self-Esteem: Client will verbalize positive statements about self.

NIC: Body Image Enhancement

1. Assist clients to review own body realistically. *Clients can confront irrational beliefs and substitute more realistic ones. External, objective feedback will help clients attain a healthier, more realistic body image.*

2. Monitor frequency of statements of self-criticism. Assist clients to identify aspects of physical appearance that they identify as positive. Help clients separate physical appearance from personal worth. *Self-criticism and negative self-perceptions promote unrealistic body images. Evaluating changes in self-comments and self-descriptions, verbalizations of self-acceptance, and willingness to focus on positive attributes provide measures to evaluate progress toward goal achievement.*

3. Work with clients to describe and discuss feelings related to body image. Help clients identify these feelings and separate them from sexual activity behaviors in a nonjudgmental manner. *Identification of feelings can assist clients to connect feelings and sexual activity.*

NIC: Self-Esteem Enhancement

1. Assist clients to acknowledge the relationship between self-expectations, sexual functioning, and feelings of inadequacy. Explore previous achievements and reasons for self-criticism or guilt. Encourage clients to identify strengths and resources. Reinforce identified strengths. *Realistic self-expectations, positive reinforcement, and ongoing feedback will increase sense of self-esteem.*

2. Determine locus of control in clients and their confidence in their own judgment. Encourage them to make independent decisions and choices. Convey confidence in their ability to handle situations.

Opportunities to practice independent functioning will help improve self-confidence and self-esteem.

3. Work with clients to determine ways to relieve anxiety and cope with feelings. Provide positive reinforcement for participation in identifying and openly expressing feelings. Teach clients about appropriate methods for problem solving. *Positive feedback and appropriate methods for problem solving promote feelings of self-worth and confidence.*

Gender Identity Disorder

Gender identity disorder refers to a person's identification with the opposite gender. This disorder leads to clinically significant distress or impaired social, occupational, or other functioning. People who identify with and live as if they are of the opposite sex are called **transsexuals**. Transsexuals are not to be confused with **transvestites**, who cross-dress for sexual arousal. Transvestites usually have no persistent desire for sex reassignment.

Assessment

DSM-IV-TR Diagnostic Criteria

- Strong and persistent cross-gender identification
- Disturbance in adolescents and adults manifested by symptoms such as:
  - Stated desire to be of other sex
  - Frequent passing as the other sex
  - Desire to live or be treated as the other sex
  - Conviction that person has typical feelings and reactions of other sex
- Persistent discomfort with or sense of inappropriateness in gender role of own sex
- Disturbance in adolescents and adults manifested by:
  - Preoccupation with removal of primary and secondary sex characteristics (via hormones, surgery, or other procedures that physically alter sexual characteristics to simulate other sex)
  - Belief that individual was the wrong sex
- Disturbance not concurrent with physical intersex condition

■ Significant distress or impairment in social, occupational, or other important area of functioning

Adapted with permission from American Psychiatric Association. (2000). *Diagnostic and statistical manual of mental disorders (4th ed., text rev.).* Washington, DC: Author.

Common History and Physical Examination Findings

- Primary and secondary sex characteristics of designated sex
- Verbalization of desire to live as opposite sex
- Dressing in clothing of opposite sex
- Behavior reflective of the opposite sex

Common Psychosocial Assessment Findings

- Insistence that individual is of the opposite sex
- Discomfort with assigned sex
- Preoccupation with appearance
- Feelings of inappropriateness with assigned sex
- Distress in social or occupational functioning
- Intense desire to become opposite sex or take on appearance of opposite sex
- Social isolation
- Relationship difficulties

Interdisciplinary Treatment Modalities

Sex Re-assignment Surgery
Hormonal Therapy
Psychotherapy

Nursing Care Planning

NURSING DIAGNOSIS: Ineffective Sexuality Pattern

Related to:	As Evidenced by:
Intense desire to be of the opposite sex	Dressing in clothing of opposite sex
	Demonstration of opposite sex behaviors
	Reports of extreme discomfort with assigned sex
	Impaired relationships

NOC: Sexual Identity; Body Image: Client will verbalize acceptance of own sexual identity.

NIC: Sexual Counseling

1. Establish rapport with clients; provide privacy and confidentiality. *Sexual information is a very private and personal matter.*

2. Provide information about sexual functioning as appropriate. When questioning clients, start by informing them that many people experience difficulties. *Sharing intimate information is difficult.*

3. Begin the discussion with the least sensitive topics and gradually proceed to more sensitive or intimate topics. *Initiating the discussion with less sensitive areas allows clients to become comfortable with the discussion.*

4. Provide facts and answer any questions that clients may have. *Facts are important to clarify any sexual myths or misconceptions that clients may have that are contributing to current feelings.*

5. Refer clients for sexual counseling as appropriate. *Expertise in sexual counseling is necessary to assist clients to cope with feelings related to sexuality.*

NIC: Body Image Enhancement

1. Use appropriate techniques to assist clients to review own body realistically. Demonstrate a nonjudgmental, positive self-image. *Realistic appraisal can help clients attain a healthier, more realistic body image.*

2. Monitor frequency of statements of self-criticism. Assist clients to identify aspects of physical appearance associated with positive feelings. Help clients separate physical appearance and feelings about gender from personal worth. *Self-criticism and negative self-perceptions promote an unrealistic body image. Evaluating changes in self-comments and self-descriptions, verbalizations of self-acceptance, and willingness to focus on positive attributes provide measures to evaluate progress toward goal achievement.*

3. Encourage continued participation in sexual counseling as appropriate; offer support, guidance, and education as necessary if clients are to receive sex re-assignment surgery or hormonal therapy. *Continued participation in sexual counseling is necessary*

for clients to adopt a positive sexual identity. Ongoing support and guidance help clients cope with anxieties associated with treatment modalities.

I NURSING DIAGNOSIS: Disturbed Personal Identity

Related to:	As Evidenced by:
Incongruence of assigned gender and desired gender	Gender of male or female at birth
	Behaviors/mannerisms/dress of opposite sex

NOC: Sexual Identity; Self-Esteem: Client will verbalize positive statements about self and sexual identity.

NIC: Self-Esteem Enhancement

1. Assist clients to acknowledge the relationship between self-image and feelings. Explore previous achievements and reasons for self-criticism or guilt. Encourage clients to identify strengths and resources. Reinforce identified strengths. *Realistic self-expectations, positive reinforcement, and ongoing feedback will increase sense of self-esteem.*
2. Determine locus of control in clients and their confidence in their own judgment. Assist clients with appropriate strategies for decision making and choices. Help them identify areas for change. Encourage clients to make decisions and choices independently. Convey confidence in their ability to handle situations. *Opportunities to practice independent functioning will help clients improve self-confidence and self-esteem.*
3. Enhance communication and socialization skills by promoting information, role-playing of appropriate behaviors, and interaction with staff. Provide ongoing, nonjudgmental support and be available for clients. *Enhanced social skills will improve relationships and contribute to enhanced self-esteem. Ongoing support and availability provide clients with a sense of security and acceptance, which can help promote feelings of self-worth.*

Sleep Disorders

S **leep disorders** involve an ongoing disruption in a person's normal sleeping and waking patterns. Disruptions in sleep can lead to excessive daytime sleepiness, napping at inappropriate times, chronic fatigue, or problems in functioning at school, work, or home. Sleep is essential to life and well-being. It is distinguished from wakefulness by perceptual disengagement from and unresponsiveness to the environment. During sleep, people are usually quiet and recumbent, with closed eyes and decreased responses to environmental stimuli. Unlike other nonwaking states (eg, coma), sleep is easily reversible.

The major categories of sleep disorders are as follows:

- Insomnia
- Sleep-related breathing disorders
  - Obstructive sleep apnea syndrome
  - Central sleep apnea syndrome
  - Central alveolar hypoventilation syndrome
- Hypersomnias
- Circadian rhythm sleep disorders
- Parasomnias
- Sleep-related movement disorders
  - Periodic limb movement disorder
  - Restless leg syndrome

- Isolated symptoms
- Other sleep disorders (eg, from a medical condition, substance abuse)

Insomnia and sleep-related breathing disorder are the most common sleep disorders.

Insomnia

Insomnia, a perception of insufficient sleep or not feeling rested after habitual sleep, is the most prevalent sleep disorder. It can range from a few days to many months or years. Clients with insomnia often report distress in social, occupational, or other areas of functioning.

Primary insomnia occurs when no cause of a sleep disturbance (eg, a psychiatric or medical diagnosis) can be identified. Primary insomnia often begins in young or middle-aged adults and tends to be more common in women. Clients with idiopathic insomnia have difficulty sleeping since childhood, and the cause is unknown. Psychophysiologic insomnia is chronic insomnia in which clients worry about sleep, are cognitively and physiologically over-aroused at bedtime, and have poor daytime functioning. This leads to further worry about sleep. This, in turn, may lead to a recurring cycle in which insomnia leads to more insomnia.

Assessment

Diagnostic and Statistical Manual of Mental Disorders, Fourth Edition, Text Revision (DSM-IV-TR) Diagnostic Criteria

---

- Difficulty initiating or maintaining sleep for at least 1 month
- Clinically significant distress or impairment of social or occupational functioning
- Disturbance not part of another sleep disorder or another psychiatric disorder
- Condition not the result of physiologic effects related to a substance or another general medical condition

Adapted with permission from American Psychiatric Association. (2000). *Diagnostic and statistical manual of mental disorders* (4th ed., text rev.). Washington, DC: Author.

Common History and Physical Examination Findings

- Reports of difficulty sleeping: difficulty falling asleep, intermittent wakefulness during sleep, nonrestorative sleep
- Falling asleep while watching television, reading, or riding in a car
- Daytime napping
- Complaints of fatigue
- Haggard appearance
- Tension headache, muscle tension, gastric distress (stress-related psychophysiologic problems)
- Maladaptive sleep habits
- Inappropriate use of medications/substances (sedatives, hypnotics, alcohol, caffeine)

Common Psychosocial Assessment Findings

- Preoccupation with sleep and inability to sleep
- Frustration
- Diminished feelings of well-being
- Decreased attention and concentration
- Anxiety

Common Laboratory and Diagnostic Test Findings

- **Polysomnography:** poor sleep continuity (increased sleep latency, increased intermittent wakefulness, decreased sleep efficiency); increased stage 1 sleep; decreased stage 3 and 4 sleep
- **Quantitative electroencephalogram:** increased muscle tension, increased amounts of alpha and beta activity during sleep

Interdisciplinary Treatment Modalities

Cognitive-Behavioral Therapy (see p. 116)

Sleep Hygiene

Psychopharmacology

- Hyponotics
  - Benzodiazepines (*see p. 150*)
  - Nonbenzodiazepines: zolpidem (*see p. 182*), zaleplon (*see p. 180*), eszopiclone (*see p. 165*)
- TCAs (*see p. 185*)

Complementary and Alternative Medicine Therapy (see p. 138)

■ Herbs: kava-kava, valerian
■ Aromatherapy: lavender, chamomile, and ylang-ylang

Nursing Care Planning

| NURSING DIAGNOSIS: Disturbed Sleep Pattern

Related to:	*As Evidenced by:*
Inappropriate sleep hygiene measures	Frequent awakenings
	Difficulty falling asleep
	Daytime fatigue
	Daytime napping

Nursing Outcomes Classification (NOC): Sleep; Rest: Client will verbalize improved sleep patterns.

Nursing Interventions Classification (NIC): Sleep Enhancement

1. Record sleep patterns and number of hours of sleep in clients; encourage them to monitor sleep patterns. *Information about current sleep patterns provides a baseline for planning appropriate interventions.*
2. Encourage clients to establish a bedtime routine. *It facilitates the transition from wakefulness to sleep.*
3. Instruct clients to avoid bedtime foods and beverages that can interfere with sleep; for example, drinking coffee in the evening may contribute to problems; discourage caffeine intake after the late afternoon. *Caffeine, a stimulant, has a half-life of 8 to 14 hours. Its effects vary. People with sleep difficulties should avoid caffeine after the late afternoon.*
4. Encourage clients to engage in activities during the day. *Activities during the day promote wakefulness and limit daytime sleep.*
5. Teach clients how to use comfort measures such as massage, positioning, and relaxation techniques. *Comfort measures help induce relaxation to promote sleep.*

6. Encourage use of sleep medications as ordered. Explain the action and effect of medication. Adjust medication administration to support sleep–wake cycle. *Short-term use of hypnotic drugs, particularly when combined with behavioral interventions, may help. The timing of drug administration should be individualized to meet the needs of clients, increasing the chances for effectiveness.*

7. Encourage clients to talk about feelings and their effects on sleep. Suggest participation in a support group. *Understanding the relationship among feelings, anxieties, fears, and sleep problems can aid in developing adaptive strategies, thus improving sleep. Participation in a support group promotes sharing of feelings and concerns.*

NIC: Environmental Management

1. Explain the need for a clean, comfortable bed and environment; encourage clients to avoid unnecessary exposure, drafts, overheating, or chilling. *Cleanliness and comfort promote relaxation, thereby facilitating the transition to sleep.*

2. Encourage clients to participate in relaxing and enjoyable activities before bedtime. Monitor participation in fatigue-producing activities during wakefulness. *Enjoyable and relaxing activities prepare the body for sleep. Overactivity can lead to being overtired.*

3. Urge clients to make the bedroom as quiet and dark as possible and to use the bed only for sleeping or sex; assist clients to control or prevent undesirable or excessive noise when possible; encourage clients to wear earplugs to decrease perceptions of noise and to consider moving items interfering with sleep to another room. *A sleep-promoting environment helps reduce stimuli that contribute to nocturnal arousal. Even low levels of movement or noise may disturb sleep.*

I NURSING DIAGNOSIS: Deficient Knowledge

Related to:	As Evidenced by:
Factors influencing sleep	Inappropriate use of medications/substances
	Preoccupation with sleep
	Environmental stimuli

NOC: Knowledge: Health Behavior: Client will identify factors contributing to sleep pattern disturbance that require modification.

NIC: Learning Facilitation

1. Assess readiness to learn; develop mutual goals. *Readiness to learn and mutual goal setting help facilitate effectiveness of teaching.*
2. Adjust instruction to client's level of knowledge and understanding. Provide information in terms they can understand. Review use of medications and comfort measures to facilitate sleep. Discourage use of caffeine late in the day. *Information provided at the appropriate level promotes better understanding and learning.*
3. Provide memory aids as appropriate; use demonstration and return demonstration as appropriate. *Memory aids and demonstration encourage client participation in learning and help provide mastery of the information.*

NIC: Teaching: Individual

1. Teach clients about how the environment can influence sleep; encourage use of sleep hygiene strategies. *Environmental stimuli can interfere with sleep–wake cycles.*
2. Explain the effects of any prescribed hypnotic. *Knowledge of the effects of prescribed drugs can help alleviate any anxiety or fears that clients may have about using the medication.*
3. Reinforce behavior, as appropriate. Work with clients to determine the most appropriate strategies. *Reinforcement provides positive feedback toward goal achievement and time for modifications if necessary. Collaboration with clients fosters empowerment.*
4. Urge clients to continue exercise and activity early in the day, encouraging clients to avoid exercise within 3 hours of bedtime. *Exercise is important; however, it acts as a stimulant and, if done too late in the day, can interfere with sleep.*

Sleep-related Breathing Disorders

Sleep-related breathing disorders involve a disruption in sleep that results from abnormal ventilation during sleep. Three forms of sleep-related disorders have been identified:

- Obstructive sleep apnea—hypopnea syndrome

- Central sleep apnea syndrome
- Central alveolar hypoventilation syndrome

The most common of these disorders is **obstructive sleep apnea—hypopnea syndrome**. This disorder is associated with repetitive episodes of reduced airflow (*hypopnea*) or cessation of airflow (*apnea*) resulting from collapse or obstruction of the upper airway.

Assessment

DSM-IV-TR Diagnostic Criteria: Sleep-related Breathing Disorder

> ▪ Disrupted sleep leading to insomnia or excessive sleepiness that results from a sleep-related breathing condition
>
> ▪ Condition not the result of physiologic effects related to a substance or another general medical condition
>
> Adapted with permission from American Psychiatric Association. (2000). *Diagnostic and statistical manual of mental disorders (4th ed., text rev.).* Washington, DC: Author.

Common History and Physical Examination Findings

- Excessive sleepiness
- Overweight
- Large neck size (greater than 17 inches in men; greater than 16 inches in women)
- Nasal airway obstruction
- Gastroesophageal reflux
- Systemic hypertension; elevated diastolic pressure
- Reports of snoring or brief gasps alternating with episodes of silence lasting 20 to 30 seconds; breathing restoration with loud gasps or snores, moans, or mumbling
- Frequent awakenings
- Reports of sleep that is not restful
- Complaints of feeling more tired on awakening
- Dry mouth
- Generalized dull morning headache
- Disrupted sleep of partner/spouse

Common Psychosocial Assessment Findings

- Memory disturbances
- Poor concentration

- Irritability
- Personality changes
- Mood changes
- Social or occupational impairment

Common Laboratory and Diagnostic Test Findings

- **Nocturnal polysomnography:** periods of apnea greater than 10 seconds (usually 20 to 30 seconds); reduction in airflow
- **Arterial blood gases:** abnormal blood oxygen and carbon dioxide levels

Interdisciplinary Treatment Modalities

Surgery
- Uvulopalatopharyngoplasty

Continuous Positive Airway Pressure (CPAP)

Weight Loss

Oral Appliances

Sleep Position changes

Nursing Care Planning

I N U R S I N G D I A G N O S I S : Risk for Impaired Gas Exchange

Related to:	As Evidenced by:
Frequent periods of apnea and hypopnea during sleep	Fatigue
	Restlessness with sleep
	Headache on awakening
	Excessive sleepiness

NOC: Respiratory Status: Gas Exchange; Respiratory Status: Ventilation: Client will demonstrate adequate oxygenation and ventilation.

NIC: Respiratory Monitoring

1. Assess rate, rhythm, depth, and effort of respiration. Note chest movement, watching for symmetry and use of accessory muscles. *Baseline data related to respiratory status is necessary to develop an appropriate plan of care.*

2. Monitor for increased restlessness or anxiety. *Restlessness or increased anxiety may provide early indications of respiratory distress.*

3. Encourage clients to use additional pillows or supports for positioning while sleeping. *An upright position facilitates the work of breathing.*

| NURSING DIAGNOSIS: Disturbed Sleep Pattern

Related to:	*As Evidenced by:*
Periods of apnea and hypopnea	Excessively loud snoring
	Periods of breathing cessation during sleep followed by loud gasps
	Disruption of partner's sleeping
	Excessive daytime sleepiness
	Waking up more tired in the morning

NOC: Sleep; Rest: Client will verbalize improved sleep with reduced daytime sleepiness.

NIC: Sleep Enhancement

1. Record sleep patterns and number of hours of sleep in clients; encourage them to monitor sleep patterns. *Information about current sleep patterns provides a baseline for planning appropriate interventions.*

2. Teach clients about appropriate measures for sleep hygiene, including environmental management, bedtime rituals, and avoidance of stimulants. *Sleep hygiene measures promote sleep.*

3. Assist with referral to sleep specialist. *Evaluation by sleep specialist is necessary to determine the most appropriate treatment.*

4. Review possible treatment measures for disorder, including surgery, CPAP, and weight reduction. *Clients need information about treatments to promote informed decision making.*

5. Assist clients to adhere to the recommended treatment. Educate client about the treatment and the need for compliance. Help clients troubleshoot problems that arise and provide supportive feedback. *Sleep disorders often require long-term behavioral changes that clients may find difficult. Assistance with treatment and supportive feedback enhance the chances for success and promote compliance.*

Somatoform Disorders

S omatoform disorders are conditions in which clients experience physical symptoms despite no underlying medical explanation for them. They complain of severe symptoms with no organic or physical basis. Although the symptoms are physical, somatoform disorders are classified as mental disorders because physical examination and laboratory tests reveal no demonstrable organic pathology.

Somatoform disorders vary in severity from mild and self-limited to chronic and disabling. Clients usually seek treatment in outpatient settings, such as primary care, but also in medical specialty practices such as dermatology and neurology. In general, somatoform disorders are diagnosed more commonly in women than in men.

Some clinicians believe that somatoform disorders provide clients with *primary gain*, meaning that symptoms block psychological conflict or anxiety from conscious awareness. They also offer *secondary gain* by relieving clients from expected responsibilities and increasing the attention they receive. Such gains may positively reinforce and help perpetuate somatic symptoms.

Somatoform disorders are categorized as follows:

- Body dysmorphic disorder
- Somatization disorder
- Undifferentiated somatoform disorder
- Conversion disorder
- Hypochondriasis

Body Dysmorphic Disorder

Body dysmorphic disorder involves a preoccupation with an imagined defect in appearance. Clients obsess about minor or nonexistent facial abnormalities, for example, wrinkles, spots on the skin, facial asymmetry, or facial hair. Other body parts, such as the genitals, breasts, buttocks, hands, or feet, may be the focus of distress and embarrassment. Clients are extremely self-conscious about the imagined defect, causing them to retreat from usual activities, become socially isolated, and display decreased academic and occupational functioning. Some clients even become housebound, and those with severe forms of body dysmorphic disorder are at risk for suicide.

Assessment

Diagnostic and Statistical Manual of Mental Disorders, Fourth Edition, Text Revision (DSM-IV-TR) Diagnostic Criteria: Body Dysmorphic Disorder

- Preoccupation with imagined defect in appearance or marked excessive concern over slight physical anomaly
- Clinically significant distress or impairment in social, occupational, or other important area of function
- Condition not better accounted for by another mental disorder

Adapted with permission from American Psychiatric Association. (2000). *Diagnostic and statistical manual of mental disorders (4th ed., text rev.).* Washington, DC: Author.

Common History and Physical Examination Findings

- Statements of being "ugly"
- Slight physical defect or anomaly
- Attempts to camouflage or hide the defect, such as with beards, hats
- Constant checking of self in mirror or other reflective surface
- Excessive grooming behavior
- Seeking out medical treatments to correct defect

Common Psychosocial Assessment Findings

- Intense preoccupation with perceived or slight defect
- Fear that defect or body part will not function or can be easily damaged

- Belief that view of defect is accurate and undistorted
- Thoughts that others focus on the defect
- Feelings of self-consciousness
- Social isolation; avoidance of interaction with others

Interdisciplinary Treatment Modalities

Psychotherapy
- Individual psychotherapy (*see p. 126*)

Group Therapy (*see p. 123*)

Cognitive-Behavioral Therapy (*see p. 111*)

Psychopharmacology
- Antidepressants: selective serotonin reuptake inhibitors (*see p. 185*)

Nursing Care Planning

NURSING DIAGNOSIS: Disturbed Body Image

Related to:	As Evidenced by:
Intense preoccupation of perceived defect or slight physical anomaly	Constant checking of defect in mirror
	Excessive grooming
	Attempts to hide defect
	Feelings of self-consciousness

Nursing Outcomes Classification (NOC): Body Image; Self-Esteem: Client will verbalize an accurate and positive description of self.

Nursing Interventions Classification (NIC): Body Image Enhancement

1. Use cognitive restructuring techniques; assist clients to review own and others' bodies realistically. *Clients can confront and substitute irrational beliefs with more rational ones. External, objective feedback will help clients attain a healthier, more realistic body image.*
2. Monitor frequency of statements of self-criticism. Assist clients to identify aspects of physical appearance about which they feel

positive. Help clients separate physical appearance from personal worth. *Self-criticism and negative self-perceptions promote an unrealistic body image. Evaluating changes in self-comments and self-descriptions, verbalizations of self-acceptance, and willingness to focus on positive attributes provide measures to evaluate progress toward goal achievement.*

NIC: Self-Esteem Enhancement

1. Assist clients to acknowledge the relationship between defect, self-expectations, and feelings of inadequacy. Explore previous achievements and reasons for self-criticism or guilt. Encourage clients to identify strengths and resources. Reinforce identified strengths. *Realistic self-expectations, positive reinforcement, and ongoing feedback will increase self-esteem.*

2. Encourage clients to engage in small activities, one step at a time. Provide positive feedback about successes. *Small, manageable activities done one step at a time prevents overwhelming clients and allows clients to achieve success, thereby promoting a positive sense of self.*

3. Determine locus of control in clients and confidence in their own judgment. Encourage clients to make decisions and choices independently. Convey confidence in their ability to handle situations. *Opportunities to practice independent functioning will help clients improve self-confidence and self-esteem.*

4. Enhance communication and socialization skills by promoting information, role-playing, and participation in group activities with peers. *Enhanced social skills will improve peer relationships and social interaction and contribute to improving clients' self-esteem.*

| NURSING DIAGNOSIS: Ineffective Coping

Related to:	As Evidenced by:
Intense preoccupation with perceived defect or slight physical anomaly	Attempts to rectify or correct defect medically
	Constant attention and focus on defect
	Belief that others are focusing on defect
	Social isolation
	Self-consciousness
	Distorted belief about defect

NOC: Coping: Client will demonstrate use of positive coping strategies.

NIC: Coping Enhancement

1. Encourage clients to discuss feelings; validate their feelings. To help clients adopt more realistic appraisals of self and events, help them identify evidence for and against their feelings. Assist clients to develop objective appraisals. Discuss the consequences of not dealing with feelings. *Feelings are real to clients but ultimately are irrational and self-defeating; validation promotes trust. Rational examination of feelings can help clients identify possible sources of anxiety and restructure faulty thought patterns.*

2. Listen to verbalizations of feelings, perceptions, and fears. Provide an accepting, calm, and reassuring atmosphere, urging clients to focus on feelings rather than the defect. *Focusing on feelings de-emphasizes the defect while addressing underlying concerns.*

3. Provide clients with opportunities to participate in activities that they can easily accomplish or enjoy. Give positive feedback for accomplishments. *Dealing with complex activities may be difficult for clients. Participating in activities that they can easily accomplish or enjoy fosters feelings of self-esteem.*

4. Encourage and assist clients gradually to limit time spent focusing on the defect. Teach methods to reduce anxiety. Assist clients to break complex goals into small, manageable steps. Encourage gradual mastery of the situation. *Gradual, controlled limit setting helps clients gain control over anxiety and behavior, reducing anxiety to a manageable level that does not interfere with ability to function. Using small, manageable steps prevents overwhelming clients and increases the chances for success.*

NIC: Counseling

1. Provide facts as necessary and appropriate; assist clients to identify the problem causing distress. Use reflection and clarification to facilitate expression of concerns. Point out discrepancies between feelings and behaviors. *Facts are necessary to help dispel irrational and self-defeating responses.*

2. Assist clients to identify strengths; encourage new skill development; reinforce new skills and use of appropriate strategies for

coping, for example, relaxation techniques. *Development of new strategies and use of appropriate coping strategies enhance abilities to deal with stress; drawing on strengths promotes feelings of control.*

Somatization Disorder

Somatization disorder at one time was also called *hysteria* or *Briquet's syndrome*. Clients with this disorder usually present exaggerated, inconsistent, and complicated medical histories. The symptoms described often involve multiple body systems. Clients often seek treatment from multiple healthcare providers (doctor shopping) when their physical complaints are not addressed to their satisfaction. Medically unexplained and unintentionally expressed physical symptoms and their relationship to psychological well-being are dramatic.

Assessment

DSM-IV-TR Diagnostic Criteria: Somatization Disorder

- Before age 30, client having had many physical complaints over several years
- Treatment sought for complaints, or material impairment of social, work, or personal functioning
- At some point, at least eight symptoms (not necessarily concurrently) from the following list, distributed as noted:
  - Pain symptoms (four or more) in different sites (eg, head, abdomen, back) or related to body functions (eg, menstruation, sex)
  - Gastrointestinal symptoms (two or more, excluding pain): nausea, bloating, vomiting (not during pregnancy), diarrhea, food intolerance
  - Sexual symptoms (at least one, excluding pain): indifference to sex, difficulties with erection or ejaculation, irregular menses, excessive menstrual bleeding, or vomiting throughout pregnancy
  - Pseudoneurologic symptoms (at least one, not limited to pain): impaired balance or coordination, weak or paralyzed muscles, lump in throat or trouble swallowing, loss of voice, urinary retention, hallucinations, numbness (to touch or pain), double vision, blindness, deafness, seizures, amnesia or other dissociative symptoms, loss of consciousness (other than with fainting)

- Each of the above symptoms meeting one of the following conditions:
  - Findings from physical or laboratory investigation unable to explain the condition as a result of a general medical condition or substance use
  - If client has a general medical condition, the impairments or complaints exceeding what would be expected, based on history, laboratory findings, or physical examination
  - Client not consciously feigning symptoms for material gain (malingering) or to occupy the sick role (factitious disorder)

Adapted with permission from American Psychiatric Association. (2000). *Diagnostic and statistical manual of mental disorders (4th ed., text rev.).* Washington, DC: Author.

Common History and Physical Examination Findings

- History of multiple physical complaints
  - Pain
  - Gastrointestinal symptoms
  - Sexual symptoms
  - Neurologic-related symptoms
- Extensive health and medical history
- Complaints of being "extremely sick"
- History of treatment by numerous healthcare providers
- Wide-ranging treatments and therapies used for complaints
- Numerous medical examinations, diagnostic tests, procedures, hospitalizations, surgeries
- Colorful and exaggerated complaints often lacking specific details
- Inability to work because of complaints

Common Psychosocial Assessment Findings

- Anxiety
- Depressed mood
- Feelings of hopelessness
- Preoccupation with complaints
- Labile mood
- Family distress
- Impaired role function; disability

Interdisciplinary Treatment Modalities

Psychotherapy
- Individual psychotherapy (*see p. 126*)

Group Therapy (*see p. 123*)

Cognitive-Behavioral Therapy (*see p. 116*)

Psychopharmacology
- Anxiolytic agents (*see p. 150*)
- Antidepressants (*see p. 185*)

Nursing Care Planning

| NURSING DIAGNOSIS: Ineffective Coping

Related to:	As Evidenced by:
Unresolved psychological issues	History of frequent bodily complaints
	unsupported by diagnostic testing
	Excessive use of medical resources
	Restricted lifestyle
	Persistent focus on/preoccupation with physical symptoms
	Inability verbally to express emotional content

NOC: Coping; Role Performance: Client will verbalize feelings about life, stressors, and physical symptoms with less time spent focusing on physical symptoms.

NIC: Coping Enhancement

1. Establish a therapeutic relationship. Provide calm reassurance and an accepting atmosphere. Show empathy for distress but focus on feelings rather than physical complaints. Recognize that physical complaints are real to clients. *Clients with possible or diagnosed somatoform disorders often have little or no trust in the healthcare system and its providers. Therapeutic intervention is possible only when providers have gained trust. Recognition is necessary to establish trust.*

2. Encourage verbalization of feelings, perceptions, and fears. Reinforce anxiety reduction strategies. Refocus clients to express

feelings rather than to describe physical complaints. *Focusing on feelings conveys interest in clients and reduces their need to garner attention through physical complaints. Refocusing provides a model for gaining insight into the behavior.*

3. Collaborate with the primary physician to coordinate physical care and appropriate use of medical services. Provide clients with realistic choices about certain aspects of care. *Care coordination is an important aspect of treatment. It helps ensure appropriate use of resources, medical screening, and care, and it conveys to clients that healthcare providers are working together to protect health.*

4. Recommend insight-oriented therapy to explore psychological motivation for somatization. Assist clients to objectively appraise events. Discuss triggering factors to help clients gain insight into patterns associated with increased somatization. *Fewer symptoms and increased functioning may result as clients gain insight into behavior patterns. Recognizing triggering events will help clients manage behavior.*

5. Encourage clients to identify strengths and abilities. Assist them to identify maladaptive strategies; provide suggestions for replacing them with appropriate ones. Support the use of appropriate defense mechanisms. Develop techniques that do not encourage focusing on bodily sensations (eg, developing an absorbing hobby, volunteering). *Clients cannot relinquish a coping strategy, no matter how dysfunctional, until they can replace it with another.*

NIC: Role Enhancement

1. Review with clients and their families tasks that need to be done. Assist clients to identify tasks in which they can participate. Encourage clients to start with small tasks and to participate in one task each week. *Identifying tasks and level of participation helps clients visualize what they can do. Keeping activities and tasks small and manageable reduces the pressure on clients to perform, allows clients to achieve success, and minimizes anxiety associated with expectations of independence.*

2. Assist clients to identify usual role in the family and specific role changes from current problems. *These measures aid in developing appropriate care strategies.*

3. Facilitate discussion of role adaptations of partner/spouse/family members to compensate for role changes in clients. *Discussion of roles helps improve everyone's understanding of the situation.*

4. Serve as a role model for learning new behaviors; facilitate opportunities for clients to role-play new adaptive behaviors. Provide positive reinforcement for use of new behaviors. *Role modeling and role playing promote increased participation in care from clients and positive coping responses. Positive reinforcement enhances the continued use of adaptive behaviors.*

| NURSING DIAGNOSIS: Caregiver Role Strain

Related to:	*As Evidenced by:*
Client's increased dependency needs and inability to provide independent self-care	Family role disruption
	Inability of client to fulfill role expectations
	Lack of social involvement
	Disability

NOC: Caregiver Physical/Emotional Health; Caregiver-Patient Relationship: Client will demonstrate participation in care activities and role function.

NIC: Caregiver Support

1. Acknowledge the difficulties of the caregiving role and of dependency of clients on family members. Encourage caregivers to give attention to clients in ways unrelated to physical complaints. *Doing so will minimize the need of clients to gain attention through a "sick role." It also will help re-establish family roles.*
2. Encourage clients to participate in one activity outside the home per week. Offer positive reinforcement for any activity performed. Encourage caregivers to slowly resume social activities with clients. *Engaging in an activity outside the home in conjunction with positive reinforcement provides an opportunity for clients to experience success at leaving home and expanding their circle of experience. Social activities help reverse the social isolation, promote a feeling of togetherness, provide an outlet for caregivers, and help clients regain a more balanced sense of self as a friend and companion of others.*
3. Monitor caregivers for indicators of stress; teach caregiver stress management techniques; encourage caregiver participation in support groups. *Stress management techniques and support groups are positive coping strategies to deal with the demands of caregiving.*

4. Provide encouragement to caregivers during setbacks for clients; support caregivers in setting limits and taking care of self. *Encouragement provides positive feedback to caregivers and helps decrease feelings of powerlessness. Limit setting and self-care are important in maintaining caregiver health and ability to function.*

NIC: Self-Care Assistance

1. Encourage clients to assist with self-care and activities of daily living to their level of ability. Break activities into manageable simple steps. Allow sufficient time for clients to complete tasks; avoid intervening when clients can perform tasks independently. *Participation in self-care promotes feelings of self-esteem. Simple manageable steps with ample time for completion minimize overwhelming clients, thereby enhancing the chances for success and increased self-esteem. Intervening when clients can perform independently reinforces dependency needs.*

2. Provide positive reinforcement and feedback for activities completed. *Positive reinforcement promotes self-esteem and continued repetition of desired behaviors.*

NIC: Respite Care

1. Monitor endurance of caregivers. Help identify other family members who can assist; arrange for substitute caregivers as necessary. *Assistance from others reduces the stress associated with the role of a constant caregiver.*

NIC: Presence

1. Demonstrate acceptance; verbally communicate empathy or understanding of experience of clients. *An accepting attitude and demonstrations of empathy are key to establishing a trusting relationship; clients need to feel that others hear complaints and understand them.*

2. Limit time spent discussing physical complaints; help clients realize that help is available, but do not reinforce dependent behaviors. Stay with clients and provide assurance of safety and security during periods of anxiety; be available for caregivers. *Limit setting helps clients focus on feelings rather than physical manifestations and aids in reducing dependency issues. This, in turn, helps alleviate some of the stress of caregivers. Being available conveys understanding of problems and caregiver's needs and helps to reduce anxiety for both.*

Substance-Related Disorders

S ubstance-related disorders involve those conditions associated with the use of a drug, including alcohol. Two major categories of substance-related disorders are identified:

- Substance use disorders
- Substance-induced disorders

Substance use disorder is a general term used to denote substance abuse and substance dependence. **Substance abuse** means the
repeated use of drugs (including alcohol) leading to functional problems. Such problems, however, involve neither compulsive use nor
withdrawal (painful physical and psychological symptoms that follow discontinuation of a drug). **Substance dependence** is the correct
term when a person uses alcohol or other drugs despite extreme negative consequences, such as significant impairments to daily living.
Substance dependence also leads to tolerance (the body becoming
less responsive to the drug with repeated exposure), as well as to
withdrawal when the client stops taking the substance.

Substance-induced disorder refers to disorders involving intoxication, withdrawal, detoxification, and specific effects such as dementia, delirium, and other disorders associated with the substance.
Intoxication refers to the set of behaviors that result specifically from
the use of the substance. **Withdrawal** involves the set of negative
reactions that occur, both physical and psychological, when substance
use is reduced or ended after heavy and prolonged use. **Detoxification**

is the process that allows an individual to safely and effectively withdraw from use of a substance; detoxification is typically accomplished under medical supervision.

Substance-related disorders are divided into twelve categories, all of which share common subdiagnostic categories (dependence, abuse, intoxication, and withdrawal) with generic diagnostic criteria:

1. **Alcohol-related Disorders**
   - Alcohol use disorders
     - Alcohol dependence
     - Alcohol abuse
   - Alcohol-induced disorders
     - Alcohol intoxication
     - Alcohol withdrawal
     - Alcohol intoxication delirium
     - Alcohol withdrawal delirium
     - Alcohol-induced: persisting dementia; persisting amnestic disorder (with delusions; with hallucinations); mood disorder; anxiety disorder; sexual dysfunction; sleep disorder; disorder not otherwise specified (NOS)

2. **Amphetamine (or amphetamine-like)-related Disorders**
   - Amphetamine use disorders
     - Amphetamine dependence
     - Amphetamine abuse
   - Amphetamine-induced disorders
     - Amphetamine intoxication
     - Amphetamine intoxication, with perceptual disturbances
     - Amphetamine withdrawal
     - Amphetamine intoxication delirium
     - Amphetamine-induced: psychotic disorder (with delusions; with hallucinations); mood disorder; anxiety disorder; sexual dysfunction; sleep disorder
     - Amphetamine-related disorder NOS

3. **Caffeine-related Disorders**
   - Caffeine-induced disorders
     - Caffeine intoxication
     - Caffeine-induced: anxiety disorder; sleep disorder
     - Caffeine-related disorder NOS

4. **Cannabis-related Disorders**
   * Cannabis use disorders
     * Cannabis dependence
     * Cannabis abuse
   * Cannabis-induced disorders
     * Cannabis intoxication
     * Cannabis intoxication, with perceptual disturbances
     * Cannabis intoxication delirium
     * Cannabis-induced: psychotic disorder (with delusions; with hallucinations); anxiety disorder
     * Cannabis-related disorder NOS

5. **Cocaine-related Disorders**
   * Cocaine use disorders
     * Cocaine dependence
     * Cocaine abuse
   * Cocaine-induced disorders
     * Cocaine intoxication
     * Cocaine intoxication, with perceptual disturbances
     * Cocaine withdrawal
     * Cocaine intoxication delirium
     * Cocaine-induced: psychotic disorder (with delusions; with hallucinations); mood disorder; anxiety disorder; sexual dysfunction; sleep disorder
     * Cocaine-related disorder NOS

6. **Hallucinogen-related Disorders**
   * Hallucinogen use disorders
     * Hallucinogen dependence
     * Hallucinogen abuse
   * Hallucinogen-induced disorders
     * Hallucinogen intoxication
     * Hallucinogen persisting perception disorder (flashbacks)
     * Hallucinogen intoxication delirium
     * Hallucinogen-induced: psychotic disorder (with delusions; with hallucinations); mood disorder; anxiety disorder
     * Hallucinogen-related disorder NOS

7. **Inhalant-related Disorders**
   * Inhalant use disorders

- Inhalant dependence
- Inhalant abuse
- Inhalant-induced disorders
  - Inhalant intoxication
  - Inhalant intoxication delirium
  - Inhalant-induced persisting dementia
  - Inhalant-induced: psychotic disorder (with delusions; with hallucinations); mood disorder; anxiety disorder
  - Inhalant-related disorder NOS

8. Nicotine-related Disorders
- Nicotine use disorder
  - Nicotine dependence
- Nicotine-induced disorder
  - Nicotine withdrawal
  - Nicotine-related disorder NOS

9. Opioid-related Disorders
- Opioid use disorders
  - Opioid dependence
  - Opioid abuse
- Opioid-induced disorders
  - Opioid intoxication
  - Opioid intoxication, with perceptual disturbances
  - Opioid withdrawal
  - Opioid intoxication delirium
  - Opioid-induced: psychotic disorder (with delusions; with hallucinations); mood disorder; sexual dysfunction; sleep disorder
  - Opioid-related disorder NOS

10. Phencyclidine (or phencyclidine-like)-related Disorders
- Phencyclidine use disorders
  - Phencyclidine dependence
  - Phencyclidine abuse
- Phencyclidine-induced disorders
  - Phencyclidine intoxication
  - Phencyclidine intoxication, with perceptual disturbances
  - Phencyclidine intoxication delirium

- Phencyclidine-induced: psychotic disorder (with delusions; with hallucinations); mood disorder; anxiety disorder
- Phencyclidine-related disorder NOS

11. Sedative–hypnotic- or anxiolytic-related Disorders
- Sedative, hypnotic, or anxiolytic use disorders
  - Sedative, hypnotic, or anxiolytic dependence
  - Sedative, hypnotic, or anxiolytic abuse
- Sedative-, hypnotic-, or anxiolytic induced disorders
  - Sedative, hypnotic, or anxiolytic intoxication
  - Sedative, hypnotic, or anxiolytic withdrawal (specify if: with perceptual disturbances)
  - Sedative, hypnotic, or anxiolytic intoxication delirium
  - Sedative, hypnotic, or anxiolytic withdrawal delirium
  - Sedative-, hypnotic-, or anxiolytic-induced: persisting dementia; persisting amnestic disorder; psychotic disorder (with delusions; with hallucinations); mood disorder; anxiety disorder; sexual dysfunction; sleep disorder
  - Sedative-, hypnotic-, or anxiolytic-related disorder NOS

12. Polysubstance-related Disorder
- Polysubstance dependence

Regardless of type and subtype, clients with substance use disorders are impaired physically, socially, and psychologically at some time during their illness. They also are at risk for social ostracization because most cultures do not tolerate or accept the behaviors that result from chronic chemical impairment.

Diagnostic and Statistical Manual of Mental Disorders, Fourth Edition, Text Revision (DSM-IV-TR) Diagnostic Criteria: Substance Disorders
**Note: These criteria apply to all twelve of the above categories.

Dependence

- Maladaptive patterns of substance use leading to clinically significant distress or impairment over a single 12-month period, as evidenced by one or more of the following:

  1. Tolerance, shown by either a markedly increased intake of the substance to achieve the same effects, or the same amount of the substance having a markedly lessened effect with continued use

2. Withdrawal, shown by either characteristic signs and symptoms associated with the substance's withdrawal syndrome, or use of the substance (or one closely related to it) to avoid or relieve withdrawal symptoms

3. Increased intake or duration of substance use beyond the client's intentions

4. Repeated unsuccessful attempts to reduce or control substance use

5. Significant time spent using, recovering from, or trying to obtain the substance

6. Reduction or abandonment of important social, occupational, or recreational activities in favor of substance use

7. Continued use despite awareness of the related physical or psychological problems

Abuse

■ Maladaptive substance use resulting in clinically important distress or impairment over a single 12-month period as shown by three or more of the following:

1. Failure to fulfill major home or work obligations because of substance use

2. Use even when physically dangerous

3. Repeated associated legal problems

4. Continued use despite awareness that substance use has caused or worsened social or interpersonal problems

5. For the class of substance in question, client never having met the criteria for dependence

Intoxication

■ Development of a reversible syndrome because of recent use of or exposure to a substance

■ During or shortly after substance use, development of clinically important maladaptive behavioral or psychological changes

■ Condition not the result of a general medical condition and not better explained by a different mental disorder

Withdrawal

■ Development of a substance-specific syndrome when client stops or reduces intake of a substance used frequently, for extended duration, or both

- Clinically important distress in or impairment of work, social, or personal functioning
- Not the result of a general medical condition and not better explained by a different mental disorder

Adapted with permission from American Psychiatric Association. (2000). *Diagnostic and statistical manual of mental disorders (4th ed., text rev.)*. Washington, DC: Author.

People with substance-related disorders can manifest a wide range of signs and symptoms based on whether the client is intoxicated or experiencing withdrawal. See Table 24.1.

Alcohol-related Disorders

Alcohol, also known chemically as ethanol, is a legal drug. Its commercial distribution differs from the more tightly regulated sale of other drugs (ie, controlled substances). The pharmacologic properties of ethyl alcohol produce mind- and mood-altering effects of central nervous system depression (similar to barbiturates). Alcohol often is mistaken for a stimulant; the reason for this misconception is that, after drinking it, some people become more talkative, hyperactive, euphoric, self-confident, or aggressive. This behavior has been attributed to the disinhibiting effect produced by low doses of alcohol.

With increasing consumption, alcohol causes the following pattern:

- Sedation
- Impaired mental and motor functioning
- Deepening stupor with a decreased stimulation response (including painful stimulus response)
- Coma
- Eventually, death from respiratory and circulatory collapse

Physical and behavioral manifestations of alcohol on the central nervous system relate directly to blood level and concentration in the brain. The blood alcohol level (BAL) is expressed as milligrams of alcohol per milliliter of blood and is determined by a laboratory blood test.

table
24.1. **Commonly Abused Controlled Substances**

Category	Examples/ Street Names	Effects of Intoxication	Health Consequences	Withdrawal Symptoms
Stimulants (*DSM-IV-TR* Categories: Amphetamine [or Amphetamine-Like]-Related Disorders and Cocaine-Related Disorders)		Increased heart rate, blood pressure, metabolism, mental alertness, energy; exhilaration	Rapid or irregular heartbeat; reduced appetite; weight loss; heart failure; nervousness; insomnia	• Fatigue • Long but disturbed sleep • Strong hangover • Irritability • Depression • Violence
Amphetamine	*Biphetamine, Dexedrine:* bennies, black beauties, crosses, hearts, LA turnaround, speed, truck drivers, uppers	See "Stimulants"; also, rapid breathing	See "Stimulants"; also, tremor, loss of coordination, irritability, anxiousness, restlessness, delirium, panic, paranoia, impulsive behavior, aggressiveness, tolerance, addiction, psychosis	See "Stimulants"
MDMA (methylenedioxy-methamphetamine)	Adam, clarity, ecstasy, Eve, lover's speed, peace, STP, X, XTC	See "Stimulants"; also, mild hallucinogenic effects, increased tactile sensitivity, empathic feelings	See "Stimulants"; also, impaired memory and learning, hyperthermia, cardiac toxicity, renal failure, liver toxicity	• Depression • Anxiety • Panic attacks • Sleeplessness • Depersonalization • De-realization • Paranoid delusions

Methamphetamine	*Desoxyn:* chalk, crank, crystal, fire, glass, go fast, ice, meth, speed	See "Stimulants"; also, aggression, violence, psychosis	See "Stimulants"; memory loss, cardiac and neurologic damage; impaired memory and learning, tolerance, addiction	Length and severity of depression is related to how much and how often drug was used; symptoms may last up to 48 hours. • Cravings • Exhaustion • Depression • Mental confusion • Restlessness • Insomnia • Deep or disturbed sleep • Irritability • Intense hunger • Moderate to severe depression • Psychotic reactions • Anxiety
Methylphenidate (safe and effective for treatment of ADHD)	*Ritalin:* JIF, MPH, R-ball, Skippy, the smart drug, vitamin R	See "Stimulants"	See "Stimulants"	• Agitation, insomnia • Abdominal cramps • Nausea • Severe emotional depression • Exhaustion • Anxiety

continued on page 466

465

table
24.1. **Commonly Abused Controlled Substances** *continued*

Category	Examples/ Street Names	Effects of Intoxication	Health Consequences	Withdrawal Symptoms
Cocaine	*Cocaine hydrochloride:* blow, bump, C, candy, Charlie, coke, crack, flake, rock, snow, toot	See "Stimulants"; also, increased temperature	See "Stimulants"; also, chest pain, respiratory failure, nausea, abdominal pain, strokes, seizures, headaches, malnutrition, panic attacks	Length varies among people and according to amount and frequency of use. • Agitation • Depression • Intense cravings • Extreme fatigue • Anxiety • Angry outbursts • Lack of motivation • Nausea/vomiting • Shaking • Irritability • Muscle pain • Disturbed sleep
Cannabinoids (*DSM-IV-TR* Category: Cannabis-Related Disorders)		Euphoria, slowed thinking and reaction time, confusion, impaired balance and coordination	Cough, frequent respiratory infections, impaired memory and learning, increased heart rate, anxiety, panic attacks, tolerance, addiction	Withdrawal first appears in chronic users within 24 hours. Marijuana withdrawal is most pronounced for the first 10 days and can last up to 28 days. • Irritability • Anxiety • Physical tension

Hashish	Boom, chronic, gangster, hash, hash oil, hemp	See "Cannabinoids"	See "Cannabinoids"	See "Cannabinoids"
Marijuana	Blunt, dope, ganja, grass, herb, joints, Mary Jane, pot, reefer, sinsemilla, skunk, weed	See "Cannabinoids"	See "Cannabinoids"	See "Cannabinoids"
Hallucinogens (*DSM-IV-TR* Category: Hallucinogen-Related Disorders)		Altered states of perception and feeling; nausea	Persisting perception disorder (flashbacks)	Psychotic-like episodes persist long after last use
LSD	*Lysergic acid diethylamide*: acid, blotter, boomers, cubes, microdot, yellow sunshine	See "Hallucinogens"; also, persistent mental disorders; increased body temperature, heart rate, blood pressure; loss of appetite, tremors, insomnia, numbness, weakness	See "Hallucinogens"	See "Hallucinogens"

continued on page 468

table
24.1. **Commonly Abused Controlled Substances** *continued*

Category	Examples/ Street Names	Effects of Intoxication	Health Consequences	Withdrawal Symptoms
Mescaline	Buttons, cactus, mesc, peyote	See "Hallucinogens"; also, increased body temperature, heart rate, blood pressure; loss of appetite, tremors, insomnia, numbness, weakness	See "Hallucinogens"	See "Hallucinogens"
Psilocybin	Magic mushroom, purple passion, shrooms	See "Hallucinogens"; also, nervousness, paranoia	See "Hallucinogens"	See "Hallucinogens"
Inhalants *(DSM-IV-TR* Category: Inhalant-Related Disorders)	*Solvents (paint thinners, gasoline, glues), gases (butane, propane, aerosol propellants, nitrous oxide), nitrites (isoamyl, isobutyl, cyclohexyl):* laughing gas, poppers, snappers, whippets	Stimulation, loss of inhibition; headache; nausea/vomiting; slurred speech, loss of motor coordination; wheezing	Unconsciousness, cramps, weight loss, muscle weakness, depression, memory impairment, damage to cardiovascular and nervous systems, sudden death	Mild withdrawal syndrome

Opioids and Morphine Derivatives (*DSM-IV-TR* Category: Opioid-Related Disorders)		Pain relief, euphoria, drowsiness	Nausea, constipation, confusion, sedation, respiratory depression and arrest, tolerance, addiction, unconsciousness, coma, death	The worst symptoms pass within a few days, but it can take months to feel normal.
Codeine	*Empirin with Codeine, Fiorinal with Codeine, Robitussin A-C, Tylenol with Codeine:* Captain Cody, schoolboy (with glutethimide); doors & fours, loads, pancakes and syrup	See "Opioids and Morphine Derivatives"; also, less analgesia, sedation, and respiratory depression than morphine	See "Opioids and Morphine Derivatives"	• Runny nose • Sweating • Muscle twitching • Muscle pain • Headaches • Irregular heartbeat • Nausea and vomiting • High blood pressure • Fever • Insomnia • Dehydration • Yawning • Weakness • Stomach cramps

continued on page 470

table
24.1. **Commonly Abused Controlled Substances** *continued*

Category	Examples/ Street Names	Effects of Intoxication	Health Consequences	Withdrawal Symptoms
Fentanyl and fentanyl analogs	*Actiq, Duragesic, Sublimaze:* Apache, China girl, China white, dance fever, friend, goodfella, jack-pot, murder 8, TNT, Tango and Cash	See "Opioids and Morphine Derivatives"	See "Opioids and Morphine Derivatives"	See "Opioids and Morphine Derivatives"
Heroin	*Diacetyl-morphine:* brown sugar, dope, H, horse, junk, skag, skunk, smack, white horse	See "Opioids and Morphine Derivatives"; also, staggering gait	See "Opioids and Morphine Derivatives"	See "Opioids and Morphine Derivatives"; also, dilated pupils; piloerection (goose bumps); watery eyes; runny nose; yawning; loss of appetite; tremors; panic; chills; nausea; muscle cramps; insomnia; stomach cramps; diarrhea; vomiting; shaking; chills or profuse sweating; irritability; jitteriness

morphine

Roxanol, Duramorph. M, Miss Emma, monkey, white stuff

See "Opioids and Morphine Derivatives"

See "Opioids and Morphine Derivatives"

...symptoms reach a peak intensity in 36 to 72 hours and cease in 5 to 7 days, even though craving may continue for months.

- Restlessness
- Lacrimation
- Rhinorrhea
- Yawning
- Perspiration
- Goose flesh
- Restless sleep
- Mydriasis
- Twitching and spasms of muscles
- Kicking movements
- Severe aches in the back, abdomen, and legs
- Abdominal and muscle cramps
- Hot and cold flashes
- Insomnia
- Nausea
- Vomiting
- Diarrhea
- Coryza
- Severe sneezing
- Increased body temperature, blood pressure, respiratory rate, and heart rate

continued on page 472

table
24.1. **Commonly Abused Controlled Substances** continued

Category	Examples/Street Names	Effects of Intoxication	Health Consequences	Withdrawal Symptoms
Opium	*Laudanum, paregoric:* big O, black stuff, block, gum, hop	See "Opioids and Morphine Derivatives"	See "Opioids and Morphine Derivatives"	• Nausea • Sweating • Cramps • Vomiting • Diarrhea • Loss of appetite • Muscle spasms • Depression • Anxiety • Mood swings • Insomnia
Oxycodone HCL	*Oxycontin:* Oxy, O.C., killer	See "Opioids and Morphine Derivatives"	See "Opioids and Morphine Derivatives"	• Perpetual fatigue • Hot/cold sweats • Heart palpitations • Joints and muscles in constant pain • Vomiting • Nausea • Uncontrollable coughing • Diarrhea • Insomnia • Watery eyes • Excessive yawning

Hydrocodone bitartrate, acetaminophen	*Vicodin:* vike, Watson-387	See "Opioids and Morphine Derivatives"	See "Opioids and Morphine Derivatives"	Withdrawal may grow stronger for 24 to 72 hours and then gradually decline over 7 to 14 days. • Restlessness • Muscle pain • Bone pain • Insomnia • Diarrhea • Vomiting • Cold flashes • Goose bumps • Involuntary leg movements • Watery eyes • Runny nose • Loss of appetite • Irritability • Panic • Nausea • Chills • Sweating
Dissociative Anesthetics (*DSM-IV-TR* Category: Phencyclidine [or Phencyclidine-Like]-Related Disorders)		Increased heart rate and blood pressure, impaired motor function	Memory loss; numbness; nausea/vomiting	Mental instability

continued on page 474

table
24.1. **Commonly Abused Controlled Substances** *continued*

474

Category	Examples/ Street Names	Effects of Intoxication	Health Consequences	Withdrawal Symptoms
Ketamine	*Ketalar SV:* cat Valiums, K, Special K, vitamin K	See "Dissociative Anesthetics"	See "Dissociative Anesthetics"; also, at high doses, delirium, depression, respiratory depression and arrest	See "Dissociative Anesthetics"
PCP and analogs	*Phencyclidine:* angel dust, boat, hog, love boat, peace pill	See "Dissociative Anesthetics"; also, possible decrease in blood pressure and heart rate, panic, aggression, violence	See "Dissociative Anesthetics"; loss of appetite, depression	See "Dissociative Anesthetics"
Depressants (*DSM-IV-TR* Category: Sedative-Hypnotic or Anxiolytic-Related Disorders)		Reduced anxiety; feeling of well-being; lowered inhibitions; slowed pulse and breathing; lowered blood pressure; poor concentration	Fatigue; confusion; impaired coordination, memory, judgment; addiction; respiratory depression and arrest; death	• Rapid heartbeat • Shaky hands • Insomnia or disturbed sleep • Sweating • Irritability • Anxiety and agitation

Barbiturates	*Amytal, Nembutal, Seconal, Phenobarbital:* barbs, reds, red birds, phennies, tooies, yellows, yellow jackets	See "Depressants"; also, sedation, drowsiness	See "Depressants"; also, depression, unusual excitement, fever, irritability, poor judgment, slurred speech, dizziness, life-threatening withdrawal	See "Depressants"
Benzodiazepines (other than flunitrazepam)	*Ativan, Halcion, Librium, Valium, Xanax:* candy, downers, sleeping pills, tranks	See "Depressants"; also, sedation, drowsiness	See "Depressants"; also, dizziness	See "Depressants"
Flunitrazepam	*Rohypnol:* forget-me pill, Mexican Valium, R2, Roche, roofies, roofinol, rope, rophies	See "Depressants"	See "Depressants"; also, visual and gastrointestinal disturbances, urinary retention, memory loss for the time under the drug's effects	See "Depressants"
GHB	*Gamma-hydroxybutyrate:* G, Georgia home boy, grievous bodily harm, liquid ecstasy	See "Depressants"	See "Depressants"; also, drowsiness, nausea/vomiting, headache, loss of consciousness and reflexes, seizures, coma, death	See "Depressants"
Methaqualone	*Quaalude, Sopor, Parest:* ludes, mandrex, quad, quay	See "Depressants"; also, euphoria	See "Depressants"; also, depression, poor reflexes, slurred speech, coma	See "Depressants"

continued on page 476

table
24.1.

Commonly Abused Controlled Substances *continued*

Category	Examples/ Street Names	Effects of Intoxication	Health Consequences	Withdrawal Symptoms
Other Compounds Anabolic Steroids	*Anadrol, Oxandrin, Durabolin, Depo-Testosterone, Equipoise:* roids, juice	No intoxication effects	Hypertension, blood clotting and cholesterol changes, liver cysts and cancer, kidney cancer, hostility and aggression, acne; in adolescents, premature stoppage of growth; in males, prostate cancer, reduced sperm production, shrunken testicles, breast enlargement; in females, menstrual irregularities, development of beard and other masculine characteristics	• Mood swings • Fatigue • Restlessness • Loss of appetite • Insomnia • Reduced sex drive • Steroid cravings • Depression • Suicide attempts If left untreated, some depressive symptoms associated with anabolic steroid withdrawal have been known to persist for 1 year or more after the abuser stops using.
Dextromethorphan (DXM)	*Found in some cough and cold medications;* Robotripping, Robo, Triple C	Dissociative effects, distorted visual perceptions to complete dissociative effects	For effects at higher doses see "Dissociative Anesthetics"	N/A

Sources: Narcanon of Southern California. (2007). *Drug withdrawal.* Retrieved April 23, 2008, from http://www.addictionwithdrawal.com/, and National Institute on Drug Abuse

Alcohol-related disorders include two major categories:

- Alcohol use disorders
- Alcohol dependence
- Alcohol abuse
- Alcohol-induced disorders
- Alcohol intoxication
- Alcohol withdrawal
- Alcohol intoxication delirium
- Alcohol withdrawal delirium
- Alcohol-induced: persisting dementia, persisting amnestic disorder (with delusions, with hallucinations), mood disorder, anxiety disorder, sexual dysfunction, sleep disorder, disorder NOS

The discussion here focuses primarily on the alcohol-induced disorders of intoxication and withdrawal, including delirium.

Assessment

DSM-IV-TR Diagnostic Criteria: Alcohol Use Disorder

Alcohol Intoxication

- Recent alcohol ingestion
- Clinically significant maladaptive behavior or psychological changes developing during or shortly after alcohol ingestion
- Development during or shortly after use of one or more of the following:
  1. Slurred speech
  2. Lack of coordination
  3. Unsteady gait
  4. Nystagmus
  5. Attention or memory impairment
  6. Stupor or coma
- Symptoms not caused by a general medical condition and not better accounted for by another mental disorder

Alcohol Withdrawal

- Cessation (or reduction) in heavy and prolonged alcohol use

---

■ Development within several hours to a few days after cessation/reduction of two or more of the following:

1. Autonomic hyperactivity

2. Increased hand tremor

3. Insomnia

4. Nausea or vomiting

5. Transient visual, tactile, or auditory hallucinations or illusions

6. Psychomotor agitation

7. Anxiety

8. Grand mal seizures

■ Clinically significant distress or impairment in social, occupational, or other important areas of function due to symptoms

■ Symptoms not due to a general medical condition and not better accounted for by another mental disorder

Adapted with permission from American Psychiatric Association. (2000). *Diagnostic and statistical manual of mental disorders (4th ed., text rev.).* Washington, DC: Author.

Common History and Physical Examination Findings

See also "Substance Disorder Assessment Tools," *p. 99–105.*

GENERAL (RELATED TO ALCOHOL USE)

• Weight loss
• Poor nutritional status
• Deconditioning
• Gastric distress
• Oral health problems, such as gum disease

INTOXICATION

• Slurred speech
• Lack of coordination
• Unsteady gait
• Nystagmus
• Flushing
• Inattention
• Blackout
• Vomiting
• Impaired motor function
• Altered level of consciousness

- Respiratory depression
- Medical complications involving any body system related to long-term use

WITHDRAWAL

Occurring 4 to 12 hours after last intake; see also "Clinical Institute Withdrawal Assessment—Alcohol, revised [CIWA-Ar]," p. 99–100.

- History of alcohol use
- Coarse hand tremors
- Sweating
- Elevated temperature, pulse, and blood pressure
- Insomnia
- Nausea and vomiting
- Seizures
- Delirium tremens

Common Psychosocial Assessment Findings
GENERAL (RELATED TO ALCOHOL USE/DEPENDENCE)

- Family dysfunction
- Occupational problems
- Withdrawal
- Reduced social, occupational, or recreational activities
- Possible guilt, embarrassment, shame, despair

INTOXICATION

- Aggressiveness
- Inappropriate sexual behavior
- Loss of inhibitions
- Irritability
- Mood swings
- Impaired judgment

WITHDRAWAL

- Anxiety
- Transient hallucinations
- Nightmares

Common Laboratory and Diagnostic Test Findings

- **BAL**: elevated above legally established limits
- **Serum gamma-glutamyltransferase**: elevated levels (indicative of heavy drinking)
- **Mean corpuscular volume**: high-normal levels
- **Liver function tests (alanine aminotransferase; alkaline phosphatase)**: evidence of liver damage (from heavy drinking)
- **Lipid levels**: elevated

Interdisciplinary Treatment Modalities

Medical Detoxification Program

Self-Help Groups

12-Step Programs

Rehabilitation

Cognitive Therapy (*see p. 111*)

Brief Therapy

Cognitive-Behavioral Therapy (*see p. 116*)

Group Therapy (*see p. 123*)

Psychotherapy

■ Individual psychotherapy (*see p. 126*)

Family Therapy (*see p. 122*)

Psychopharmacology

■ Long-term maintenance therapy: disulfiram (*see p. 296*); naltrexone; acamprosate; baclofen

■ Acute withdrawal management: benzodiazepines: diazepam (*see p. 162*); chlordiazepoxide (*see p. 159*); lorazepam (*see p. 169*)

Nursing Care Planning*

Note: The information that follows could be adapted to any other substance use or induced disorder.

| NURSING DIAGNOSIS: Risk for Injury

Related to:	As Evidenced by:
Impending alcohol withdrawal	BAL
	Time of last ingestion
	Evidence of alcohol intoxication
	Increased hand tremor
	Insomnia
	Nausea and vomiting
	Brief hallucinations
	Elevation in vital signs
	Anxiety

Nursing Outcomes Classification (NOC): Risk Control: Alcohol Use: Client will exhibit minimal effects associated with alcohol withdrawal during the first week of detoxification.

Nursing Interventions Classification (NIC): Substance Use Treatment: Alcohol Withdrawal

1. Minimize environmental stimuli during detoxification. Speak in a low, calm, reassuring voice. *A comfortable, quiet, nonthreatening environment reduces anxiety-provoking stimuli.*

2. Assess vital signs; look for indicators of impending withdrawal: tachycardia, hypertension, tremors, anxiety, sweating, hallucinations, and psychomotor agitation. *Assessing vital signs and monitoring for the onset of withdrawal symptoms allows for timely intervention.*

3. Institute seizure and fall precautions. *These actions promote client safety.*

4. Administer sedatives and other medications as ordered. *Sedatives help control the exaggerated sympathetic activity associated with withdrawal. Other medications may be needed for long-term maintenance.*

5. Monitor for covert alcohol consumption during detoxification. *Having to deal with uncomfortable feelings during sobriety may increase anxiety and emotional discomfort, which may lead to relapse.*

6. Continue frequent monitoring of vital signs, sensorium, and other variables. Provide verbal reassurance and reality orientation as appropriate. Report worsened conditions immediately. Institute emergency procedures if clients show signs of delirium. *Preventing alcohol-withdrawal delirium is critical because of the associated mortality rate. Verbal reassurance and reality orientation help reduce anxiety associated with withdrawal and detoxification.*

7. Listen to clients' concerns about alcohol withdrawal. Encourage them to discuss feelings; assist with measures for effective coping. *Listening provides support and helps reduce anxiety and stress. Adaptive coping strategies must replace maladaptive ones for recovery.*

NURSING DIAGNOSIS: Ineffective Denial

Related to:	As Evidenced by:
Dysfunctional defense mechanisms associated with alcohol abuse	Continued use of alcohol despite problems with work and family
	Minimization of effects of alcohol on self and others

NOC: Knowledge: Substance Use Control; Coping: Client will acknowledge problem with alcohol and the need for treatment, developing adaptive coping strategies to manage stressors without alcohol.

NIC: Substance Use Treatment

1. Establish a therapeutic relationship, maintaining a nonjudgmental attitude. *Development of a trusting relationship is the first step in helping the clients relinquish denial.*

2. Discuss with the clients the effects of alcohol use on family health and daily functioning. Point out evidence of severe dysfunction. Assist clients to evaluate how much time is spent consuming alcohol and usual daily patterns. Firmly remind clients that problems are the result of alcohol abuse. *Identifying problem areas and effects of alcohol use (including time spent on use) is necessary to dispel probable rationalizations for problems and aids in confronting denial.*

3. Inform clients that alcohol abuse is a disease, not a character flaw. Encourage use of a 12-step program. *Education about the*

facts of the disorder can help reduce feelings of guilt and weakness, thus lessening the need for denial. A 12-step program reinforces the disease concept of alcohol abuse, and hearing the stories of others in recovery helps the clients relinquish denial.

4. Encourage clients to have an open mind about feedback from staff, family, and others and to speak openly about this feedback. *Speaking openly with others reduces the risk for continued rationalization and denial and helps expose maladaptive thinking patterns associated with alcohol use.*

NIC: Coping Enhancement

1. Determine usual methods of coping and problem solving in clients. Help identify maladaptive strategies. *Identification of maladaptive coping methods is necessary for client recovery and growth.*

2. Provide suggestions for replacing maladaptive coping methods with appropriate ones. Teach cognitive restructuring techniques to reappraise the situation. *These interventions help clients determine and substitute the most beneficial strategies for maladaptive ones. Cognitive restructuring helps clients reappraise situations in a less ego-threatening way, thereby diminishing their need to over-defend themselves.*

3. Rehearse with clients various strategies to cope with anxiety. *Rehearsing enhances the chances for success when clients use these techniques.*

4. Refer clients to appropriate community agencies. Suggest that they consider joining a support group. *Community agencies and support groups are tremendous resources for people who feel alone with their disorder.*

NURSING DIAGNOSIS: Chronic Low Self-Esteem

Related to:	As Evidenced by:
Doubts and anxiety about self-worth and abilities	Use of alcohol to cope with stressors
	Reduced activities
	Family dysfunction
	Damaged relationships

NOC: Self-Esteem: Client will identify positive aspects about self.

NIC: Self-Esteem Enhancement

1. Assist clients to acknowledge the relationship between alcohol use and feelings. Explore previous achievements and reasons for self-criticism or guilt. Encourage clients to identify strengths and resources. Reinforce identified strengths. *Realistic self-expectations, positive reinforcement, and ongoing feedback will increase self-esteem.*

2. Assist clients to minimize negative self-talk and rumination; encourage the use of thought-stopping techniques. Assist clients to set realistic goals; offer praise and encouragement for achievements. *Negative self-talk and rumination are sources for poor self-esteem. Thought-stopping techniques help to move the focus of thinking to more positive thoughts.*

3. Focus clients on the present. Discuss ways to change current status. *Focusing on the past only helps reinforce low self-esteem.*

4. Determine locus of control for clients and their confidence in their own judgment. Encourage clients to make independent decisions and choices as appropriate. Convey confidence in their ability to handle situations. *Opportunities to practice independent functioning will help improve self-confidence and self-esteem.*

5. Enhance communication and socialization skills by promoting information, role-playing, and participation in group activities. Suggest that clients find personally rewarding activities. Encourage participation in recovery program. *Enhanced social skills will improve relationships and contribute to improving self-esteem. Personally rewarding activities promote feelings of accomplishment. Participation in recovery programs promotes sharing of feelings and support.*

| NURSING DIAGNOSIS: Dysfunctional Family Processes: Alcoholism

Related to:	*As Evidenced by:*
History of long-term alcohol abuse	Episodes of intoxication/withdrawal
	Signs and symptoms of intoxication/withdrawal
	Problems with work, relationships

NOC: Family Coping; Role Performance: The family will demonstrate balanced and adaptive family functional and mature interpersonal relationships.

NIC: Family Integrity Promotion

1. Identify typical family relationships and coping mechanisms. Identify conflicting priorities among family members. *The family's relationships and coping mechanisms provide clues to develop an individualized plan of care.*

2. Teach family members effective communication skills and assertiveness. Help them clarify what they want, expect, and need from one another. Encourage family members to participate in support groups and family therapy as appropriate. *Behavior that respects the rights and feelings of others leads to increased trust and intimacy. Participation in support groups and family therapy helps family members adjust to client sobriety and develop a less vigilant, more interdependent relationship.*

3. Explore topics to determine how each member can support and meet the needs of others. Help clients recognize excessive dependency or unrealistic expectations. Refer family to support group for those dealing with similar problems. *Self-awareness and insight into others improve relationships. Providing client and family support services and new tools for interaction will help them abandon older, less functional behaviors.*

NIC: Role Enhancement

1. Help clients and families explore appropriate expression of anger or other negative emotions. Collaborate with them in problem solving. Teach problem-solving skills and conflict management techniques. Assist with conflict resolution. *Appropriate use of problem-solving and conflict resolution techniques help build trust and respect for improving relationships.*

2. Encourage clients to assume functional family roles. Facilitate opportunity for clients to role-play new behaviors; facilitate discussion of expectations among family members in reciprocal roles. Explore potential problems (eg, power struggles) as clients become more functional. *Other family members have been the responsible partner for many years. Although they may welcome*

sobriety and involvement from clients, these events represent a change in roles, which may be difficult for the family.

| NURSING DIAGNOSIS: Ineffective Health Maintenance

Related to:	As Evidenced by:
Continued alcohol use and abuse	Deterioration in physical health status
	Underweight status
	Deconditioning
	Medical complications associated with long-term use

NOC: Personal Health Status; Substance Addiction Consequences: Client will demonstrate improved overall health status with adoption of health-seeking behaviors.

NIC: Nutrition Management

1. Obtain an initial weight and periodically weigh clients. Encourage calorie intake appropriate for body type and lifestyle. *Weight is a valuable indicator of health status. These measures assist with tailoring a nutritional plan to individual clients.*
2. Provide vitamin and mineral supplements. Encourage consumption of well-balanced meals with little refined sugar or caffeine. *Alcohol depletes essential nutrients, which must be replaced. Refraining from sugar and caffeine helps manage anxiety and mood swings.*
3. Offer snacks as appropriate; provide easy-to-consume nutritious foods and drinks. *Snacks, liquids, and easily prepared foods facilitate intake and enhance the chances for success.*
4. Monitor clients' tolerance to intake; note any nausea or vomiting and characteristics of emesis. Consider small frequent meals. *Alcohol is highly irritating to the gastrointestinal tract, and clients are at risk for esophageal varices secondary to prolonged alcohol use.*

NIC: Exercise Promotion

1. Assist clients to develop an appropriate and appealing exercise program; inform clients about health benefits and physiologic effects of exercise. *Physical exercise increases stamina, helps*

balance mood, and aids in managing anxiety and stress. It also provides clients with an activity that can occupy time previously spent with alcohol use.

2. Provide positive feedback for efforts. *Positive feedback promotes self-esteem and motivation for continued participation.*

NIC: Oral Health Restoration

1. Instruct and assist clients to perform oral hygiene after eating and as often as necessary. Encourage frequent rinsing of the mouth, using a soft toothbrush, and flossing between teeth twice daily. *Proper oral hygiene reduces the risk of further oral health problems.*

2. Assist clients to select soft, bland, and nonacidic foods. *These food types prevent exacerbation of the already irritated oral mucosa.*

3. Monitor clients at least every shift for dryness of the oral mucosa. Monitor for signs and symptoms of glossitis and stomatitis. Arrange for dental care. *Gum disease places a burden on the immune system.*

Thought Disorders

T hought disorders are serious and often persistent mental illnesses characterized by disturbances in reality orientation, thinking, and social involvement. Major categories of thought disorders include schizophrenia, schizophreniform disorders, brief psychotic disorders, schizoaffective disorders, delusional disorders, and shared psychotic disorders.

Schizophrenia

Schizophrenia is a common and serious neurobiologic illness; it is the most prevalent thought disorder. General hallmarks include disturbed thinking and preoccupation with frightening inner experiences (eg, delusions, hallucinations). Marked disturbances occur in affect (eg, flat, inappropriate), behavior (eg, unpredictable, bizarre), and social interactions (eg, isolation). These disturbances seem related to problems with brain circuitry.

Schizophrenia occurs in all cultures, races, and social classes. It is thought to have multiple causes; its exact cause is unknown. People with schizophrenia manifest alterations in cognitive functioning.

Three dimensions of psychopathology have been identified in schizophrenia:

- *Disorganized dimension*: formal thought disorder that affects the relationships and associations among the words people use to express thoughts (ie, the verbal form of thoughts); disorganized speech, disorganized or bizarre behavior, and incongruous affect

- *Psychotic dimension*: two classic symptoms that reflect confusion about the loss of boundaries between self and the external world; delusions and hallucinations
- *Negative dimension*: reflection of a deficiency in normal mental functioning; alogia, affective blunting, avolition, anhedonia, and attentional impairment

Assessment

Diagnostic and Statistical Manual of Mental Disorders, Fourth Edition, Text Revision (DSM-IV-TR) Diagnostic Criteria: Schizophrenia

---

- Two or more of the following *characteristic symptoms* for a significant portion of 1 month (or less if successfully treated):
  - Delusions
  - Hallucinations
  - Disorganized speech (eg, frequent derailment or incoherence)
  - Grossly disorganized or catatonic behavior
  - Negative symptoms (ie, affective flattening, alogia, or avolition)
- Significant social/occupational dysfunction since the disturbance began, markedly below the client's level before onset; when onset is in childhood or adolescence, failure to achieve expected interpersonal, academic, or occupational achievement
- Signs of disturbance continuous for at least 6 months, including at least 1 month of symptoms (or less if successfully treated); during any prodromal or residual periods, possibly only negative symptoms or two or more symptoms listed in the first criterion in an attenuated form (eg, unusual perceptual experiences)
- Schizoaffective disorder and mood disorder with psychotic features ruled out because either no mood episodes have accompanied the active-phase symptoms or total duration of accompanying mood episodes has been brief relative to the active and residual periods
- Disturbance not caused by a substance or general medical condition
- For a client with a history of a pervasive development disorder, the additional diagnosis of schizophrenia made only if prominent delusions or hallucinations also present for at least 1 month (or less if successfully treated)

- Subtypes:
  - **Paranoid**: preoccupation with delusions of persecution or grandeur (organized around a coherent theme), ideas of reference, or frequent auditory hallucinations; client may appear tense, suspicious, guarded, reserved, hostile, or aggressive
  - **Disorganized**: markedly regressed, disorganized, silly, inappropriate, and uninhibited behavior; disorganized speech; flat or inappropriate affect; poor reality contact; poor grooming and social skills; a prominent thought disorder; and possibly grimacing, strange mannerisms, or other odd behaviors
  - **Catatonic**: motor immobility or stupor, rigidity, excessive motor activity, extreme negativism, stupor, and peculiarities of movement, such as posturing, echolalia and echopraxia, mutism, and waxy flexibility
  - **Undifferentiated**: behavior and speech clearly indicative of schizophrenic psychosis but fail to meet the criteria of paranoid, disorganized, or catatonic types
  - **Residual**: absence of active, positive symptoms, such as hallucinations and delusions, but continued demonstration of negative symptoms, such as withdrawal from others or flat affect

Adapted with permission from American Psychiatric Association. (2000). *Diagnostic and statistical manual of mental disorders (4th ed., text rev.)*. Washington, DC: Author.

Common History and Physical Examination Findings

- Bizarre or inappropriate clothing or appearance
- Decreased spontaneous movements
- Poor eye contact
- Impaired grooming and hygiene
- Inattentiveness
- Difficulty in following language content, rambling speech
- Speech disturbances: clang associations, neologisms, verbigeration, echolalia, stilted language, perseveration, word salad
- Sleep disturbances
- Decreased appetite
- Somatic complaints such as headache, malaise, constipation
- Short attention span
- Restlessness, agitation, aggressiveness
- Unmoving (catatonia)
- Purposeless gestures
- Odd facial expressions
- Imitation of movements (echopraxia)

- Slowing of movements
- Waxy flexibility
- Polydipsia, water intoxication

Common Psychosocial Assessment Findings

- Delusions
- Hallucinations
- Inappropriate affect
- Loss of interest or pleasure
- Distorted thought processes: though blocking, thought broadcasting, thought withdrawal, thought insertion
- Impaired judgment
- Lack of insight
- Depersonalization, derealization
- Inability to function in role
- Social isolation
- Possible substance abuse

Common Laboratory and Diagnostic Test Findings

- **Serum sodium levels:** below 135 mEq/L, indicating water intoxication
- **Urine specific gravity:** below 1.011 as a result of water intoxication
- **Positive emission tomography scanning:** relative metabolic underactivity of the frontal lobes; decreased basal ganglia activity

Interdisciplinary Treatment Modalities

Psychotherapy
- Individual psychotherapy (*see p. 126*)

Milieu Therapy (see p. 130)

Group Therapy (see p. 123)

Cognitive-Behavioral Therapy (see p. 116)

Electroconvulsive Therapy (see p. 146)

Social Skills Training

Vocational Rehabilitation

Psychopharmacology

- A typical antipsychotics: clozapine (Clozaril [*see p. 242*]), risperidone (Risperdal [*see p. 258*]), olanzapine (Zyprexa [*see p. 251*]), quetiapine (Seroquel [*see p. 256*]), ziprasidone (Geodon [*see p. 266*]), aripiprazole (Abilify [*see p. 238*]), and paliperidone (Invega)

- Traditional antipsychotics: chlorpromazine (Thorazine [*see p. 240*]), fluphenazine (Prolixin [*see p. 246*]), haloperidol (Haldol [*see p. 248*]), trifluoperazine (Stelazine [*see p. 264*]), thioridazine (Mellaril [*see p. 260*]), thiothixene (Navane [*see p. 262*]), and perphenazine (Trilafon [*see p. 254*])

Nursing Care Planning

| NURSING DIAGNOSIS: Disturbed Thought Processes

Related to:	As Evidenced by:
Possible neurochemical dysregulation	Non–reality-based thinking
	Thought blocking, broadcasting, withdrawal, insertion
	Hallucinations
	Delusions
	Speech disturbances
	Depersonalization
	Derealization

Nursing Outcomes Classification (NOC): Distorted Thought Self-Control: Client will demonstrate increased reality-based thinking with fewer hallucinations and delusions.

Nursing Interventions Classification (NIC): Delusion Management

1. Focus on underlying feelings about the delusion, not the content. For example, avoid arguing about false beliefs; state doubt in a matter-of-fact manner. Avoid reinforcing delusions. Involve clients in present-oriented conversations and activities, describing real events and clarifying facts. Encourage clients to validate delusions with trusted others, such as staff (reality testing), and to verbalize delusions to caregivers before acting on them. *Focusing on*

nondelusional content (eg, feelings) and discouraging animated discussions of delusions (which would only reinforce them) will help clients see that their thoughts are not real. Asking clients to bring delusional content to the caregivers' attention provides opportunities for reinforcing reality-based thinking and may prevent bizarre or possibly violent behavior generated by delusions.

2. Provide recreational, diversionary activities that require attention or skill. Engage clients in reality-based activities, such as looking at pictures in a magazine or taking a walk. If clients cannot interact, stay with them. *They help clients focus on something other than the delusions. Reality-based activities are therapeutic because they allow clients to interact in a satisfying interpersonal relationship and diminish time spent in poor contact with reality. Staying with clients who cannot interact provides a vital link with the real world.*

3. Monitor delusions for self-harmful or violent content; protect clients and others from potentially harmful delusional-based behaviors. *Monitoring is important for safety.*

4. Administer medications as ordered and needed, observing for any side effects and desired therapeutic effects. *Antipsychotics are the most powerful tool in the treatment of schizophrenia.*

NIC: Hallucination Management

1. Keep clients in a safe, protected, and restricted environment. Provide appropriate surveillance and supervision. Do not leave clients who are hallucinating alone. Encourage clients to tell staff when they are hallucinating and to reveal the hallucinatory content. Monitor hallucinations for harmful content. *Close observation of clients with active hallucinations in a secure environment is essential to maintain overall safety. Staying with clients provides reassurance and a potentially calming force. Staff should be aware of any hallucinatory content, especially if it is potentially harmful.*

2. Avoid excessive activity or stimulation. Maintain a consistent routine; assign consistent caregivers daily. *Excessive sensory stimulation or changes in routine could overwhelm and agitate clients.*

3. Encourage clients to discuss rather than act on feelings and impulses. Focus on feelings about, rather than details of, the hallucination (eg, "You seem to be afraid," not "Why would the voices tell you to hurt yourself?"). *Focusing on feelings, which are real, minimizes emphasis on the hallucination.*

4. Do not argue with clients about whether hallucinations are real; state, if asked, that you do not perceive the stimuli that clients perceive. *Arguing or expressing skepticism does not affect the belief of clients in the reality of the hallucination and can disrupt trust and the therapeutic relationship. Expressing that you do not see, hear, or otherwise experience the hallucinatory stimuli indirectly encourages clients to question the reality of the experience.*

5. Use limit setting, area restriction, or other measures when clients cannot control behavior. *Measures to control behavior promote the safety and comfort of clients and others.*

6. Engage clients in reality-based activities. *Activities help to distract clients from the hallucinations and promote reality-based thought.*

| NURSING DIAGNOSIS: Disturbed Sensory Perception, Auditory/Visual

Related to:	As Evidenced by:
Hallucinations associated with disturbed thought processes	Statements of hearing voices Statements of seeing things

NOC: Distorted Thought Self-Control; Cognitive Orientation: Client will demonstrate fewer hallucinations.

NIC: Reality Orientation

1. Approach clients calmly, slowly, and from the front. Speak to them in a calm, unhurried, distinct manner using concrete, specific terms and repeating information as necessary. Avoid using gestures or objects when communicating. *A calm, unhurried approach prevents overwhelming clients. Concrete specific terms and avoidance of gestures or objects are necessary to prevent misinterpretation by clients who cannot think abstractly. Repetition is important to help clients refocus or maintain focus.*

2. Provide simple tasks and activities that clients can realistically complete. Limit questions and give simple directions one at a time. *Simple tasks and activities help to maintain reality focus*

without overwhelming clients. Limiting questions and directions to one at a time prevents overwhelming clients and adding to their frustration and anxiety level.

3. Attempt to determine the content of hallucinations. Provide realistic reassurance, informing clients that you are aware that the voices or images are very real to them but that you are not experiencing them. Communicate concern that clients are bothered, upset, or frightened. *Determining the content of the hallucinations is important in identifying the type of stimuli that clients are receiving. Providing realistic reassurance validates the feelings of clients without reinforcing their hallucinations. Concern fosters the development of trust.*

| NURSING DIAGNOSIS: Risk for Self-directed or Other-Directed Violence

Related to:	As Evidenced by:
Distorted thought processes	Auditory hallucinations
	Delusions
	Agitation
	Aggressiveness
	Depressed mood
	Anhedonia

NOC: Suicide Self-Restraint; Impulse Self-Control: Client will refrain from harming self or others.

NIC: Behavior Management: Self-Harm

1. Assess the potential for violent behavior in clients. Ask them directly if voices tell them to hurt themselves or anyone else. Communicate risks to other care providers. Maintain ongoing surveillance of clients and environment. *Preventing self- or other-directed violence is possible if healthcare providers heed warnings (eg, intimidating behaviors, threats). Continuing evaluation of clients and environment reduces the potential for injury.*

2. Administer medication as ordered and needed. Monitor for side effects and desired therapeutic effects. *Antipsychotic drugs are the most powerful tools in the treatment of schizophrenia. Even if*

clients receive depot injections, they may require more medication if psychotic symptoms escalate.

3. Assist clients to identify situations or feelings that may prompt self-harm. Give reassurance, comfort, and opportunity to discuss delusions. *Caring interventions help build a therapeutic relationship and may increase the likelihood that clients will reveal the content of their auditory hallucinations.*

4. Communicate behavioral expectations and consequences. *Clear communication helps foster a therapeutic relationship and enhances awareness and knowledge.*

5. Instruct clients in appropriate coping strategies; teach and reinforce effective behaviors and appropriate expression of feelings. *Knowledge and reinforcement of coping strategies and behaviors help promote continued use by clients.*

6. Place clients in a more protective environment if impulses/behaviors escalate. *Doing so can ensure the safety of clients and others.*

NIC: Suicide Prevention

1. Be alert for signs of self-harm; keep clients in a protected environment with frequent observation until delusions and hallucinations subside. Determine the degree of suicidal risk and whether clients have available means to follow through with a suicide plan. *Warning signs of self-directed violence may be covert; protecting, observing, and asking clients about them and any means to accomplish them may be the only preventive tools available.*

2. Assign clients to a room near the nursing station. *Doing so facilitates observation.*

3. Contract with clients as appropriate for "no self-harm." Implement necessary actions to reduce immediate distress. Identify immediate safety needs when negotiating the contract; assist clients to discuss feelings about the contract. Observe for signs of incongruence that may indicate lack of commitment. *Contracting reinforces behavioral expectations, promotes trust, and enhances overall safety. Identification of signs of incongruence aids in early detection and prevention of harm.*

4. Interact with clients regularly; use a direct, nonjudgmental approach in discussing suicide; discuss plan for dealing with future suicidal ideation. *Frequent direct interaction helps convey*

caring and openness and provides an opportunity for clients to talk about feelings.

NIC: Impulse Control Training

1. Be alert to inappropriate and possibly pre-violent behaviors such as irritability, intimidating behavior, refusal to cooperate with unit routines, motor restlessness, intense staring, loud speech, or overt threats. *Identifying potential behaviors allows for early intervention to prevent escalation of behavior.*

2. Use a behavior modification plan; assist clients to identify problems or situations that require thoughtful action. Teach them to "stop and think" before acting impulsively. *Behavior modification helps reinforce positive problem-solving strategies to deal with hallucinations and delusions.*

3. Provide opportunities to practice problem solving; provide positive reinforcement for successful outcomes. *Positive reinforcement promotes continued and appropriate use of strategies in the future.*

NIC: Environmental Management: Violence Prevention

1. Determine with other team members a plan of action if violence appears imminent. Discuss the plan with clients; ask them to tell staff when or if they feel they may harm themselves or others. *Having a plan will help staff more effectively manage violence. Engaging clients in the plan may help them gain control over thought processes, increase the likelihood that they will comply with the plan, and help build a therapeutic relationship.*

2. Place clients in the least restrictive environment that permits necessary observation. Remove other people from the vicinity of a violent or potentially violent client. *Use of the least restrictive environment protects the client's rights while maintaining unit safety.*

| N U R S I N G   D I A G N O S I S : Ineffective Management of Therapeutic Regimen

Related to:	As Evidenced by:
Exacerbation and relapse of thought disorder	Failure to take prescribed medications
	Behavior escalation
	Reappearance of hallucinations and delusions

NOC: Compliance Behavior: Client will take prescribed medications.

NIC: Patient Contracting

1. Encourage clients to identify strengths and abilities; assist them to set realistic, attainable goals and to break them into small, manageable steps. Help clients recognize even small successes. *Identification and participation enhance feelings of control. Breaking down goals prevents overwhelming clients and promotes feelings of accomplishment as they achieve each step.*

2. Facilitate involvement of significant others in the contracting process if clients agree; facilitate negotiation of contract terms if necessary. *Participation from others provides additional support for clients. Flexibility in contract terms is necessary to meet changing needs.*

3. Explain the rationale for medications. Discuss the possible use of depot injections to manage short-term medication compliance. *Inability to maintain medication therapy suggests that adherence most likely will remain an issue. Depot injections ensure the maintenance of therapeutic levels of neuroleptic medication for 2 weeks at a time.*

4. Encourage clients to identify appropriate meaningful reinforcers or rewards. *Appropriate rewards enhance the chances that clients will follow the contract.*

NIC: Self-Responsibility Facilitation

1. Encourage verbalizations of feelings, perceptions, and fears about assuming responsibility. *Underlying knowledge of status is important in individualizing strategies.*

2. Initiate medication adherence therapy. Help clients achieve insight into the benefit of taking the drugs by helping them review the history of their illness, symptoms, and medication side effects; encourage them to consider benefits *versus* drawbacks of drug treatment. Encourage compliance and provide information about neuroleptic medication. *Medication adherence therapy, which involves medication education, support, and insight into the disorder, has been shown to increase long-term use of pharmacologic therapy.*

3. Encourage independence, but assist clients with things they cannot perform. Set limits on manipulative behavior; refrain from

arguing or bargaining about established limits. *Encouraging independence along with assistance and limit setting promotes responsibility for actions and enhances clients' feelings of control over the situation.*

4. Teach clients and their families about the disorder and need to follow the treatment plan, including medication regimen and follow up. *Such instruction promotes improved understanding, which increases the chance for the plan to succeed.*

| NURSING DIAGNOSIS: Interrupted Family Processes

Related to:	As Evidenced by:
Effects associated with the chronic nature of the disorder	Long-term need for antipsychotic therapy
	Increased potential for exacerbations and relapses

NOC: Family Coping; Family Normalization; Family Resiliency: Client and family will demonstrate positive behaviors to cope with client's disorder.

NIC: Family Process Maintenance

1. Identify effects of role changes on family processes. Promote family cohesion. Help family members, including clients, identify their feelings about role and health status changes. Help them resolve any feelings of guilt. Identify effective coping mechanisms; encourage their use as family adjusts to changes. Discuss strategies for normalizing family life. *Open communication about the effects of schizophrenia will help family members. Clients may feel guilty about not being able to help more or about becoming a "burden" on the family; caregivers may have resentment about increased responsibilities.*

2. Minimize disruptions by facilitating family routines and rituals. *Encouraging normal activities reduces guilt or anxiety related to the condition of clients.*

3. Discuss existing social support mechanisms; assist the family to use them. Help them resolve any conflicts; suggest attending a

support group. *Helping the family resolve feelings and identify appropriate coping behaviors will decrease stress. Support groups are a tremendous resource for sharing feelings and gaining insight and help.*

NIC: Family Support

1. Appraise the family's emotional reaction to the condition; listen to the family's concerns, feelings, and questions. Foster realistic hope. Facilitate communication of concerns and feeling between clients and family and between family members. *The diagnosis of schizophrenia is associated with the stigma of shame and family burden. Family members must understand that schizophrenia is a "no-fault" brain disease (ie, no reason for blame). Listening to clients and their families fosters a therapeutic relationship and provides them with a source of support.*

2. Provide information about the diagnosis, progress, and plan of care. Encourage family decision making that involves clients when appropriate. Encourage family to seek out information. *Information and decision making foster empowerment. Providing education to clients and their families and promoting increased involvement by clients usually result in increased adherence to medication regimens.*

3. Determine the level of knowledge and acceptance of roles among all family members. Provide practical support. Explore reaction and help identify stressors, tasks, or behaviors that are most frustrating or anxiety producing. Help families develop a plan for managing them. Provide support for decision making. Give information about the disease and local support groups. *Helping caregivers become aware of their feelings, strengths, the chronicity of schizophrenia, and available supports will empower the family to manage the demands of care while protecting the family's emotional state. Thinking through and planning ahead will help manage responsibilities.*

4. Explore how each family member is coping; teach stress management techniques and healthcare maintenance strategies to sustain each member's physical and mental health. *Determining coping techniques and providing instruction about stress management*

and health maintenance strategies enhance a family's ability to provide the necessary care.

5. Give encouragement to families during clients' setbacks. *Setbacks can promote guilt, frustration, and anxiety. Encouragement helps preserve a family's self-esteem.*

Emergency Situations

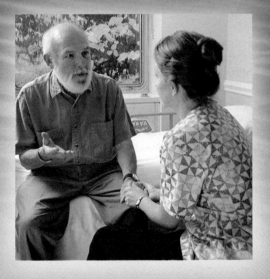

Anger and Aggression

A ggressive behavior usually involves anger and physical or verbal threats or actions. **Anger** is an emotional response to perceived frustration, shame, or humiliation. It can be positive when people direct it toward actual injustices or if it motivates them to organize and institute constructive and beneficial change. Anger loses any positive effect when it turns inward, flails ineffectively with little or no cause, bullies those with less strength or power, harms or hurts the self or others physically or emotionally, or rages out of control.

Aggression is intentional behavior with the potential to cause destruction or harm; it may manifest as verbal threats or attacks, negative use of objects, or physical assaults on known people, strangers, or self (eg, suicidal gestures, self-harm). Aggression against others ranges from verbal threats to homicide.

Factors Contributing to Anger and Aggression

Possible contributors include the following:

- Psychiatric illnesses (Box 26.1)
- Medical conditions (Box 26.2)
- Traumatic life events (eg, direct threats of death, severe bodily harm, psychological injury)

box
26.1 Psychiatric Diagnoses and Patterns of Aggression or Violence

- **Antisocial personality disorder (adults):** Callous, cynical, contemptuous of the feelings and rights of others, irresponsible, exploitative, lacks empathy, often violent

- **Attention-deficit hyperactivity disorder:** Predominantly hyperactive-impulsive type with low frustration tolerance, temper outbursts, intrusive, oppositional behavior

- **Bipolar disorders (especially bipolar I manic episodes):** Irritability, agitation, and violent behavior during manic or psychotic episodes; highly co-morbid with alcohol abuse, which worsens the prognosis

- **Conduct disorder (children):** Aggressive conduct that threatens or causes physical harm to other people or animals

- **Delusional disorder, persecutory type:** Persecutory delusions (eg, of being conspired against, cheated, spied on, maliciously maligned, poisoned or drugged); often resentful and angry and may become violent toward those whom they believe are threatening or harmful to them

- **Dementia:** Generalized irritability and low frustration tolerance, confusion, destructive attempts at self-protection

- **Dissociative identity disorder:** Aggressive behavior toward self (self-mutilation, suicide attempts) and toward others

- **Impulse-control disorders** (eg, intermittent explosive disorder): Discrete episodes of failure to resist aggressive impulses resulting in serious injury to self, assaults on others, or destruction of property

- **Oppositional defiant disorder** (children): Negativistic, hostile, defiant, spiteful, blaming behavior directed at adults or peers, primarily by verbal aggression

- **Paranoid personality disorder:** Pervasive distrust and suspiciousness that others will exploit, harm, or deceive oneself even with no evidence of such; overly vigilant; holds grudges, unwilling to forgive perceived insults or slights; may attack others suddenly

- **Post-traumatic stress disorder:** Irritability, hypervigilance, and outbursts of anger

- **Schizophrenia, paranoid type:** Persecutory ideation, which may predispose the person to suicidal behavior, or anger and violence toward others

- **Substance-related disorders:** Aggressive episodes that result from the direct physiologic effects of the drugs of abuse or the medication

Source: American Psychiatric Association. (2000). *Diagnostic and statistical manual of mental disorders* (4th ed., text rev.). Washington, DC: Author.

box

26.2 Selected Medical Conditions Associated With Aggression and Violence

Chronic Pain

Bone and joint diseases (eg, severe arthritis, rheumatism)

Neurobiologic Disorders

Brain tumors

Traumatic brain injury

Neurotransmitter imbalances

Seizure disorder

Parkinson's disease

Multiple sclerosis

Huntington's disease

Dementia

Infectious Diseases

Neurosyphillis

Meningitis

Herpes simplex encephalitis

HIV encephalopathy

Endocrine Disorders

Hyperthyroidism

Hypothyroidism

Hyperparathyroidism

Hypoparathyroidism

Adrenal disorders

Diabetes mellitus

Pancreatic tumors

Progressive hypoglycemia

Metabolic Disorders

Hyponatremia

Hypernatremia

Chronic renal failure

Hepatic encephalopathy

Porphyria

Systemic lupus erythematosus

Vitamin Deficiencies

Wernicke's encephalopathy

Pernicious anemia

Folate deficiency

Exogenous Toxins

Alcoholic hallucinosis

Hallucinogens

Illicit stimulants

Amphetamine-induced psychosis

Inhaled solvents

Heavy metals

Medications

- Biological factors and temperament (negative emotionality)
- Social-environmental factors (eg, exposure to aggressive models, random positive reinforcement of direct experience)

Phases of Aggression

Anger expressed inappropriately can lead to hostility and aggression. Although aggression may occur suddenly, it typically progresses through five phases (Table 26.1).

Interdisciplinary Management

- Verbal interventions: communication to prevent escalation:
  - Making personal contact
  - Discovering the source of distress
  - Relieving the distress

table
26.1. **Five-Phase Aggression Cycle**

Phase	Definition	Signs, Symptoms, and Behaviors
Triggering	An event or circumstances in the environment initiates the client's response, which is often anger or hostility	Restlessness, anxiety, irritability, pacing, muscle tension, rapid breathing, perspiration, loud voice, anger
Escalation	Client's responses represent escalating behaviors that indicate movement toward a loss of control	Pale or flushed face, yelling, swearing, agitated, threatening, demanding, clenched fists, threatening gestures, hostility, loss of ability to solve the problem or think clearly
Crisis	During period of emotional and physical crisis, the client loses control	Loss of emotional and physical control, throwing objects, kicking, hitting, spitting, biting, scratching, shrieking, screaming, inability to communicate clearly
Recovery	Client regains physical and emotional control	Lowering of voice, decreased muscle tension clearer, more rational communication, physical relaxation
Postcrisis	Client attempts reconciliation with others and returns to the level of functioning before the aggressive incident and its antecedents	Remorse, apologies, crying, quiet, withdrawn behavior

Adapted from Keltner, N. L., Schwecke, L. H., & Bostrom, C. E. (2003). *Psychiatric nursing* (4th ed.). St. Louis: Mosby, Inc.

- Keeping everyone safe
- Assisting with alternative behaviors and problem solving
- Limit setting (*see p. 127*)
- Cognitive-behavioral therapy (*see p. 116*)
- Guided discovery
- Anger management training
- Behavioral therapy: token economy (*see p. 108*)
- Group therapy (*see p. 123*)
- Family therapy (*see p. 122*)
- Prevention of vapor lock and meltdown
- Pharmacological therapy
  - Antipsychotics (*see Chapter 10*)
  - Sedatives/hypnotics (*see Chapter 7*)
  - Antidepressants (*see Chapter 8*)
  - Mood stabilizers (*see Chapter 9*)
  - Anticonvulsants
  - Others
- Restraint and seclusion (*see p. 134*)

Nurse's Role

- Maintaining the safety of clients and staff
- Assisting with defusing anger and aggression through verbal interventions
- Setting limits to prevent violent behavior
- Teaching anger management and coping skills

Abuse and Violence

A **buse** is defined as the wrongful use or maltreatment of a person by another. **Violence** refers to threatened or actual physical force by one person or group against another. Abuse and violence are likely to result in psychological or physical injury or death.

Factors contributing to abuse and violence can be categorized as:

- Societal and macrosystem factors
  - Societal beliefs
  - Cultural norms
  - Formal and informal social structures
  - Societal influences that make up children's and their families' world: neighborhood, schools, workplaces, churches, and social service agencies
- Microsystem factors
  - Family environment: family dynamics, parenting style, and socioeconomic status (Box 27.1)
- Individual factors: biologic and neurodevelopmental factors within people

Types of abuse and violence include the following:

- Youth violence
- Family violence
  - Intimate partner violence

box
27.1 Characteristics of Families with Abuse and Violence

REGARDLESS OF THE TYPE OF ABUSE THAT OCCURS IN A FAMILY, CERTAIN CHARACTERISTICS HAVE BEEN IDENTIFIED:

- Social isolation: members keep to themselves
- Abuse of power and control: person who is abusing exerts physical, economic, and social control; the only individual making the decisions
- Substance abuse, especially alcohol abuse
- Intergenerational transmission process: perpetuation of abuse and violence from one generation to the next *via* role modeling and learning

- Child maltreatment
- Elder abuse
- Rape and sexual assault (*see p. 519*)

Youth Violence

Violence among U.S. youth has reached almost epidemic proportions. Four categories of risk factors have been identified: individual, family, peer/school, and environment (Table 27.1). Experts agree that one factor in isolation rarely causes a teen to pick up a gun and shoot someone. Rather, the risk factors are additive: the more that a person is exposed to violence from various categories, the greater is the likelihood of violence erupting.

Children do overcome adversity and develop resiliency. Protective factors allow them to thrive even in adverse life conditions. These factors include the following:

- Innate characteristics, such as solid intelligence
- Acquired features
  - Self-regulatory abilities
  - Self-esteem
  - Strong parental monitoring
  - Secure parental attachment and emotional security

table
27.1. **Risk Factors for Youth Violence**

Factor	Examples
Individual	• Biological predisposition, i.e., low serotonin levels • Early-onset behavior problems, particularly involving temperamental, physiologic, and attentional factors • Early experiences of neglect and abuse possibly causing changes in brain chemistry and the neurotransmitters crucial to behavioral regulation • Behavioral influences, i.e., aggressive youths' predispositions to particular cognitive biases, such as the belief that violence is a legitimate method of handling conflict, or misreading of situations so as to attribute hostile intent to benign situations
Family	• Attachment problems • Family stress • Inappropriate parenting styles • Neglectful or disengaged parents • Poor monitoring of children • Exposure to violence • Poor family functioning
Peer/school	• Frequently use of aggression for control and social gain • Association with teens who condone antisocial or aggressive behavior, including gang involvement (associated with both gun involvement and disproportionate criminal and violent offenses)
Environment	• Living in a violent neighborhood • Frequent exposure to community violence • Poverty • Disconnection from social support systems

• Community *via* provision of good schools, recreational outlets, and laws and surveillance that limit youths' access to guns, alcohol, and drugs

Intimate Partner Violence

Intimate partner violence (IPV), also called domestic violence, is one of the most common forms of violence against women, having reached epidemic proportions. IPV is the predominant cause of injury to women, more common than rapes, muggings, and automobile accidents combined.

Violent acts include physical and sexual violence, as well as threats and psychological–emotional abuse. Physical violence includes acts with enough force to potentially cause death, disability, or injury, as well as scratching, pushing, shoving, burning, or using restraint on another's body.

Cycle of Violence

A typical pattern of abuse exists, consisting of three phases (Box 27.2):

- Tension building
- Eruption of violence
- Remorse (honeymoon)

box
27.2 **The Cycle of IPV**

Phase 1: Tension Building

- Minor incidents
- Perpetrator establishes total control of victim by psychological and emotional means.
- Perpetrator demands total acquiescence from victim; verbal abuse and accusations follow.
- Perpetrator isolates victim by approving/disapproving social contacts.
- Perpetrator monitors victim's activities, phone calls, mail, and travel and demands explanations.
- Perpetrator degrades and demoralizes victim by scrutinizing victim's physical and mental characteristics (unattractive, stupid) and functions and assaulting victim's self-esteem (worthless, "no good").

Phase 2: Violence Erupts

- Perpetrator causes severe injury to victim and children.
- Victim may incite violence as a way to control mounting terror.
- Period of relative calm follows battering.

Phase 3: Remorse Ensues

- Perpetrator becomes kind, contrite, and loving, begging for forgiveness and promising never to inflict abuse again.
- Tension builds; the cycle repeats.

As the abuse progresses, these phases are more frequent and become more intense and severe.

Indicators of IPV

- Partner (person doing the abusing)
  - Belief of owning individual
  - Demonstration of increased violence when individual attempts independence
  - Exhibiting of:
    - Strong feelings of inadequacy
    - Low self-esteem
    - Poor problem solving and social skills
    - Emotional neediness
    - Irrational jealousy
    - Possessiveness
- Victim (*see Chapter 4, Assessment Tools, Abuse and Violence Assessment Tools, page 67*)
  - Dependency
  - Inability to function without partner
  - Low self-esteem
  - Blaming of self
  - Fear of partner
  - Physical evidence of injury
  - Seeking of medical care for problems not related to abuse

Child Maltreatment

Child maltreatment is a major public health crisis. Maltreatment is behavior toward another person that is outside the norms of conduct and involves a significant risk of physical or emotional harm.

Types of Child Maltreatment

Four categories of child maltreatment are recognized, the various forms of which often do not occur in isolation but overlap:

- Physical abuse: scaldings, beatings with objects, severe physical punishment, and Münchhausen syndrome by proxy

- Sexual abuse: incest, sexual assault by a relative or stranger, fondling of genitals, exposure to indecent acts, sexual rituals, or involvement in pornography
- Neglect: deficiencies in caretaker obligation that harm the child's psychological health, physical health, or both
- Emotional maltreatment: acts such as verbal abuse and belittlement, acts designed to terrorize a child, and lack of nurturance or emotional availability

Indicators of Child Maltreatment

Box 27.3 lists assessment findings that might lead to the suspicion of child neglect or abuse.

Effects on Child Functioning

Child maltreatment affects all aspects of a child's ability to function socially, behaviorally, emotionally, intellectually, and physically.

Socially, maltreated children:

- Tend to be attached less securely to their mothers or primary caregivers

box
27.3 **Warning Signs of Abused/Neglected Children**

- Serious injuries such as fractures, burns, or lacerations with no reported history of trauma
- Delay in seeking treatment for a significant injury
- Child or parent gives a history inconsistent with severity of injury, such as a baby with *contrecoup* injuries to the brain (shaken baby syndrome) that the parents claim happened when the infant rolled off the sofa
- Inconsistencies or changes in the child's history during the evaluation by either the child or the adult
- Unusual injuries for the child's age and level of development, such as a fractured femur in a 2 month old or a dislocated shoulder in a 2 year old
- High incidence of urinary tract infections, bruised, red, or swollen genitalia, tears or bruising of rectum or vagina
- Evidence of old injuries not reported, such as scars, fractures not treated, multiple bruises that parent/caregiver cannot explain adequately

- Have increased difficulties with peers
- Generate fewer quality solutions to interpersonal problems
- Have difficulty understanding complex social roles
- Exhibit decreased social involvement and sophistication in play, with decreased socially competent behaviors in interactions
- Initiate fewer positive interactions with peers
- Are both withdrawn and aggressive with other children
- Show inappropriate responses to peer distress

Because of these difficulties, maltreated children are not popular; they have fewer friends and their peer group is more likely to reject them.

Behaviorally, maltreated children:

- Display significant oppositional and aggressive behavior
- Demonstrate fewer peer interactions
- Engage in fewer prosocial behaviors
- Display more developmental delays as infants
- Have increased sensitivity to aggressive stimuli
- Have a greater frequency of running away, being expelled, and using drugs
- Are diagnosed more frequently with oppositional or conduct disorders

Emotionally, maltreated children:

- Display more emotional maladjustment and psychiatric symptoms (in older maltreated children)
- Tend to be more depressed or hopeless
- More commonly experience symptoms of post-traumatic stress disorder
- Show difficulty with empathy and emotional recognition

Intellectually, maltreated children seem to demonstrate lower scores on cognitive measures, especially related to verbal intelligence and language.

Physically, maltreated children:

- Demonstrate an increased risk for impaired physical growth and development
- Show evidence of increased heart rate in response to everyday scenes

- Exhibit an increase in documented scars, skin wounds, and neurologic soft signs
- Show an increase in drug use
- Frequently have a history of feeding and sleeping problems, physical handicaps, and serious health problems at birth; early developmental delays; developmental disabilities or mental retardation; and more illnesses, "accidents," and hospitalizations early in life
- Demonstrate an increased risk for various somatic symptoms as adults
  - Nightmares
  - Back pain
  - Frequent or severe headaches
  - Pelvic pain
  - Eating binges or self-induced vomiting
  - Fatigue
  - Breast pain
  - Abdominal pain
  - Sleeping difficulties
  - Irritable bowel syndrome
  - Fibromyalgia

Elder Abuse

Elder abuse is the mistreatment of older adults, found in all socioeconomic groups. It occurs in homes and institutional settings, including hospitals and long-term care facilities. Elder abuse may include one or a combination of the following: physical abuse, physical neglect, sexual abuse, psychological abuse or neglect, financial abuse, and violation of personal rights (Table 27.2).

Nurse's Role

- Participating in violence prevention programs at all levels
- Screening and identifying individuals at risk at each health encounter
- Adhering to legal mandates for reporting suspected abuse

table
27.2. **Types of Elder Abuse**

Type	Definition	Manifestations
Physical abuse	Intentional infliction of bodily harm	Bruises, burns, lacerations, dislocations, sprains, or fractures
		Frequent visits to emergency departments with unexplained traumatic injuries
		Unreasonable descriptions of how injuries happened
		Depressed, anxious, withdrawn, or confused behavior
		Passivity or anxious behavior to please healthcare providers
Physical neglect	Intended or unintended failure by a caregiver to meet the older adult's basic needs	Malnourishment, dehydration, poor hygiene, pressure ulcers, contractures, perineal excoriation, fecal impaction, signs of overmedication or undermedication, and untreated health problems
		Reports from clients that caregivers leave them in unsafe situations or that they cannot obtain medical care or medications
		Substandard housing in disrepair with poor housekeeping
		Depression, poor self-esteem, and apathy
Sexual abuse	Sexual activity without consent or the ability to provide consent	Reddened or traumatized genitals, genital pain, sexually transmitted infections, bruises, scratches, or abrasions
		Depression, anxiety, and withdrawal

continued on page 518

table
27.2. **Types of Elder Abuse** *continued*

Type	Definition	Manifestations
Psychological abuse	Infliction of mental anguish by yelling, verbally assaulting, or threatening, humiliating, and intimidating the person	Restlessness, insomnia, hand tremors, or worsening chronic health conditions Depression, anxiety, paranoia, and confusion Fear of strangers in their home environment
Psychological neglect	Failure of the caregiver to meet the older adult's emotional needs	Isolating the elder from contact with other people or not providing a stimulating environment, socially and cognitively Similar behaviors to victims of psychological abuse
Financial abuse or material exploitation	Use of, or taking the possessions of, an older adult for personal or monetary gain without consent or through unwarranted power	Theft, mismanagement of funds, improper financial advice, or use of the older adult's money for personal benefit
Violation of personal rights	Taking unlawful advantage of the older adult's rights	Loss of privacy Not being given opportunities to be involved in decision making

- Educating families about firearm safety, substance abuse, and violence prevention
- Assisting in rehabilitation as appropriate

Rape and Sexual Assault

Rape is forced or coerced sexual penetration (oral, anal, or vaginal) of a nonconsenting person. **Sexual assault** is forced or coerced sexual acts on a nonconsenting person. Statutory rape is rape of a minor (age varies among states). With statutory rape, consent is not an issue; minors are considered incapable of giving consent because of their vulnerability and dependence on adults or older peers.

Rape and sexual assault are acts of violence. These forced sexual behaviors shatter the victim's sense of self, safety, and predictability.

Types of rape include the following:

- Rape by a stranger
- Date rape and acquaintance rape
- Marital rape

Rape Trauma Syndrome

Rape trauma syndrome is a two-phase process experienced by all rape survivors. The first phase, which may last days or weeks, is the acute phase of disorganization characterized by:

- Fear, anxiety, disbelief, anger, and shock
- Sleep disturbance, nightmares, body aches and pains related to the rape, fatigue, and loss of appetite (variable according to the nature of the rape and the victim's perception of the incident)
- Emotional responses such as increased irritability, difficulty concentrating, and obsessive thoughts about the rape or some aspect of it; shame, guilt, self-blame
- Ritual behaviors associated with ensuring safety (eg, checking window and door locks repeatedly), hyperalertness to potential danger (eg, scanning the environment continually for the rapist), and an increased startle response

Some survivors openly express their feelings; others exhibit a controlled response. Both responses are normal.

The second phase is the long-term process of reorganization. In this phase, clients work toward integration and resolution of the experience. Healthy integration and resolution involve regaining empowerment and reconnecting with others. Most survivors benefit substantially from professional help during this phase. In therapy, they can learn ways to feel safe again and to manage disturbing symptoms. Furthermore, they can remember and work through associated feelings. Gradually, survivors begin to reassert control and gain a new sense of relative safety, a new worldview.

Nurse's Role and Nursing Care Planning

| NURSING DIAGNOSIS: Rape Trauma Syndrome

Related to:	As Evidenced by:
Experience of rape, sexual assault	Feelings of guilt
	Self-blame
	Hyperalertness
	Fear

Nursing Outcomes Classification (NOC): Abuse Recovery: Client will begin to demonstrate measures to integrate the trauma of rape into her personal history and take steps toward resolution.

Nursing Interventions Classification (NIC): Rape Trauma Treatment

1. Provide for a support person to stay with clients; demonstrate an accepting and caring attitude. *Support is key to assisting clients to cope with the trauma and feel safe. Acceptance and concern are necessary to establish trust and to help clients express feelings.*
2. Explain rape protocol and obtain consent to proceed with protocol; implement protocol, including assistance with obtaining samples for legal evidence (Box 27.4). *Thorough explanation and informed consent are necessary to prevent additional trauma; proper specimen collection is essential to ensure evidence for legal proceedings.*
3. Implement crisis intervention counseling (*see Chapter 29*); assist clients to use techniques to reduce anxiety and fear. Ensure that

box
27.4 Evidence Collection

MOST AGENCIES HAVE A SEXUAL ASSAULT NURSE EXAMINER (SANE), A SPECIALLY TRAINED NURSE WHO IS RESPONSIBLE FOR CONDUCTING THE PHYSICAL EXAMINATION AND COLLECTING EVIDENCE FROM A RAPE VICTIM. IN ADDITION, A SPECIAL SEXUAL ASSAULT EVIDENCE COLLECTION KIT, WHICH CONTAINS ALL THE ITEMS NECESSARY FOR SPECIMEN COLLECTION BASED ON LOCAL LAW ENFORCEMENT REQUIREMENTS, MAY BE AVAILABLE.

WHEN ASSISTING WITH THE COLLECTION OR COLLECTING SPECIMENS:

- Ensure the client's privacy and ask the client if there is someone, such as a friend, family member, or staff member, whom she would like to have stay with her during the examination and specimen collection.
- Always wear gloves and change them frequently.
- Place each specimen obtained into the appropriate bag, envelope, or other designated container.
- Never leave a specimen or item considered to be evidence unattended.
- Place clothing only in a paper bag, using a separate bag for each piece of clothing.
- Document the collection of each specimen on the specimen collection device and required form; include documentation in the medical record of the client's initial appearance, condition during specimen collection, and after collection. Initial, sign, and date all specimens.

SPECIMENS TO BE COLLECTED:

- Articles of clothing, each removed one at a time and placed in a separate paper bag
- Vaginal or cervical secretions: swabs of the area are applied to slides (in the kit) and allowed to dry; slides are then placed in cardboard sleeves, closed, taped shut, and placed in an envelope that is then sealed and labeled
- Anal or penile secretions: swab of the area that is allowed to air dry and then placed in an envelope that is sealed and labeled
- Pubic hair: comb pubic hair with collection of approximately 20 to 30 hairs; place the hairs in an envelope that is sealed and labeled
- Blood samples
- Urine specimens: random specimen

WHEN ALL SPECIMENS ARE COLLECTED, GIVE THE KIT TO LAW ENFORCEMENT OFFICERES UPON THEIR ARRIVAL.

clients have support people available to stay with them. *Rape trauma is a crisis. Crisis intervention counseling promotes positive coping and helps clients regain functioning. Techniques to reduce anxiety and fear help calm the autonomic nervous system, which causes many unpleasant physical symptoms and is overly sensitive during emotional trauma. Support people help promote feelings of safety and security.*

4. Use strategies from cognitive-behavioral therapy to address fears. Have clients talk through and gradually re-expose themselves to the assault. Teach the cognitive technique of challenging automatic thoughts to help manage and defeat guilt and fear. *Cognitive-behavioral therapy has demonstrated effectiveness in short-term reduction of fear-related symptoms. Helping clients remember and visualize the rape can aid in gradually reducing anxiety and distress. Helping them recognize how automatic thoughts contribute to guilt, fear, and anxiety and to use more positive self-talk will empower clients and decrease self-blame and guilt.*

5. Refer clients to a rape advocacy program; involve them in a rape survivors' support group. *Such participation can help clients understand that they are not to blame for the trauma. The ability to share experiences with others who have experienced similar events will be a source of support and compassion for clients who need a place to express feelings safely.*

6. Include supportive partners in counseling sessions, if clients agree. Help partners work through feelings of isolation, confusion, anger, powerlessness, and frustration. *The willingness of partners to participate is crucial for clients to positively cope with the trauma. Partners of rape survivors often experience distress and frustration. They can be greater resources for clients if their feelings are addressed.*

NIC: Crisis Intervention

1. Re-inforce anxiety-reduction techniques; assist in redirecting focus. *Increased anxiety interferes with the ability to focus and cope.*

2. Assist in identifying past/present coping skills and their effectiveness, as well as personal strengths and abilities that clients can use to resolve the crisis. *Determining a baseline helps nurses*

suggest skills that would be appropriate for use in this situation. Identifying and then using personal strengths and abilities to resolve a crisis promote empowerment. Use of positive coping skills, strengths, and abilities aids in crisis resolution and fosters growth.

3. Assist clients to develop new coping and problem-solving skills. *Development of new strategies enhances the ability to deal with stress; drawing on strengths promotes feelings of control.*

NIC: Coping Enhancement

1. Encourage clients to discuss feelings of guilt. To help them adopt a more realistic appraisal, help clients identify evidence for and against these feelings. Assist them to objectively appraise the event. Discuss consequences of not dealing with guilt and shame. *Emotional responses are common but irrational and self-defeating. Asking clients to rationally examine emotional responses will reveal no basis in reality for self-blame.*

2. Encourage clients to talk about the event. Encourage verbalization of feelings, perceptions, and fears. Provide an atmosphere of acceptance; use a calm, reassuring approach. *All forms of avoidance behaviors are common and an attempt to reduce stress. Fear levels will remain high, however, until clients confront the fear often enough for it to dissipate. Talking about the event is a form of exposure therapy.*

Suicide

A lthough the definition of **suicide** is simple (the voluntary and intentional act of taking one's own life), the processes surrounding it are complex. The actions associated with suicide are termed **suicidal behaviors**. Suicide or death by suicide describes the act of killing oneself.

Risk Factors for Suicide

- Genetic factors
  - Family history of suicide
  - Individual predisposition because of personality traits
  - Reduced serotonergic function and alterations in noradrenergic function in the central nervous system
- Psychological factors
  - Some forms of psychiatric illness
    - Depressive disorders (*see Chapter 19*)
    - Substance abuse disorder (*see Chapter 24*)
    - Bipolar disorder (*see Chapter 19*)
    - Schizophrenia (*see Chapter 25*)
    - Personality disorders (borderline, antisocial, histrionic and narcissistic) (*see Chapter 20*)
    - Anxiety disorders (panic and obsessive compulsive) (*see Chapter 14*)

- Somatoform disorders (*see Chapter 23*)
- Eating disorders (anorexia nervosa and bulimia) (*see Chapter 17*)
- History of previous suicide attempt
- Psychological pain
- Hopelessness
- Physical factors
  - Epilepsy
  - Spinal and brain injury
  - HIV infection/AIDS
  - Pain
- Environmental factors
  - Loss of job with a resultant loss of status, relationships, and social contacts
  - Other losses, such as the death of loved ones, divorce, financial problems, or other major stresses

Protective Factors

Although numerous factors can increase risk for suicidal behavior, protective factors can help prevent death by suicide. People can increase their resilience and decrease their risk by improving social support, strengthening coping skills, and decreasing stigma associated with seeking help for mental health problems. Additional protective factors may include the following:

- Effective clinical care for mental, physical, and substance abuse disorders
- Easy access to various clinical interventions and support for help-seeking
- Close familial/friend relationships, which foster better coping with stress
- Restricted access to highly lethal means of suicide
- Strong connections to family and community support
- Support through ongoing medical and mental healthcare relationships
- Skills in problem solving, conflict resolution, and nonviolent handling of disputes
- Cultural and religious beliefs that discourage suicide and support self-preservation

Warning Signs of Suicide

Determining suicide risk begins with understanding common warning signs of suicide (Box 28.1). Many experts agree that suicide does not happen without some type of indication or warning.

box
28.1 **Warning Signs of Suicide**

Emotional/Psychological Signs
- Feelings of hopelessness and helplessness
- Frequent mood changes
- Feelings of being a burden to others
- Anxiety and agitation
- Fatigue and tiredness
- Sadness
- Depression
- Inability to find enjoyment in anything
- Feelings of guilt
- Feelings of worthlessness
- Feelings of failure
- Feelings of isolation

Behavioral Signs
- Making a will
- Putting one's affairs in order
- Giving away prized possessions
- Making suicide threats
- Talking of wanting to kill oneself
- Talking about death, dying, or suicide
- Planning for death (stockpiling pills, seeking access to firearms)
- Previous suicide attempts
- Loss of interest in usual activities (sports, work, hobbies)
- Decreased interest in school (drop in grades and decreased achievement)
- Skipping school
- Running away from home
- Acting reckless or engaging in risky behaviors seemingly without thinking (such as careless use of firearms, driving)
- Sexual promiscuity

- Withdrawal from friends and family
- Increased use of substances (alcohol or drugs)
- Change in sleep habits (difficulty sleeping or sleeping a great deal of the time)
- Change in eating habits (eating more or less with resultant weight changes)

Several suicide prevention organizations, such as the National Suicide Prevention Lifeline (www.suicidepreventionlifeline.org), use a mnemonic developed by the American Association of Suicidology to help remember the warning signs of suicide:

- I   Ideation   (threatened or communicated)
- S   Substance Abuse   (excessive or increased)
- P   Purposelessness   (feels no reason for living)
- A   Anxiety   (agitation/insomnia)
- T   Trapped   (feels there is no way out)
- H   Hopelessness   (feels there is no hope, nothing to look forward to)
- W   Withdrawal   (withdraws from family, friends, society)
- A   Anger   (uncontrolled rage, seeking revenge)
- R   Recklessness   (risky behavior, without thinking)
- M   Mood Change   (severe and dramatic)

None of the warning signs alone is predictive of risk. A key to understanding a client's specific risk is to understand behaviors in terms of the person's normal context. (*see Chapter 4, Assessment Tools, Suicide Assessment, page 91*).

Assessment of Suicide Lethality

Lethality assessment is part of conducting a risk assessment. When it is determined that someone is considering suicide, a lethality assessment is necessary. It is an attempt to predict how likely a person is to die by suicide. Although there is no sure way to predict suicide, a few factors can assist nurses in helping plan appropriate and informed interventions. The more lethal the method that the person is thinking about, the higher at risk he or she is (Table 28.1).

table
28.1. **Lethality of Suicide Attempts by Method**

Less Lethal Methods	More Lethal Methods
Overdose of nonprescription drugs (except for acetaminophen and aspirin)	Firearms Hanging Overdose of antidepressants
Wrist slashing	Overdose of barbiturates and sleeping pills Overdose of aspirin and Tylenol Jumping Carbon monoxide poisoning

Nurse's Role

- Using sensitivity and empathy to gather information, engage clients, and develop the therapeutic relationship
- Establishing a therapeutic alliance with clients
- Assessing clients at risk
- Actively listening with a nonjudgmental attitude
- Reviewing the client's history of suicidality
- Determining the method and lethality of the plan
- Removing the means of suicide
- Instituting suicide precautions
- Ensuring client safety
- Encouraging compliance with medication therapy
- Providing client and family support
- Advocating for suicide prevention activities
- Offering comfort and support to survivors of suicide to come to terms with the loss
- Encouraging survivors to seek out counseling services

CHAPTER

29

Crisis and Disaster

A **crisis** involves a threat to homeostasis. The magnitude of the problem and the immediate resources available to deal with them are imbalanced, with resultant confusion and disorganization. No person can tolerate such imbalance for long. The active crisis state usually is short, approximately 4 to 6 weeks.

Phases of a Crisis

During a traumatic or overwhelming event, people move through phases or steps that determine the level of the crisis state (Table 29.1).

Types of Crisises

There are three types of crises:

- Maturational (developmental): results from normal life events that cause stress
  - Mastering control of body functions
  - Starting school
  - Experiencing puberty
  - Getting married
  - Becoming a parent or grandparent
  - Retiring

table
29.1. **Phases of a Crisis**

Phase	Characteristics
Phase 1: Problem or trauma arises, causing increased anxiety.	• A person tries to use familiar mechanisms to cope. • If effective, no crisis develops; if ineffective, person enters next phase.
Phase 2: Anxiety levels continue to increase.	• Usual problem-solving methods are ineffective. • Person uses methods of trial and error to cope.
Phase 3: Anxiety continues to escalate.	• Trial and error methods continue to fail. • Person usually feels compelled to reach out for assistance. • Those who are emotionally or socially isolated before the trauma usually experience a crisis at this point.
Phase 4: Person is in the active state of crisis.	• Inner resources and support systems are inadequate. • The precipitating event is not resolved. • Stress and anxiety mount intolerably. • The person has a short attention span, ruminates, and looks inward for possible reasons for the trauma and how he or she might have changed or avoided it. • Anguish, apprehension, and distress accompany this rumination. • Behavior becomes increasingly impulsive and unproductive. Relationships with others usually suffer. • The person becomes less aware of the environment and begins to view others in terms of ability to help solve the problem. • The high anxiety level may make the person feel like he or she is "losing my mind" or "going crazy." • The person in crisis often needs others to explain the difference and to give reassurance that when anxiety dissipates, he or she will be able to think clearly again.

• Situational: develops as a response to a sudden and unavoidable traumatic event that dramatically alters a person's identity and roles; usually follows the loss of an established support, affects self-perception, and threatens self-image

- Death of a spouse
- Divorce
- Job or academic failure
- Birth of a child with a disability
- Diagnosis with a chronic or terminal illness
- Adventitious: results from an outside external event that causes trauma and disruption, usually to many people
  - Terrorism
  - Natural disasters
  - Hurricanes
  - Fires
  - Floods
  - Earthquakes
  - Riots
  - Unusual media events
  - Kidnappings
  - Wars
  - Bombings

Crisis Intervention

Crisis intervention focuses on the problem or stressor that precipitated the crisis, viewing people in crisis as normal and capable of problem solving and growth. Nevertheless, assistance from others is needed. The goal is to assist people in distress to resolve the immediate problem and regain emotional equilibrium. Problem solving should lead to enhanced coping to deal with future stressful events.

Crisis intervention is a partnership between intervener and client. The intervener actively participates in helping the client problem solve. The person acting as the intervener must possess good communication skills, be an active listener, demonstrate keen assessment skills, and act nonjudgmentally and collaboratively, advocating, consulting, teaching, and coaching the client. The intervener assists the client in the following:

- Analyzing the stressful event
- Expressing feelings without probing
- Exploring ways to deal with stress and anxiety
- Problem solving and identifying actions and strategies

- Seeking support from family, friends, and community resource groups
- Averting possible future crises through anticipatory guidance

Nurse's Role

- Assisting with evaluating the client's feelings
- Determining the client's perception of the event
- Assessing the client's support systems and coping skills
- Determining the potential for self-harm
- Demonstrating nurturing, caring, listening, and a willingness to help
- Helping the client to communicate directly with significant others and to recognize interdependence
- Teaching the client how to ask for help
- Assisting with the development of healthier coping skills
- Keeping the client focused on the problem and goals leading to its resolution

Special Populations

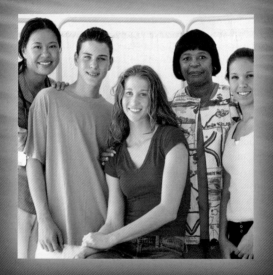

Forensic Clients

F orensic clients are those people with mental illness who have been involved with courts of law and legal proceedings. They share distinct and common legal, ethical, political, administrative, and professional concerns. Forensic clients are treated in secure environments, which may belong to the mental health system, criminal justice system, or both. Various settings may include the following:

- Community-based outpatient clinics
- Secure units in general hospitals
- State psychiatric hospitals
- Forensic psychiatric hospitals
- Custodial-type settings (e.g., young offender facilities, jails, prisons)

Characteristics of the Forensic Population

Forensic clients present with complex and multifaceted issues further complicated by the unique environmental and social factors of their milieu. Generally, forensic clients demonstrate poor judgment, limited reasoning, and a history of not learning from mistakes. They also report an exceptionally high level of substance abuse at the time of arrest. Forensic populations may include the following:

- Suspects or convicts
- Those sentenced or unsentenced

- Those not guilty by reason of insanity or incompetent to stand trial
- Those not criminally responsible because of mental disorders

Other classifications may include the following:

- Mentally ill offenders (predominant client group)
- Violent offenders
- Special populations
  - Juvenile offenders
  - Female offenders
  - Older adult offenders
  - Offenders with HIV infection/AIDS or hepatitis
  - Offenders with a terminal illness

Effects of Incarceration on Mental Health

In addition to offenders who enter correctional systems with mental disorders, forensic psychiatric nurses care for people who become mentally ill while incarcerated. Daily living conditions affect all forensic clients. Creating a healing therapeutic environment in a forensic setting is a challenge. The physical conditions, client population, and authoritarian interpersonal atmosphere contribute to society's most extreme and stressful living environment (Box 30.1).

Strategies to Maintain Boundaries

Establishing and maintaining therapeutic nurse–client relationships in forensic settings are trying and difficult tasks. Issues surrounding treatment boundaries frequently prevail (Box 30.2).

Nurse's Role

- Establishing a therapeutic relationship
- Promoting health
- Maintaining an interdisciplinary approach
- Focusing on the family
- Ensuring continuity of care
- Acting as an advocate

box
30.1 Common Stressors to Mental Health in Secure Environments

Stressors That Affect the Client

- Loss of freedom
- Overcrowding
- Double stigmatization
- Grief, isolation, loneliness
- Gang violence
- Institutional violence: stabbing, beating, sexual assault
- Deteriorating living conditions
- Lack of privacy
- Protective custody
- Segregation
- Fear of the unknown
- Separation from loved ones
- Cumulative effects of losses

Stressors That Affect the Nurse

- Actual or implied threats of violence/personal safety
- Constant barrage of swearing
- Need to be constantly on guard against manipulation
- Dual responsibility of providing custody and caring
- Role confusion and ambiguity
- Professional isolation
- Stigma of "second-class nurse"
- Institutionalization
- Antagonistic relationships with correctional staff
- Fear of the unknown
- Ethical dilemmas
- Secondary trauma
- Understaffing

box
30.2 Boundary Maintenance Strategies

- **Be aware of red flags of caution such as:**
  - "You are such a good nurse."
  - "You are the only one who understands me."
  - "I would never have gotten into trouble if I had someone like you in my life."
- **Do not become dependent on your clients to meet your social needs.** Have a good, intact, and separate social life.
- **Avoid inappropriate self-disclosure.** Self-disclosure that

meets the needs of the nurse, not of the client, can lead to role reversal.

- **Engage in boundary violation "spot checks."** Ask yourself the following questions:
  - "What do I do when I am attracted to a client, or when a client is attracted to me? How do I set the boundaries?"
  - "Am I having my intimacy needs met through my relationship with my clients?"
  - "Would I say or do this in front of my other clients? My colleagues? My supervisor?"

- "Am I doing this for the client's benefit or to meet a need of my own? And if I think I am doing this for the client's benefit, am I fooling myself?"
- **Talk to trusted colleagues.** Be honest with yourself regarding your feelings about clients. Talking to trusted colleagues and supervisors will assist in effective boundary maintenance.
- **Seek clinical supervision.** This is an effective risk management

strategy that can assist with the management of feelings related to the nurse–client relationship and prevent the gradual erosion of boundaries.

- **Contribute to meaningful practice guidelines.** Realistically, guidelines for every situation are unlikely. Hypothetical scenarios, however, can be used to educate team members and invite differing views and recommendations for practice.

For further information, see Peternelj-Taylor, C., & Yonge, O. (2003). Exploring boundaries in the nurse–client relationship: Professional roles and responsibilities. *Perspectives in Psychiatric Care, 39*(2), 55–66.

Children and Adolescents

C hildren and their behavior must be viewed within a developmental context. Providers must approach pediatric clients with an understanding of where they are in their developmental trajectory and what influences are affecting that development.

Developmental Perspectives

Many theories of child development exist, and new ones emerge constantly, questioning and building on earlier discoveries. The field has evolved greatly in the past 20 years. Traditionally, past theorists view development as linear (Table 31.1).

Global stages, however, are no longer current thinking in the field. Rather, scholars recognize that children have different domains of functioning, which develop optimally, suboptimally, or not at all, depending on many variables and environmental factors. Moreover, past conceptualizations were inadequate because they were not culturally appropriate for many people.

Temperament Theory

Temperament theory views humans as being born with certain temperaments. The focus is on the "how," or style of behavior, as opposed to the "why," or its motivation.

table
31.1.

Overview of Traditional Developmental Theories

Theory	Summary	Era	Proponents
Maturationist	Development is a biologic automatic process with predictable, sequential stages over time.	Very early to mid-20th century	Sigmund Freud Erik Erikson
Environmentalist	The child's environment shapes learning and behavior; in fact, human behavior, development, and learning are thought of as reactions to the environment.	Early to mid-20th century	John Watson B. F. Skinner Albert Bandura
Constructivist	Learning and development happen when children interact with their environments. Young children are active participants in the learning process and initiate most of the activities required for learning and development.	Later 20th century	Jean Piaget Maria Montessori Lev Vygotsky
Information Processing	Children are active, sense-making beings who modify their own thinking in response to environmental demands. Thought processes are similar for people of all ages. The same thought processes in adults are found in children but to a lesser degree. Development is continuous.	Mid-20th century	George A. Miller

continued on page 540

table
31.1. **Overview of Traditional Developmental Theories** *continued*

Theory	Summary	Era	Proponents
Ethology	Adaptation, survival, and the value of behavior in ensuring survival are prominent. This field has its origins in zoology and has become more influential in child development research in recent years. Observations of ethology scholars have led to the important concept of the *critical period*, which refers to a limited time span during which a child is prepared biologically to acquire certain adaptive behaviors but needs the support of appropriate environmental stimuli to do so.		Konrad Lorenz Donald Dewsbury
Ecological Systems Theory	The child develops within complex environmental systems. Environment is a series of nested structures that includes, but extends beyond, home, school, and neighborhood.	Late 20th century	Uri Bronfenbrenner

- Easy temperament: fairly regular feeding schedule and sleep–wake cycles; quickly adaptable to change; predominantly positive mood or mild or moderate intensity
- Difficult temperament: biologic irregularity; withdrawal tendencies to the new; slow adaptability to change; frequent negative emotional expressions of high intensity
- Slow to warm up: withdrawal tendencies to the new; slow adaptability to change; frequent negative emotional expressions of low intensity; often labeled as "shy"

Moral Development Theory

Moral development theory, proposed by Lawrence Kohlberg, focuses on "moral reasoning," defined as judgments about right and wrong (Box 31.1).

Cognitive Theory

Cognitive theory, developed by Jean Piaget, focuses on intelligence, defined as the person's adaptation to the environment. The theory has two main components: the process of coming to know and the stages people move through as they gradually acquire this ability (Table 31.2).

Attachment Theory

Attachment theory, developed by John Bowlby, focuses on attachment, defined as the strong emotional bond that develops between infant and caregiver and provides babies with emotional security. By the second half of the first year, infants have become bonded to familiar people who have responded to their needs for physical care and stimulation.

- Infant and parent relationship beginning as a set of innate signals that call the adult
- Over time, development of affection supported by new cognitive and emotional capacities and a history of consistent, sensitive, responsive parental care
- Formation of enduring bond with caregivers, relying on this attachment as a base of security across time and distance
- Inner representation of the parent–child bond as an important part of personality, serving as an internal working model, or set

box
31.1 **Kohlberg's Stages of Moral Development**

- **Level 1–Preconventional:** People make judgments based solely on their own needs.
  - *Stage I: Punishment-obedience orientation.* People obey rules to avoid punishment. They determine good or bad actions based on physical consequences.
  - *Stage II: Personal reward orientation.* Personal needs determine right or wrong, along the lines of "You scratch my back, I'll scratch yours."
- **Level 2–Conventional:** People consider society's expectations and laws when making moral decisions.
  - *Stage III: Good boy–nice girl orientation.* "Good" means "nice." People determine behaviors on the basis of what pleases and is approved of by others.
  - *Stage IV: Law-and-order orientation.* Authority must be respected and social order maintained; when deciding punishment for wrongdoings, laws are absolute.
- **Level 3–Postconventional:** People base judgments on abstract personal principles not necessarily defined by society's laws.
  - *Stage V: Social contract orientation.* People determine "good" by a socially agreed upon standard of individual rights (eg, the U.S. Constitution). People operating in this moral stage believe that different societies have different views of what is right and wrong.
  - *Stage VI: Universal ethical principle orientation:* What is right and good are matters of individual conscience and involve abstract concepts of justice, human dignity, and equality. People believe that there are universal points of view on which all societies should agree.

of expectations about the availability of attachment figures, the likelihood of receiving support from them during times of stress, and ongoing interactions
- Image as the basis for all future close relationships throughout a person's life

Pediatric Mental Illness

Pediatric mental illness has staggering effects. Untreated psychiatric problems in childhood often result in long-term mental disorders in

table
31.2. Piaget's Cognitive Development

Stage	Explanation
Sensorimotor (infancy)	People demonstrate intelligence through motor activity without using symbols. Knowledge of the world is limited (but developing) because it is based on physical interactions and experiences. Children acquire *object permanence* (the ability to recognize that things still exist even if they are not directly visible) at approximately 7 months (memory). Physical development (mobility) allows them to gain new intellectual abilities. They have attained some symbolic (language) abilities at the end of this stage.
Preoperational (toddler and early childhood)	Children show intelligence through the use of symbols. Language use matures, and memory and imagination are developed, but thinking is nonlogical and nonreversible. Egocentric self-centered/self-referential thinking predominates during this period. Play is frequently parallel (side-by-side) rather than cooperative.
Concrete operational (elementary and early adolescence)	People demonstrate intelligence through logical and systematic manipulation of symbols related to concrete objects. Operational thinking develops (mental actions that are reversible). Egocentric thought diminishes. Group activity and cooperative play and projects emerge.
Formal operational (adolescence and adulthood)	In this stage, people use symbols related to abstract concepts logically. Early in the period, there is a return to egocentric thought. Only 35% of high school graduates in industrialized countries reach this stage; many people do not think formally during adulthood.

adulthood. Psychiatric problems occur in children from all socioeconomic backgrounds. Children and teens have unique developmental needs, which providers must assess in terms of each client's familial, social, and cultural backgrounds.

Risk Factors

No single cause can explain child and adolescent psychopathology. Risk factors that may increase susceptibility include the following:

* Biologic influences
  * Family history of mental illness
  * Immature development of the brain
  * Brain abnormality
* Familial and societal influences
  * Family problems and dysfunction
  * Poverty
  * Mentally ill or substance-abusing parents
  * Teen parents
* Stressors
  * Abuse (*see Chapter 27*)
  * Discrimination based on race, creed, or color
  * Chronic parental conflict or divorced parents
  * Chronic illness or disability

Therapeutic Modalities

Several different forms of intervention are available for children and families. Types vary based on the specific disorder and the child himself or herself. Types include the following:

* Individual psychotherapy (*see page 126*)
* Behavioral therapy (*see page 108*)
  * Token economies
  * Time-out (from positive reinforcement)
  * Rewards for and reinforcements of desired behaviors
* Cognitive therapy (*see page 111*)
  * Problem solving
  * Positive self-talk
  * Cognitive problem skills training
  * Multisystem therapy
* Brief psychotherapy
* Play therapy
* Family therapy (*see page 122*)

- Parent management training
- Group therapy (*see page 123*)
- Milieu therapy (*see page 130*)
- Pharmacologic therapy (*see Section 4*)
  - Antidepressants: selective serotonin reuptake inhibitors (SSRIs) (*see page 185*); imipramine (*see page 204*), amitriptyline (*see page 187*)
  - Atypical antipsychotics: risperidone (Risperdal; *see page 258*), quetiapine (Seroquel; *see page 256*), and olanzapine (Zyprexa; *see page 251*)

General Nursing Care

When working with children with mental health and psychiatric disorders, nursing care generally involves psychiatric-mental health nursing assessment and interventions that address common needs or clinical situations.

- Assessment
  - Family assessment: family functioning, family relationships, concern for one another's, roles, empathy, decision making, and degree of autonomy or enmeshment
  - Current problems, including any significant concomitant events
  - History, including:
    - *Previous treatment*: type, length, and outcomes; testing results and diagnoses
    - *Family history*: any medical and mental health problem or symptoms in immediate and extended family members
    - *Developmental history*: prenatal history (maternal health or illness, substance use, or physical abuse), neonatal history (birth complications), developmental milestones (sitting, walking, talking, self-care)
    - *Social history*: names, ages, and relationships of people with whom the child lives; relationships with parents, siblings, other relatives, and peers; activities or hobbies; legal charges against the child
    - *Abuse history*: exposure to physical, sexual, or emotional abuse, whether Child Protective Services was notified, and any treatment; exposure to family or community violence

- *Chemical history*: use of substances by the child or adolescent, as well as by parents and other caretakers
- *Medical history*: history of seizures, head injuries, acute illnesses, other injuries and accidents, surgeries, loss of consciousness, asthma and other chronic illnesses, and vision and hearing deficits; current medications, their effects and side effects, and the names and effects of prior medications; drug, food, and seasonal allergies
- *School history*: current grade, regular or special education, any learning difficulties, and any behavior problems in school
- Mental status examination *via* observation, appropriate use of play, and questioning for:
  - Behavior
  - Orientation
  - Memory
  - Attention and concentration
  - Speech
  - Thought content and process
  - Hallucinations, delusions
  - Suicidal ideation
  - Self-harm or homicidal thinking or actions
  - Judgment
  - Insight
- Physical examination
- Interventions
  - Providing medication education
  - Meeting family's needs
  - Promoting the rights of children in treatment settings:
    - To be treated with dignity and not to be abused or mistreated in any way
    - To receive treatment in the least restrictive setting
    - To be free of physical restraints unless every other method to provide safety for the child and others has been tried and failed; if use of restraints or seclusion is necessary, children should never be left alone during that restriction of their freedom
    - To be treated in a developmentally appropriate way

- To receive an individualized treatment plan that includes aftercare or follow-up measures
  - To have access to an advocacy group
  - To expect confidentiality and access to their records
- Avoiding seclusion and restraint
- Providing advocacy

Common Psychiatric Disorders in Children and Adolescents

Many psychiatric illnesses affect children and adolescents. Some of these disorders are primarily identified during infancy, childhood, or adolescence; others are diagnosed across the lifespan, but manifestations, treatments, or both for children and adolescents may differ from that for adults. The most common disorders include the following:

- Adjustment disorders
- Anxiety disorders
  - Obsessive-compulsive disorder
  - Separation anxiety disorder
  - Phobias
  - Social anxiety disorder (social phobia)
  - Generalized anxiety disorder
  - Post-traumatic stress disorder
- Disruptive behavior disorders
  - Attention-deficit hyperactivity disorder (ADHD)
  - Oppositional defiant disorder (ODD)
  - Conduct disorder
- Autism-spectrum disorders
- Mood disorders
  - Depression
  - Bipolar disorder
  - Comorbidities

Adjustment Disorders

An adjustment disorder is marked by clinically or behaviorally significant symptoms within 3 months of the onset of an identifiable stressor. Stress temporarily overwhelms the client's capacity to solve problems, resulting in impaired functioning. The course of an adjustment disorder may be acute or chronic. It may accompany depression, anxiety, or conduct disturbances.

Assessment

Manifestations may include the following:

- Difficulty at school or with peers or family members
- Increased risk of suicidal actions
- Response to stressor greater than normally expected, such as regressed, fearful, or acting-out behavior.

Interdisciplinary Treatment Modalities

Treatment requires understanding, support, and encouragement for the youth to move beyond the event as he or she works through feelings associated with the stressor.

Nurse's Role

- Teaching and reinforcing adaptive coping skills
- Administering prescribed medications for cormorbid conditions of depression or anxiety

Anxiety Disorders

Children and adolescents with anxiety disorders often have symptoms of fear, anxiety, physical complaints, and sleep disturbances, including nightmares and night terrors. In all age groups, sleep problems are associated with mental illness (Table 31.3). (*See also Chapter 14.*)

Attention-Deficit Hyperactivity Disorder (ADHD)

ADHD is characterized by inattention, impulsivity, and hyperactivity. It is diagnosed through comprehensive clinical evaluation, as well as parents' and teachers' ratings of inattention, hyperactivity, and impulsivity. The cause of this disorder most likely involves a complex combination of genetic and environmental factors.

table
31.3. **Anxiety Disorders in Children**

Disorder	Assessment Findings	Interdisciplinary Treatment Modalities
Obsessive-compulsive disorder (OCD)	Recurrent intrusive thoughts (obsessions) and repetitive behaviors (compulsions) that the client recognizes as senseless but feels must be performed; obsessions and compulsions consuming hours of the day and causing great distress	Behavioral techniques: • Exposure (deliberately confronting the client with stimuli that trigger obsessions and provoke the urge to perform rituals) • Response prevention (either instructing the client to delay the ritual or blocking the child from performing it) Psychopharmacology: • Clomipramine (*see page 192*) • Fluoxetine (*see page 201*) • Sertraline (*see page 217*)
Separation anxiety disorder	Severe anxiety to the point of panic when apart from a parent or attachment figure When threatened with parental separation, the child possibly fearing accidents or injuries befalling the parent, clinging to or shadowing the parent, having nightmares, and refusing to attend school or spend the night away from home. During actual separation, complaints of headaches and stomachaches, severe homesickness, and vomiting	Psychopharmacology: SSRIs (*see page 185*) Behavioral therapy (*see page 108*) • Imagery • Self-talk • Cognitive techniques

continued on page 550

table
31.3. **Anxiety Disorders in Children** *continued*

Disorder	Assessment Findings	Interdisciplinary Treatment Modalities
	Sleep disturbances (eg, inability to fall asleep apart from the parent) Usual teenager complaints of physical ailments and refusal to attend school	
Phobias	Morbid, irrational, and persistent fears Possible expression of anxiety of a specific phobia by crying, clinging, or having tantrums Asking repeated questions about illness or death, kidnappers, or criminals	Pharmacotherapy: SSRIs *(see page 185)* Preparation of children for traumatic experiences Behavioral training • Relaxation • Desensitization *(see page 137)* • Modeling Psychotherapy for youths who have experienced traumatic events
Social anxiety disorder (social phobia)	Avoidance of contact with unfamiliar people and performing or speaking in front of others Interference with typical functioning, such as with peers or at school Social withdrawal, embarrassment, shyness, self-consciousness, and anxiety if asked to interact with strangers Avoidance and anxious anticipation causing marked distress in new or feared social situations	Social skills training Psychopharmacology: SSRIs (paroxetine [Paxil], *see page 212*)

Generalized anxiety disorder	Excessive or unrealistic fears Worrying about past and future events, the weather, their own school performance or health, the family's finances, and the welfare of others	Relaxation techniques Psychopharmacology • Anxiolytic buspirone (BuSpar; *see page 155*) • SSRI paroxetine (Paxil, *see page 221*)
Post-traumatic stress disorder	Exposure to traumatic event Re-experiencing of event Avoidance of stimuli associated with trauma Hyperarousal (*see PTSD, page xx*)	Psychotherapy Psychopharmacology • Antipsychotics for auditory hallucinations • Antidepressants for depressive symptoms and thoughts of self-harm • Combination of both types of drugs

Assessment

Diagnostic and Statistical Manual of Mental Disorders, Fourth Edition, Text Revision (DSM-IV-TR) Diagnostic Criteria: ADHD

- For at least 6 months, client exhibits at least six of the following symptoms of **inattention**, which are maladaptive and inconsistent with developmental level:
  - Fails to pay attention to details or makes careless mistakes in school or activities
  - Has difficulty sustaining attention in tasks or at play
  - Fails to listen when spoken to directly
  - Fails to follow instructions and finish schoolwork or chores (not as a result of oppositional behavior or inability to understand instructions)
  - Has difficulty organizing tasks and activities
  - Avoids, dislikes, or is reluctant to engage in tasks that require sustained mental effort
  - Loses necessary items (eg, toys, books)
  - Is easily distracted by extraneous stimuli
  - Shows forgetfulness in daily activities

OR
- For at least 6 months, client exhibits at least six of the following symptoms of **hyperactivity-impulsivity** to a degree that is maladaptive and inconsistent with developmental level:

Hyperactivity

  - Fidgets or squirms
  - Leaves seat when remaining seated is expected
  - Runs about or climbs excessively in inappropriate situations
  - Has difficulty playing or resting quietly
  - Is "on the go" or acts as if "driven by a motor"
  - Talks excessively

Impulsivity

  - Blurts out answers
  - Has difficulty awaiting turn
  - Interrupts others
- Some hyperactive-impulsive or inattentive symptoms developing before age 7 years

- Impairment from symptoms occurring in at least two settings (eg, both school and home)
- Social, academic, or occupational functioning clearly impaired
- Symptoms not occurring exclusively during the course of and not better explained by another psychiatric disorder

Types:

- Combined type
- Predominantly inattentive type
- Predominant hyperactive-impulsive type

Adapted with permission from American Psychiatric Association. (2000). *Diagnostic and statistical manual of mental disorders (4th ed., text rev.)*. Washington, DC: Author.

Common History and Physical Examination Findings

- Inability to follow instructions
- Constant moving; inability to sit still; hyperactivity
- Excessive talking
- Problems with submitting homework or assignments
- Academic deficits
- Accidental injuries

Common Psychosocial Assessment Findings

- Restlessness
- Inattention
- Impulsiveness, impatience
- Low frustration level
- Temper outbursts
- Mood lability
- Rejection by peers
- Poor self-esteem

Interdisciplinary Treatment Modalities

Behavioral Therapy (see page. 108)

- Parent management training
- Problem-solving skills training

Psychopharmacology

■ Stimulants: methylphenidate (Ritalin, Concerta; *see page 283*), dextroamphetamine (Dexedrine; *see page 280*), and a combination of mixed amphetamine salts (Adderall; *see page 286*)

■ Bupropion (Wellbutrin; *see page 188*), clonidine, and tricyclic antidepressants (*see page 185*)

Nursing Care Planning

NURSING DIAGNOSIS: Deficient Knowledge

Related to:	As Evidenced by:
Diagnosis and initiation of medication therapy	Numerous questions from child and family
	First experience with medication therapy
	New diagnosis of disorder

Nursing Outcomes Classification (NOC): Knowledge: Disease Process; Knowledge: Medication: The family will verbalize an understanding of ADHD and its treatment, including medication name, purpose, desired effects, side effects, action, dosage, route, and duration of the therapy.

Nursing Interventions Classification (NIC): Teaching: Disease Process

1. Explain the cause, signs and symptoms, treatments, and outcomes of ADHD. *Providing information about the biologic basis of ADHD will improve the family's understanding to help them better manage the client's care.*

2. Reassure the family about the child's condition; discuss potential lifestyle changes. Explain various potentially effective behavioral strategies, emphasizing the importance of focusing on only one or two behaviors at a time. *Information about ADHD and possible changes in lifestyle can improve understanding of the condition and necessary treatments. Behavioral strategies diminish disruptive behavior and encourage positive activity. Focusing on one to two behaviors at a time avoids overwhelming the client.*

3. Explore possible additional resources/support, as appropriate. Assist the family to develop positive coping skills; encourage the parents to take time for themselves. *The family may experience*

disrupted routines and strains associated with caretaking. Finding assistance and other outlets helps preserve the health and functioning of all members.

NIC: Teaching: Prescribed Medication

1. Discuss the medication's name, purpose, desired effects, and side effects. Teach its action, dosage, route, and duration. Instruct on proper administration and appropriate actions to take for side effects. *Stimulants can greatly increase attentiveness and ability to focus; however, the parents need to know what therapeutic and side effects to look for to ensure a therapeutic dosage. Changing dosing times can manage some side effects.*

2. Assist the family to develop a written medication schedule. *Doing so helps facilitate medication administration and promotes compliance.*

3. Provide written information about the action, purpose, and side effects. *Written information provides an additional source for teaching and reinforcement and a ready reference for future use.*

NIC: Developmental Enhancement: Child

1. Explore the family's feelings about the client's behavior. *Doing so promotes awareness of the condition and helps parents understand that the client "just can't behave" like other children.*

2. Role-model appropriate interaction skills; teach the child about sharing and taking turns; provide activities that encourage inter- action among children. *Role-modeling promotes appropriate social skills and fosters the development of relationships.*

3. Encourage parents to be consistent and structured with behavior management/modification strategies. *Consistency is essential in ensuring reinforcement of appropriate behavior.*

NURSING DIAGNOSIS: Social Isolation

Related to:	As Evidenced by:
Effects of disorder and inappropriate social skills	Poor academic interactions
	Difficulties with peers and classmates
	Lack of peers for play
	Few friends
	Others' view of child as a problem

NOC: Social Interaction Skills; Play Participation: Client will demonstrate appropriate social skills with others and engage in cooperative play with others, reporting positive experiences.

NIC: Socialization Enhancement

1. Teach parents how to help their child improve social skills. Develop role-playing scenarios in which the child practices positive, socially acceptable interactions and responses. Encourage patience in developing relationships. *Practicing difficult social situations increases the client's ability to respond appropriately.*

2. Discuss with the client how aggression affects others. Review how body language and facial expressions are clues to feelings. Encourage respect for the rights of others and honesty in presenting oneself to others. Help client increase self-awareness of strengths and limitations in communicating. *Increasing the client's sensitivity to others and teaching how to interpret nonverbal communication provide tools for more effective interactions with his peers.*

NIC: Therapeutic Play

1. Provide a quiet environment free from interruptions. *Such an atmosphere allows the child to focus on the task at hand.*

2. Provide sufficient time for effective play; structure play sessions to facilitate the desired outcome. *Sufficient time is necessary to prevent overwhelming the child. Effective play enhances positive feelings of self-esteem.*

3. Promote activities that require the child to use energy productively and focus on skills and accomplishments. *Finding and focusing on a child's strengths promote a sense of self-pride.*

4. Encourage the child to share feelings, knowledge, and perceptions. Validate and communicate acceptance of feelings that the child expresses during play. *Play helps the child communicate perceptions of the world and gain mastery of the environment.*

5. Facilitate interactions with other children as appropriate; provide positive reinforcement for effective interactions. *Such interactions help the child become more aware of behaviors and their effects on others. Positive reinforcement promotes a more positive self-image.*

6. Develop a reward system based on a daily report from the client's teacher. For example, clients can earn tokens for each day they come home with a good report on behavior with classmates. They

can later trade the tokens for time on the computer or some other preferred activity. *Establishing a reward system will reinforce positive behaviors.*

Autism-Spectrum Disorders

Autism-spectrum disorders, also called pervasive developmental disorders, have three core features: impairments in socialization, impairments in communication, and restricted repertoire of behavior. Two major types include autism and Asperger's syndrome (Table 31.4).

Conduct Disorder

Adolescents with **conduct disorder** are often unmanageable at home and disruptive in the community. Risk factors for conduct disorder include physical and sexual abuse, inconsistent parenting with harsh discipline, lack of supervision, early institutional living or out-of-home placement, association with a delinquent peer group, and parental substance abuse.

Assessment

DSM-IV-TR Diagnostic Criteria: Conduct Disorder

- Repeated and persistent violation of basic rights of others or major age-appropriate societal norms or rules, as manifested by at least three of the following in the past 12 months (at least one criterion in the past 6 months):

Aggression to People and Animals

- Bullying, threatening, or intimidating others
- Initiation of physical fights
- Use of a weapon that can seriously harm others (eg, bat, knife, gun)
- Physical cruelty to people
- Physical cruelty to animals
- Stealing while confronting a victim (eg, mugging, purse snatching)
- Forcing someone into sexual activity

Destruction of Property: Deliberate setting of fires or destruction of property (other than setting fires)

Deceitfulness or Theft

- Breaking into a house, building, or car
- Lying to obtain goods or favors or to avoid obligations (eg, "cons" others)

- Stealing of items of nontrivial value without confronting a victim (eg, shoplifting, but without breaking and entering; forgery)

Serious Violations of Rules

- Staying out at night, despite parental prohibitions, before age 13 years
- Running away from home overnight at least twice while living in parental or parental surrogate home (or once without returning for many days)
- Truancy from school, beginning before age 13 years
- Significant impairment of social, academic, or occupational functioning
- Not meeting the criteria for antisocial personality disorder if client age 18 years or older

Adapted with permission from American Psychiatric Association. (2000). *Diagnostic and statistical manual of mental disorders (4th ed., text rev.).* Washington, DC: Author.

Other assessment findings include the following:

- Little empathy or concern for others
- Callousness; lacking appropriate feelings of guilt; possible remorse to avoid punishment
- Blaming of others for own actions
- Risk-taking behaviors such as drinking, smoking, using illegal substances, experimenting with sex, and participating in crime

Interdisciplinary Treatment Modalities

- Behavioral therapy (*see page 108*)
  - Behavior modification techniques
  - Parent management training
- Psychopharmacology (for aggression and impulsivity)
  - Atypical antipsychotics (*see page 237*)
  - Lithium (*see page 231*)
  - Valproic acid (*see page 227*)

Nursing Care Planning

See ADHD, pages 554–557; see also Chapter 18.

Oppositional Defiant Disorder (ODD)

ODD is marked by negativistic, defiant behaviors such as stubbornness, resistance to directions, and unwillingness to negotiate with adults or peers. Youth with ODD are at risk for conduct disorder. Although teens are typically oppositional, those with ODD show more severe behaviors with more serious consequences and impairments in home, school, and social functioning.

Clients with ODD persistently test limits, usually by ignoring rules, arguing, or failing to accept responsibility for behavior. They direct hostility at adults or peers through verbal aggression or deliberately annoying actions. They do not see themselves as defiant but justify their behavior as a response to unreasonable demands. Symptoms may be present at home but not seen at school. School-aged children exhibit mood lability, low frustration tolerance, swearing, precocious substance abuse, and interpersonal conflicts. Parents and affected clients often bring out the worst in one another.

Assessment

DSM-IV-TR Diagnostic Criteria: ODD

- For at least 6 months, client with a pattern of hostile, negative, and defiant behavior, with at least four of the following:
  - Frequent loss of temper
  - Arguments with adults
  - Active defiance or refusal to follow rules
  - Deliberate annoyance of others
  - Frequent blaming of others for mistakes or misbehavior
  - Touchiness or easily annoyed by others
  - Anger and resentment often
  - Spitefulness or vindictiveness
- Significant impairment of social, academic, or occupational functioning
- Not occurring exclusively during a psychotic or mood disorder
- Not meeting the criteria for conduct disorder, or, if older than 18 years, antisocial personality disorder

Adapted with permission from American Psychiatric Association. (2000). *Diagnostic and statistical manual of mental disorders (4th ed., text rev.).* Washington, DC: Author.

Interdisciplinary Treatment Modalities

- Behavior modification techniques
- Family therapy (*see page 122*) to improve communication between parents and children
- Psychopharmacology to treat comorbidities (*see Section 4*)

Nursing Care Planning

See ADHD, page 548

Depression

Childhood depression is real, serious, and takes a serious toll on youth in the United States. Depression affects all areas of physical, emotional, and cognitive development. Duration and intensity of symptoms differentiate depression from sadness. Depressive behavior differs significantly from the child's usual behavior and interferes with his or her family, schoolwork, and friends.

Assessment

Depression in children and adolescents is easily confused with other childhood disorders, such as ADHD. Because children often cannot tell adults what they are feeling, they communicate by acting out. Prepubertal children with depression often exhibit irritability and separation anxiety; adolescents may be negative, antisocial, defiant, socially withdrawn, and failing at school.

Signs of depression in children and adolescents are as follows:

- Depressed or irritable mood, low frustration level, overreaction to simple requests, loss of joy, and moodiness
- Psychomotor agitation or retardation; the child may talk slowly and pause before responding
- Changes in appetite and sleep; the child may eat everything or very little, not sleep restfully, have trouble falling or staying asleep, or awaken very early
- Physical complaints such as headache, stomach ache, fatigue, and loss of energy

table
31.4. **Autism-Spectrum Disorders**

Disorder	Description
Autism	• Genetic disorder of neuronal organization • Slow or no language development • Use of words without attaching meaning to them or communication only by gestures or noises • Time spent alone; little interest in making friends • Isolation from the world around them; detachment, aloofness • Decreased responsiveness to social cues (eg, smiles, eye contact) • Some sensory impairment, including sensitivity in sight, taste, hearing, touch, or smell • No spontaneous or imaginative play • No imitation of others' actions or participation in pretend games • Possible aggressive action, tantrums for no obvious reason • Perseveration (showing an obsessive interest in some item or activity and engaging in ritualistic behavior) • Adherence to routines; inability to tolerate change well
Asperger's syndrome	• Major difficulties with social interaction and restricted, unusual interests and behaviors • Monotone speech and rigid vocabulary • Inability to understand jokes; easily taken advantage of • Little desire to meet people and make friends • Obsession with facts about circumscribed and odd topics • Perfectionists

- Depressive themes expressed in play, dreams, or verbalizations; examples include feeling worthless or guilty, minimizing strengths and maximizing failures, and blaming self over family problems
- Social withdrawal
- Intense anger or rage
- Anhedonia, or loss of pleasure in hobbies or activities of interest
- Acting-out behaviors: substance abuse, truancy, dropping out of school, running away, antisocial behaviors, self-injury, or sexual promiscuity
- Decreased ability to think, concentrate, or make decisions, often manifested in poor academic performance

- Thoughts of and verbalizations about death or wishing one had never been born; teens may express their thoughts through music, films, or writing with morbid themes
- Stressors, such as a breakup with a boyfriend or girlfriend, which may trigger suicidal thoughts

Interdisciplinary Treatment Modalities

The goal of treatment is to help children or teens become well. Modalities may include the following:

- Cognitive-behavioral therapy (*see page 116*)
  - Self-talk
  - Active participation in planning activities
  - Self-monitoring by writing about moods or feelings in a journal
- Family consultation
- Psychopharmacology
  - SSRIs (*see page 185*)
  - Atypical antipsychotics (to treat aggression, severe agitation, or delusions and hallucinations): risperidone (Risperdal, *see page 258*), quetiapine (Seroquel; *see page 256*), and olanzapine (Zyprexa; *see page 251*)

Nurse's Role

- Staying abreast of the latest research on the efficacy, utility, and risk of psychotropic medications with children
- Educating the child and family about the disorder and treatment
- Monitoring for possible suicide
- Teaching family about warning signs for increasing depression and suicide (*see also Chapter 19*)
- Offering support and guidance to child and family

Older Adult Clients

Older adults are defined as people 65 years or older. To attempt more precision regarding the relationship between age and particular needs, the older adult cohort can be further subdivided into chronological categories of young old (65 to 74 years), middle old (75 to 84 years), old old (85 to 94 years), and elite old (95 years and older).

Normal Age-Related Changes

Although highly variable, some physiologic changes are normal in older adults. These include changes in the major body systems:

- Nervous and sensory systems
  - The central nervous system (CNS) loses neurons, dendrites, and pigment; brain plasticity and functional reserve decrease.
  - All five senses decline.
  - Cognitive changes include a slowed reaction time and difficulty retaining new material unrelated to previous learning.
  - Memory loss is not a normal part of aging.
- Cardiovascular system
  - Blood pressure increases; cardiac contractile function and reserve decrease.
  - Most cardiovascular changes result from disease, not from disability.

- Respiratory system
  - Lung function decline is mild.
  - Disease is usually associated with a disability in this system.
- Renal and urinary systems
  - Changes in the kidneys are significant.
  - Peak bladder capacity diminishes, renal blood flow is halved, and renal tubules are less able to concentrate urine.
- Musculoskeletal system
  - Loss of muscle by up to 30% may be related to deconditioning.
  - Universal changes in bone structure and composition result in a decline in bone density. Osteoarthritis is common.
- Gastrointestinal system
  - Peristalsis is reduced
  - Acid secretion is decreased.

Influences on Mental Health

Various biologic, psychosocial, and sociopolitical aspects and issues can influence older adults' overall health and function.

- Biologic issues
  - Chronic illness
  - Medications
    - Changes in pharmacokinetics
    - Changes in pharmacodynamics
    - Polypharmacy
- Psychosocial influences
  - Retirement
  - Relocation
  - Bereavement
  - Responses to life transitions
- Sociopolitical issues
  - Ageism
  - Myths and prejudices
  - Healthcare fragmentation

Older adults also face numerous stresses related to these influences that place them at risk for mental health disorders (Box 32.1).

box
32.1 Stressors for the Older Adult

Loss of physical or mental ability
- Loss of independence
- Worries about being a "burden"
- Worries about the future

Death of a spouse
- Loss of companion
- Loss of sexual partner
- Feelings of emptiness, loneliness, grief
- Changes in responsibility
- Dependency on others

Death of a friend or loved one
- Loss of companion
- Emptiness, loneliness, grief
- Worries about own health

Retirement
- Loss of income
- Loss of purpose in life
- Loss of identity
- Loss of contact with others
- Loss of structure or schedule

Move to a long-term care facility
- Loss of independence
- Loss of space
- Movement away from friends/familiar neighborhood

Psychiatric Disorders in Older Adults

Many mental health disorders occur across the lifespan. As clients age, some disorders become more prevalent, and the resulting prognoses are more serious (Table 32.1).

table
32.1. **Common Psychiatric Conditions in Older Adults**

Disorder	Onset	Symptoms	Assessment and Treatment	Prognosis
Delirium	Rapid (from hours to days)	Fluctuating loss of concentration, confusion, disorientation, disturbed sleep, impaired memory and cognition, incoherent speech, good insight when lucid	Score on Mini-Mental Status Examination improves as condition improves. Treatment should address underlying medical condition as indicated.	Reversible
Dementia, Alzheimer's type	Gradual (from months to years)	Confusion, disorientation, labile affect, impaired memory and cognition, disorganized speech and behavior, delusions, poor insight and judgment	Score on Mini-Mental Status Examination decreases over time. Treatment aims at controlling psychosis.	Irreversible: mental condition deteriorates, as does physical condition eventually.
Vascular dementia	Rapid—immediately after vascular incident (eg, cerebrovascular accident and transient ischemic attack)	Confusion, disorientation, labile affect, impaired memory and cognition, delusions, poor insight and judgment	Score on Mini-Mental Status Examination decreases over time. Treatment aims at controlling psychosis. Condition remains the same over time, unless there is an additional vascular incident.	Irreversible: initial improvement is possible with therapeutic intervention, but condition tends to stabilize and becomes irreversible after 3 to 6 months.

				Reversible
Delusional disorder	Fluctuates: can be gradual or rapid	Possible visual or auditory hallucinations, often paranoia, difficulty distinguishing between reality and delusions	Thorough physical examination is necessary to rule out medical conditions (usually infections). Treatment aims at eliminating the delusions through medication and reality orientation.	
Depression	Usually gradual, unless there is a sudden personal loss	Sleep disturbance, appetite changes, decreased pleasure in usual activities, feelings of sadness, worthlessness, and guilt	Use of a depression scale is essential, as is assessment of suicidal ideation and lethality. Treatment may include antidepressants, psychotherapy, and various somatic therapies.	Improvement occurs with medication and psychotherapy; somatic therapies also may be needed. Without treatment, deterioration to the point of suicide is a risk.
Anxiety disorders	Usually rapid	Feelings ranging from apprehension, to dread, to panic	Treatments include psychotherapy, antianxiety agents, and biofeedback.	Improvement occurs with treatment but can recur with increased stressors.
Late-onset schizophrenia	Usually develops over 6 months; usually first noted in client's early 20s	Delusions, hallucinations, flat affect, disorganized speech and behaviors	Mini-Mental Status Examination is necessary. Treatment includes antipsychotic medication and psychotherapy aimed at adherence to medication regimen.	Remission is possible with adherence to treatment plan.

continued on page 568

567

table
32.1.

Common Psychiatric Conditions in Older Adults *continued*

Disorder	Onset	Symptoms	Assessment and Treatment	Prognosis
Substance abuse (drugs, alcohol, caffeine, tobacco)	May be rapid or gradual	Inability to hold a job or meet obligations, substance use in dangerous situations (driving, caring for children, operating machinery), legal problems related to substance use	Thorough psychosocial assessment, history, and physical examination are needed to rule out emergency and other secondary medical conditions. Treatment includes detoxification, psychotherapy, and medication management.	Remissions are possible with treatment; however, relapses are common. There can be long-term medical consequences of any substance abuse. Suicidal and homicidal ideation is not uncommon during initial treatment.
Elder abuse	May be rapid or gradual	Unexplained bruising, malnutrition, social isolation, and withdrawal	A detailed history and physical examination are necessary, as is a psychosocial assessment. Treatment can include removal of client from residence and appropriate medical and legal interventions.	With quick, appropriate interventions, prognosis is positive. There may be long-term consequences of injuries and malnutrition.

Adaptations for Assessment

Assessment of an older client must be modified to meet the client's special needs. Atypical presentations of illness are common in older adults, and physical and psychiatric illnesses are interwoven.

- Perform a comprehensive assessment to pursue a multidisciplinary approach.
- Include family members because they bring practical expertise and knowledge.
- Determine how illness affects daily functioning (*see Chapter 4, Mental Status Examination, page 53, and Global Assessment of Functioning, page 51*).
- Be alert to individual differences in energy levels.
- Use appropriate communication techniques.
  - Use direct eye contact and maintain a position within the client's view.
  - Speak in a calm, clear, slightly lower-pitched voice.
  - Eliminate background noise.
  - Ensure adequate lighting.
  - Use larger-type reading and teaching materials.
  - Ask one question at a time and allow a longer time for the client to respond.
  - Do not interrupt the client.
  - Listen attentively and actively.
  - Use nonverbal language to denote undivided attention.
- Obtain a complete medication history including over-the-counter medications and herbal supplements.

Nurse's Role

- Assisting with managing all of the client's medications
  - List of all general medications and psychotropic agents
  - Possible interactions
  - Possible adverse effects
  - Scheduling and reminders
- Preparing the client for and assisting with somatic therapies
- Implementing appropriate psychosocial interventions
- Implementing measures to promote mental health and wellness in older adults

Homeless Clients

C lients who are homeless are those people who lack a regular and adequate nighttime residence. Consequently, homeless people spend nighttime hours in a shelter, institution, or nonresidential location under temporary conditions. For most affected people, homelessness is a short-term situation. For some, however, including many people with concomitant mental illness, homelessness is a long, difficult, and frequently chronic state.

Homelessness and Mental Health and Illness

People with serious mental illness account for a significant percentage of the homeless population. Clients with serious mental illness have great difficulty escaping homelessness. Compared with those who are mentally healthy, people with psychiatric problems often are homeless for longer periods, have less contact with family, encounter more barriers to obtaining employment, display poorer physical health, and have more encounters with the legal system.

Common psychiatric diagnoses in the homeless population include the following:

- Alcohol dependence
- Alcohol-related disorder
- Amphetamine abuse

- Antisocial personality disorder
- Bipolar I disorder
- Bipolar II disorder
- Borderline personality disorder
- Delusional disorder
- Hallucinogen-related disorder
- Nicotine dependence
- Obsessive-compulsive disorder
- Opioid dependence
- Major depressive disorder
- Personality disorder not otherwise specified
- Polysubstance dependence
- Post-traumatic stress disorder
- Psychotic disorder not otherwise specified
- Schizoaffective disorder
- Schizophrenia (paranoid, disorganized, undifferentiated, residual)

Even when clients are homeless but not experiencing a psychiatric disorder, they are at risk for problems. Homelessness adversely affects mental health. People who become homeless because of economic stressors, unemployment, domestic violence, or eviction are prone to anxiety, depression, substance abuse problems, and other health concerns (Box 33.1).

box
33.1 **Stressors of Homelessness That Influence Mental Health**

- The effect of constant vigilance for safety, resulting in lack of sound sleep, fearfulness, suspicion, and insecurity
- Social isolation, being shunned by others, or feelings of "invisibility"
- Use of drugs or alcohol in a futile attempt to create comfort or a sense of community
- Poor diet, which may contribute to biochemical imbalances and mood changes
- Susceptibility to physical illness
- Constant uncertainty and disruptions
- Lack of medical, psychiatric, or other needed assistance
- Pervasive sense of hopelessness and uncertainty

From Haus, A. (1988). *Working with homeless people.* New York, NY: Columbia University Press.

Adaptations for Assessment

Assessment of clients who are homeless presents special challenges because of the lack of privacy, noise level, and clients' fear of being stigmatized. Assessment may involve sensitive questioning, particularly with clients who have psychiatric disorders (Box 33.2).

box
33.2 Suggestions for Communicating With Homeless Mentally Ill Clients

- Be aware of your own feelings, fears, and even your breathing.
- Create physical space so that both you and the client can leave the room if either of you decide to do so; it creates a safety zone.
- Involve significant others in communication if it facilitates a client's sense of security; don't involve others until you have asked the client's permission to do so.
- Discuss basic needs—it may be the best starting place for communication.
- Promote the client's sense of control and choice within the current environment; it may simply involve giving the client a choice of placement for his or her bedroll or whether you should give an injection in the left or right side.
- Be mindful and respectful of confidentiality issues.
- Be sensitive to possible feelings of not wanting to be identified with a psychiatric nurse or program.
- Be concrete in your interactions, avoiding metaphors, until you understand the client's cognitive functioning.
- For clients experiencing psychotic symptoms, let them know that you are not afraid of them and that your presence is not intrusive or demanding.
- For clients responding to internal stimuli, it may be helpful to ask if you could have their attention for a little while.
- For clients with delusions, let them experience that you have some sensitivity and understanding of the situation (or desire understanding); attempt to connect with the symbolism of the delusion.
- For clients with paranoia, it may be helpful to sit side by side rather than in front of them; it is possible to identify with the feeling more than the content of the paranoia and let clients know you understand that feeling.
- For clients who are suicidal, be direct in your concern and your questions in assessing for suicidality.
- Be aware of clients' varying insights into their illness.
- It may be helpful to summarize with clients, expressing your observations of their situation, then assessing with them if your observations are congruent with theirs.

Priorities for Care

Priorities for clients who are homeless focus on the basic needs: food, clothing, and shelter or assistance with housing. Care for mental health issues is secondary.

Key interventions include the following:

- Forming a therapeutic alliance
  - Homeless mentally ill clients may distrust anyone who represents the mental health system.
  - The nurse initiates the helping relationship in a nonthreatening manner, giving clients as much control as possible, possibly postponing interventions (or even discussions of them) for the most disturbing symptoms to avoid creating a negative therapeutic experience for clients.
- Managing medication compliance
  - Homeless mentally ill clients have special medication management needs.
  - Many psychotropic drugs have sedative or otherwise unwanted side effects that place clients in danger in relation to life on the streets.
  - Issues of access and storage of medications pose another problem.
  - Specific instructions to clients are necessary for taking certain medications.
- Teaching clients
  - Homeless clients need information to promote health and to use pertinent healthcare resources.
  - Client education may include topics such as personal hygiene, recognizing and treating infestation, thermoregulatory disorders, tuberculosis screening, respiratory problems, sexually transmitted infections, signs of domestic violence, emergency services, and substance abuse issues.
  - Education also includes information about the nature of mental illness; symptoms to expect; side effects, risks, and benefits of prescribed medications; and ways to negotiate the complexities of the mental health system.
- Providing case management

- Service coordination is necessary to ensure that clients receive the structure and support needed to achieve and maintain optimal functioning.
- Case management encompasses health teaching, crisis intervention, symptom monitoring, assistance with federal or local entitlements, assistance with transportation, teaching about money management, and consumer advocacy.
- Becoming politically involved
  - Responsibilities involve interventions in the lives of homeless mentally ill clients.
  - Knowledge about governmental influences on healthcare and willingness to testify from their knowledge and experience are important aspects

Appendices

Quick Reference to Disorders

Quick Reference to Therapeutic Modalities

Internet Resources

Alzheimer's Association
www.alz.org
Alzheimer's Disease Education and Referral (ADEAR) Center
www.nia.nih.gov/alzheimers
American Academy of Addiction Psychiatry
www.aaap.org
American Academy of Child and Adolescent Psychiatry
www.aacap.org
American Association of Intellectual and Developmental Disability
www.aamr.org
American Association of Sex Educators, Counselors, and Therapists
www.aasect.org
American Association of Suicidology
www.suicidology.org
American Autism Society
www.autism-society.org
American Foundation for Suicide Prevention
www.afsp.org
American Holistic Nurses' Association
www.ahna.org
American Psychiatric Association
www.psych.org
American Psychological Association
www.apa.org
American Red Cross Disaster Services
www.redcross.org/services/disaster/0,1082,0_319_,00.html

American Society of Addiction Medicine
www.asam.org
Anxiety Disorders Association of America
www.adaa.org
Autism Online
www.autismonline.org
Borderline Personality Disorder Research Foundation
www.borderlineresearch.org
Borderline Personality Disorder Sanctuary
www.mhsanctuary.com/borderline
Canadian Association for Suicide Prevention
www.suicideprevention.ca
Center for the Prevention of Sexual and Domestic Violence
www.cpsdv.org
Child Abuse Prevention Network
www.child-abuse.com
Child & Adolescent Bipolar Foundation
www.bpkids.org
Children and Adults with Attention Deficit/Hyperactivity Disorder
www.childwelfare.gov
Children of Aging Parents (CAPs)
www.aoa.dhhs.gov/coa/dir/77.html
Depression and Bipolar Support Alliance (DBSA)
www.dbsalliance.org
Eating Disorder Referral and Information Center
www.edreferral.com
Eating Disorders Resources
www.bulimia.com
Eldercare Locator
www.aoa.dhhs.gov/elderpage/locator.html
Family Violence Prevention Fund
www.endabuse.org
The Gender Identity Disorder Reform Organization
www.gidreform.org
The International Society for the Study of Trauma and Dissociation
www.isst-d.org
Mental Health America
www.mentalhealthamerica.net

Mental Health Net
www.cmhc.com
National Alliance for the Mentally Ill
http://www.nami.org/Content/NavigationMenu/Inform_Yourself/
About_Mental_Illness/About_Mental_Illness.htm
National Anxiety Foundation
http://lexington-on-line.com/naf.html
National Association for Anorexia and Associated Disorders
www.anad.org
National Center for Learning Disabilities
www.ncld.org
National Center on Elder Abuse and the Clearinghouse on Abuse and
Neglect of the Elderly
www.elderabusecenter.org
National Center for Posttraumatic Stress Disorder: Guidelines for Mental
Health Professionals' Response to Recent Tragic Events in the US
http://www.ncptsd.va.gov/ncmain/ncdocs/fact_shts/fs_guidelines_
disaster.html
National Center for Posttraumatic Stress Disorder: Treatment–Natural
Disasters and Terrorism
http://www.ncptsd.va.gov/ncmain/providers/fact_sheets/treatment/
disaster/index.jsp
National Clearinghouse for Alcohol and Drug Information
http://ncadi.samhsa.gov
National Coalition for the Homeless
www.nationalhomeless.org
National Committee for the Prevention of Elder Abuse
www.preventelderabuse.org
The National Council on Alcoholism and Drug Dependence
www.ncadd.org
The National Data Resource Center on Homelessness and Mental Illness
www.nrchmi.com
National Depressive and Manic Depressive Association
http://ndmda.org
National Domestic Violence Hotline
www.ndvh.org
National Eating Disorders Association
www.nationaleatingdisorders.org

National Foundation for Depressive Illness
www.depression.org
National Institutes of Health: National Center for Complementary and Alternative Medicine
http://nccam.nih.gov
National Institutes of Health: National Institutes of Mental Health
http://www.nimh.nih.gov/healthinformation/index.cfm
National Institute on Alcohol Abuse and Alcoholism
www.niaaa.nih.gov
National Institute on Drug Abuse
www.nida.nih.gov
Obsessive-Compulsive Foundation, Inc.
www.ocfoundation.org
Obsessive Compulsive Information Center
www.miminc.org/aboutocic.asp
Postpartum Education for Parents
www.sbpep.org
Postpartum Support International
www.postpartum.net
Recovery, International
www.recovery-inc.com
Quackwatch
www.quackwatch.org
The Schizophrenia Society of Canada
www.schizophrenia.ca
Schizophrenics Anonymous
www.sanonymous.com
Sex and Love Addicts Anonymous
www.slaafws.org
Sex Addicts Anonymous
www.sexaa.org
Sexaholics Anonymous
www.sa.org
Sexual Compulsives Anonymous
www.sca-recovery.org
Sexuality Information and Education Council of the United States
www.siecus.org

Society for Light Treatment and Biological Rhythms
www.sltbr.org

Stop Family Violence
www.stopfamilyviolence.org

Systematic Treatment Enhancement Program for Bipolar Disorder Study (STEP-BD)
www.stepbd.org

Substance Abuse and Mental Health Services Administration
www.samhsa.gov

Suicide Prevention Advocacy Network USA
www.spanusa.org

United States Drug Enforcement Administration
www.usdoj.gov/dea/concern/concern.htm

VA Homeless Assistance Information
www.va.gov/homeless

INDEX

Note: Page numbers followed by *f, t,* and *b* indicate figures, tables and boxed text, respectively.